HOLE IN THE HEART

Hole in the Heart

BRINGING UP BETH

Henny Beaumont

First published in 2016 by

Myriad Editions
59 Lansdowne Place
Brighton BN3 1FL, UK

www.myriadeditions.com

First printing

1 3 5 7 9 10 8 6 4 2

A CIP catalogue record for this book is available from
the British Library.

ISBN: 978-1-908434-92-0
E-ISBN: 978-1-908434-93-7

Printed by Jelgavas Tipografija on paper sourced from
sustainable forests.

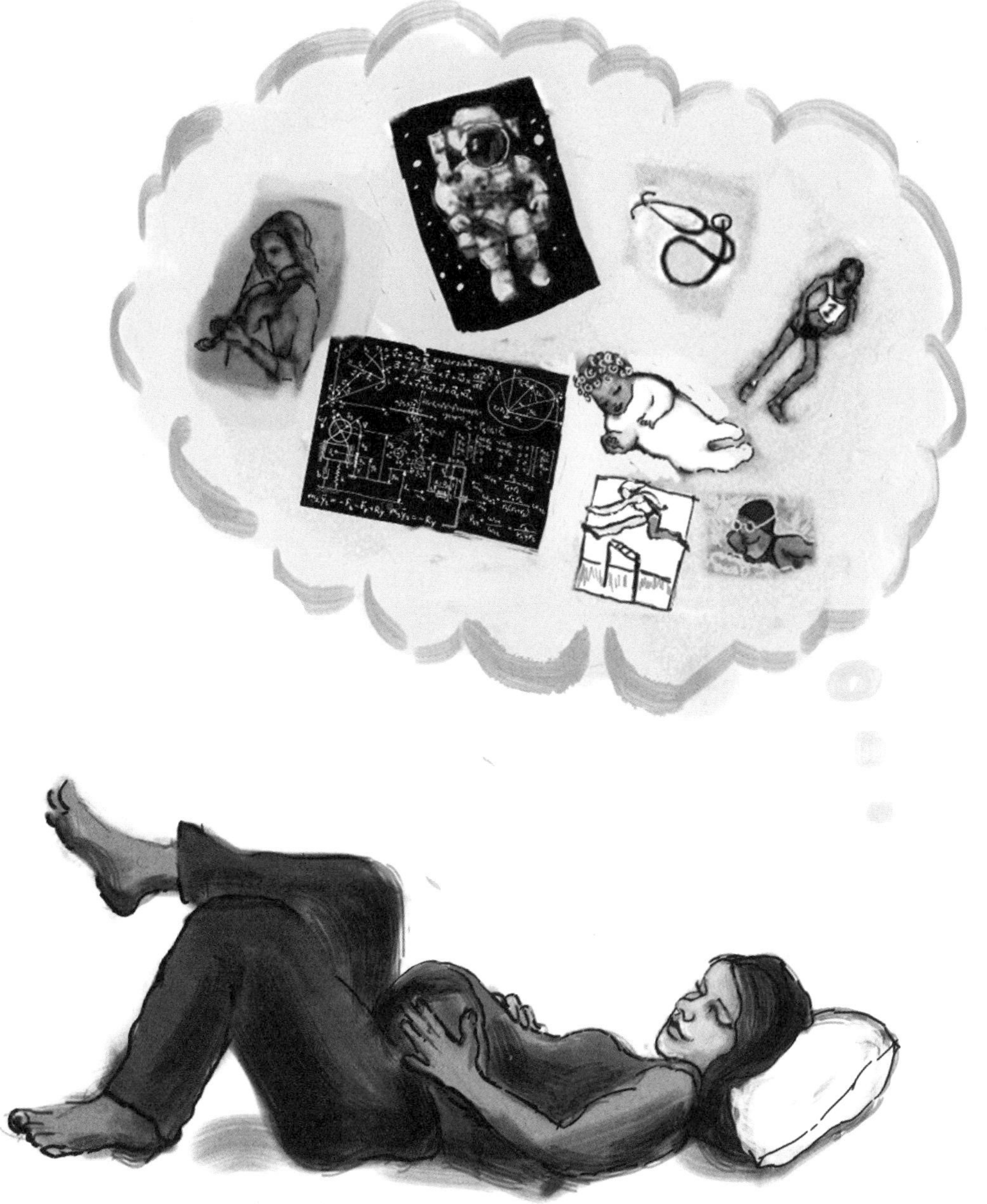

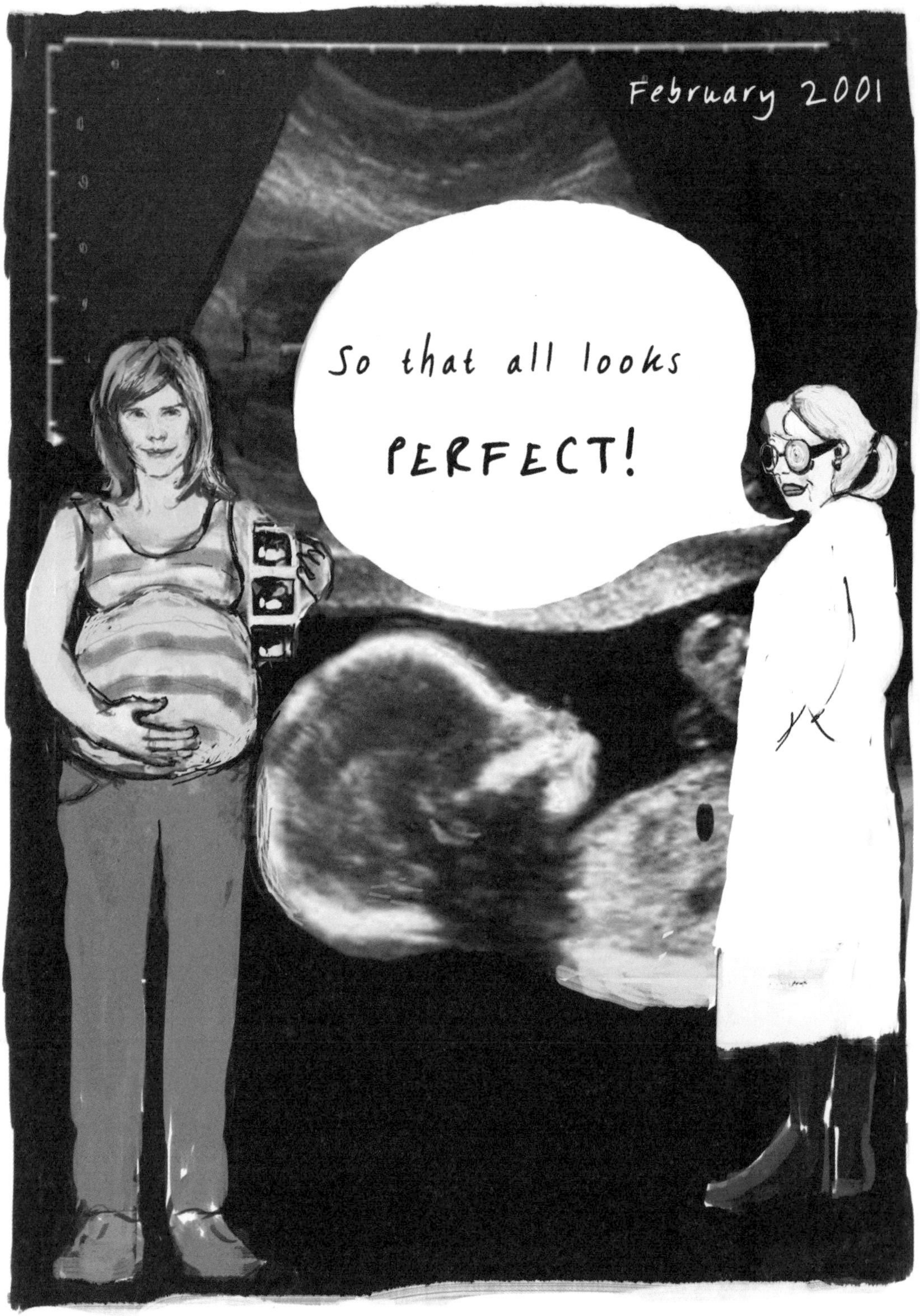
February 2001
So that all looks PERFECT!

For Steve, Matty, Bridie, Beth and Karl

Part One

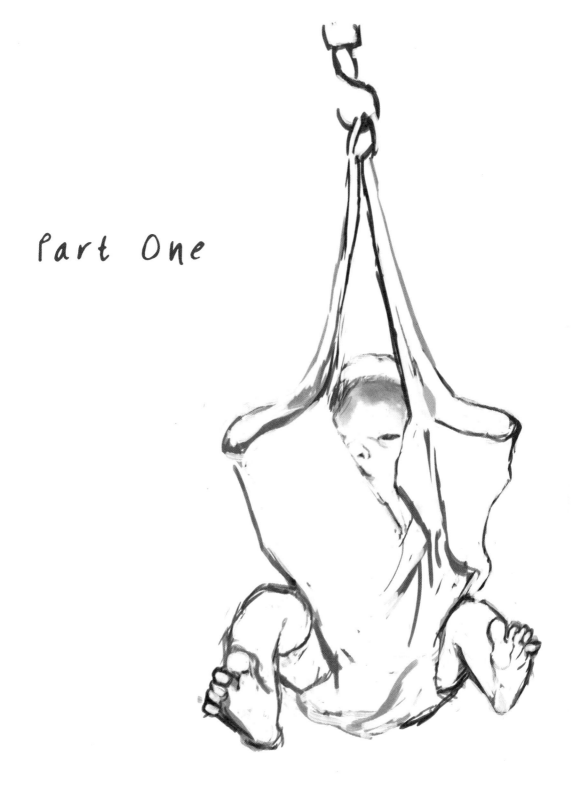

25 March 2001

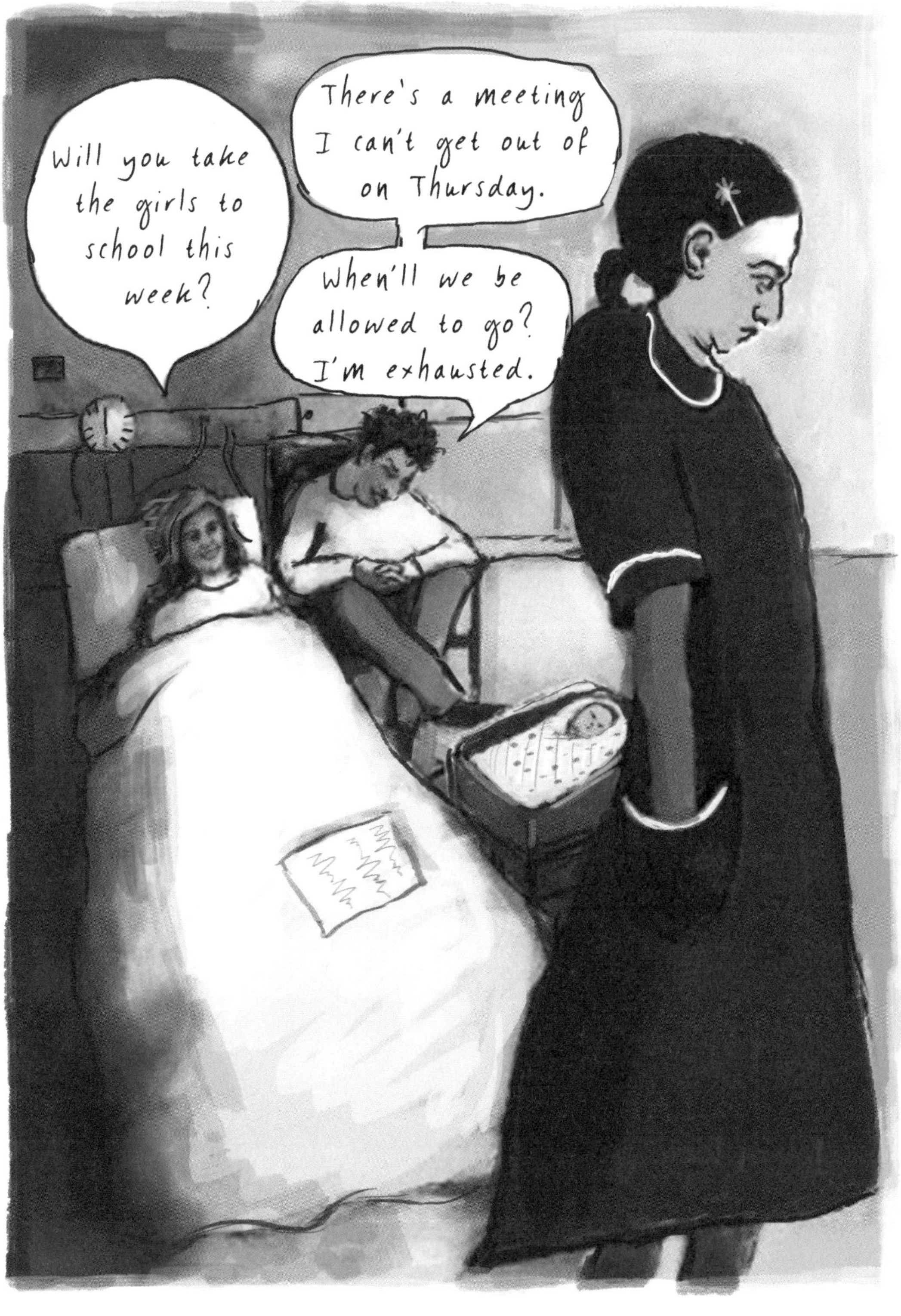
Will you take the girls to school this week?
There's a meeting I can't get out of on Thursday.
When'll we be allowed to go? I'm exhausted.

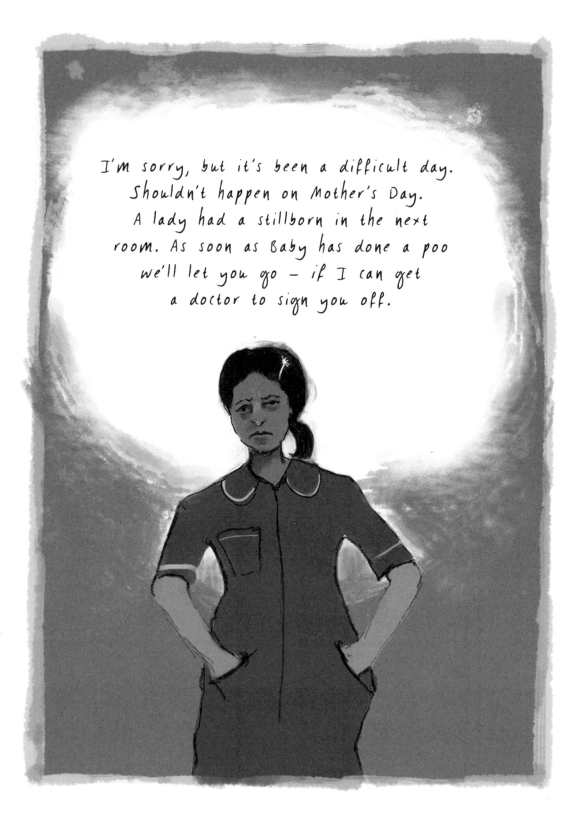

I'm sorry, but it's been a difficult day.
Shouldn't happen on Mother's Day.
A lady had a stillborn in the next
room. As soon as Baby has done a poo
we'll let you go — if I can get
a doctor to sign you off.

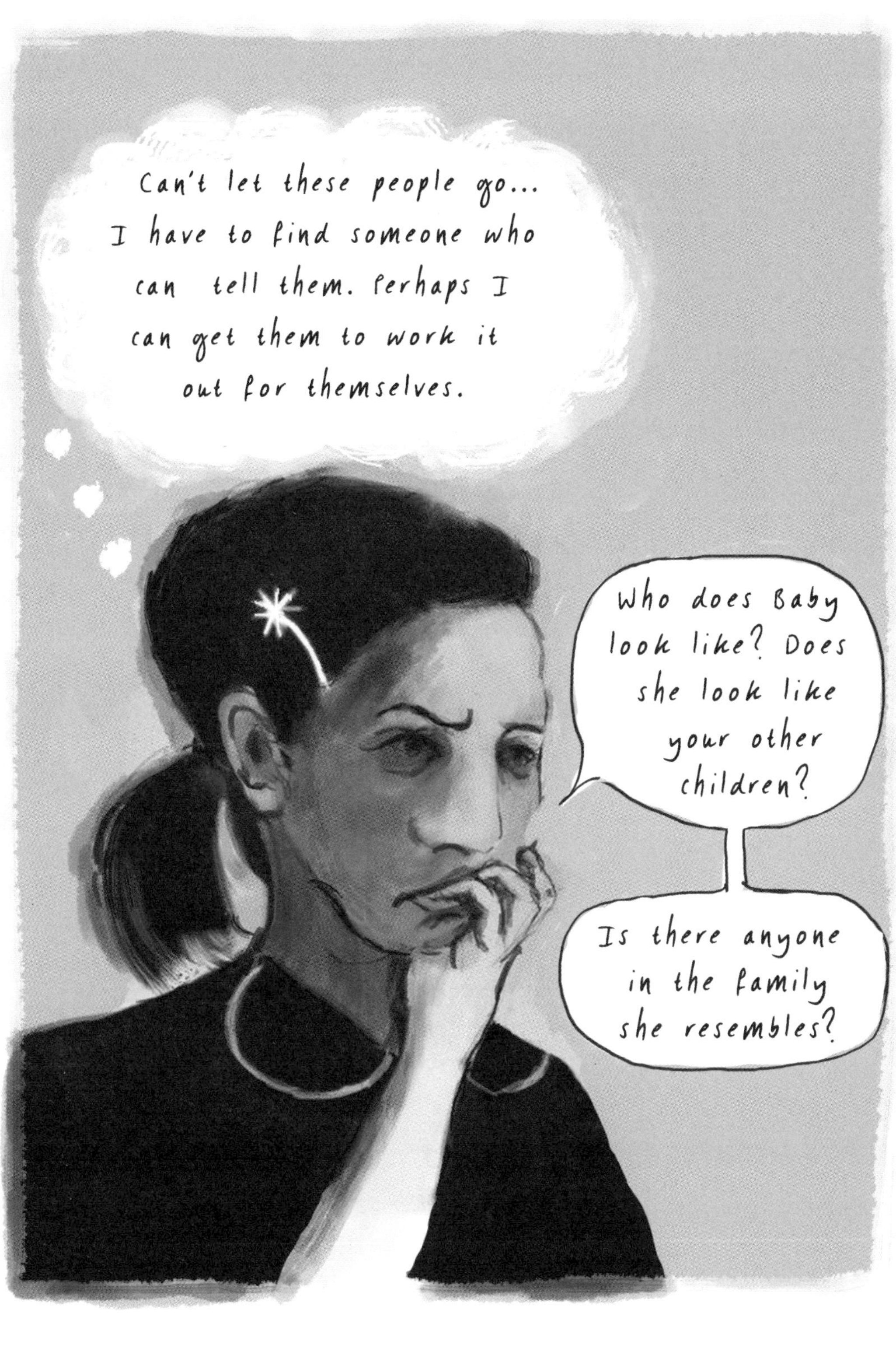
Can't let these people go... I have to find someone who can tell them. Perhaps I can get them to work it out for themselves.
Who does Baby look like? Does she look like your other children?
Is there anyone in the family she resembles?

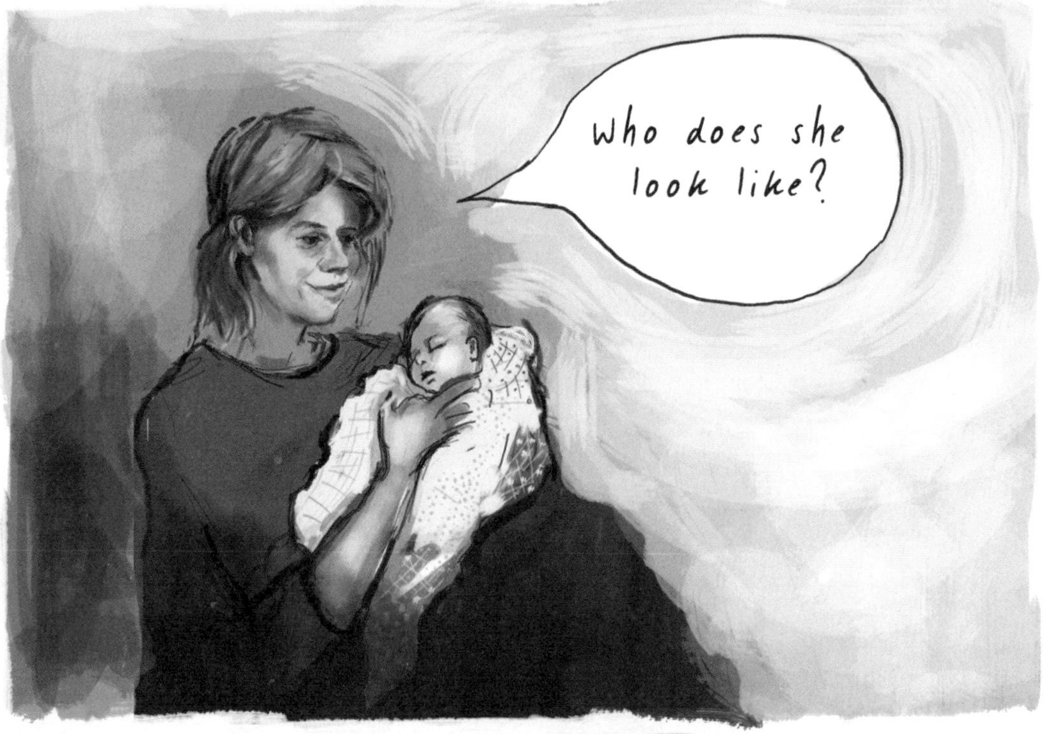

Who does she look like?

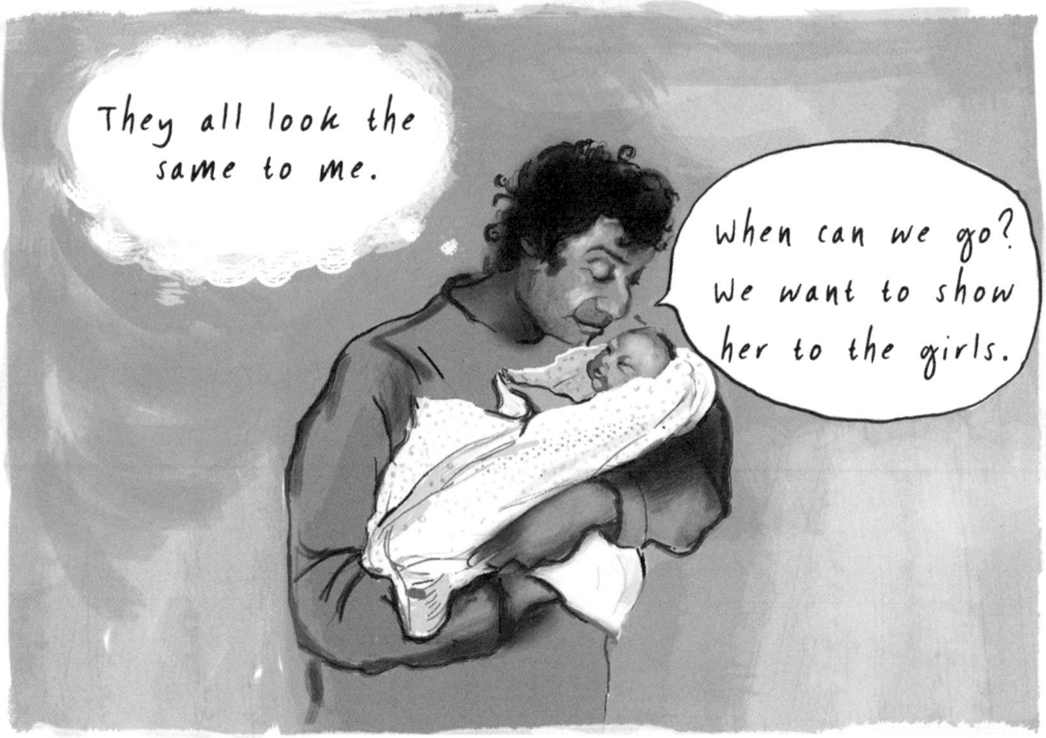

They all look the same to me.
When can we go? We want to show her to the girls.

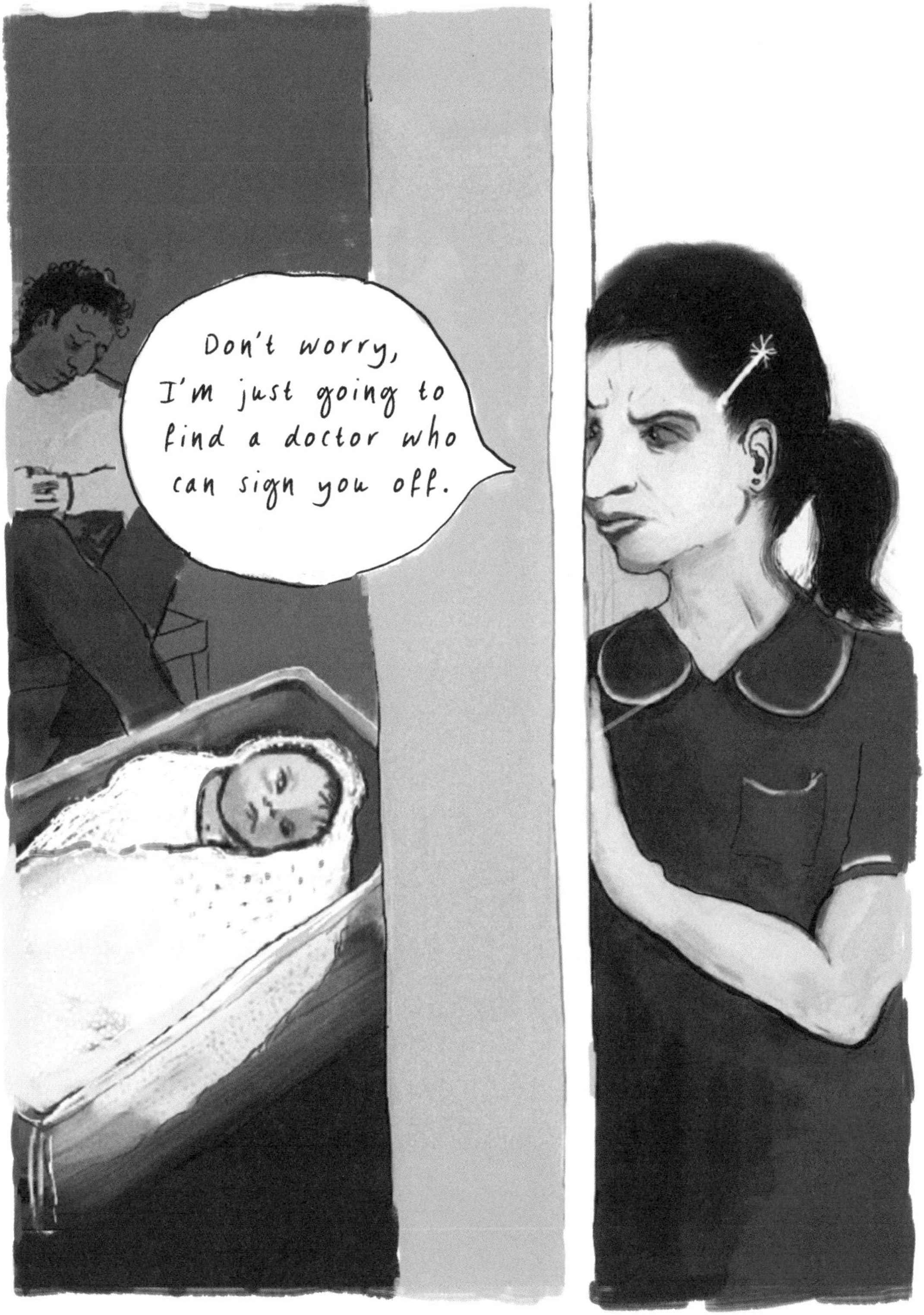
Don't worry, I'm just going to find a doctor who can sign you off.

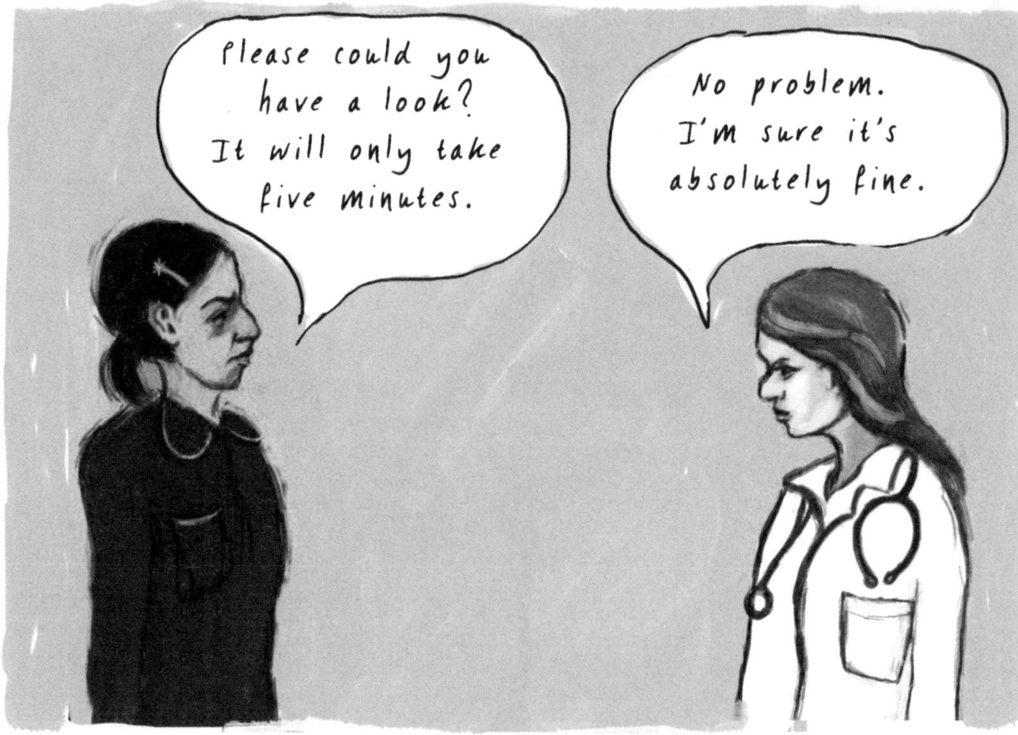
Please could you have a look? It will only take five minutes.
No problem. I'm sure it's absolutely fine.

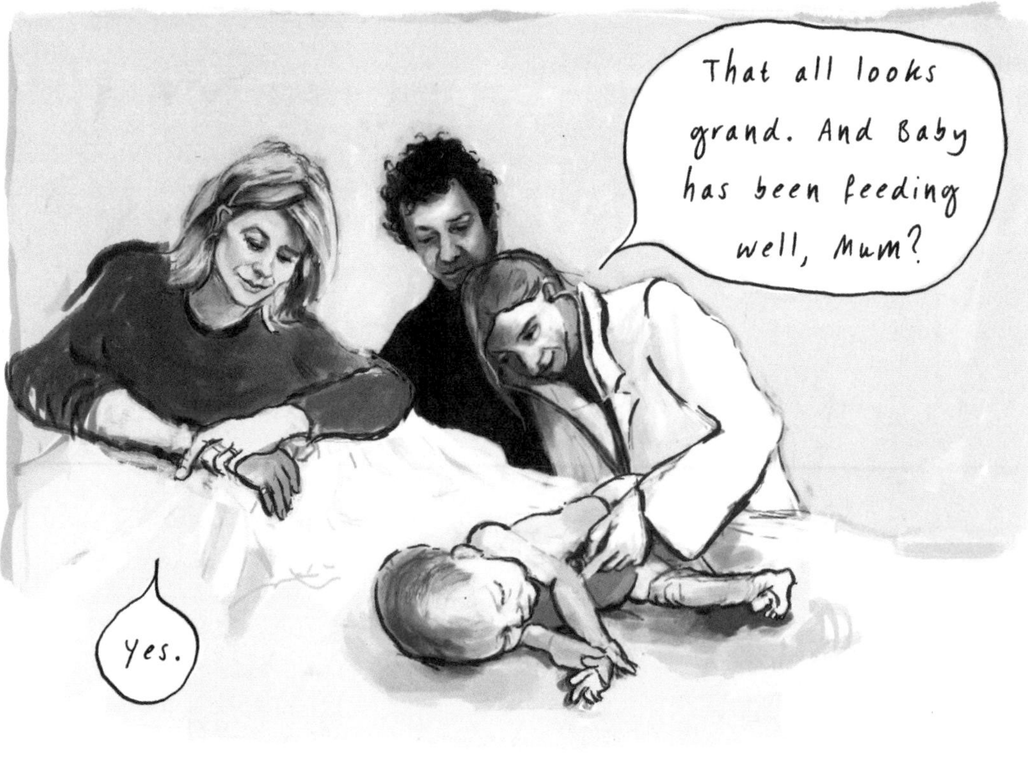
That all looks grand. And Baby has been feeding well, Mum?
Yes.

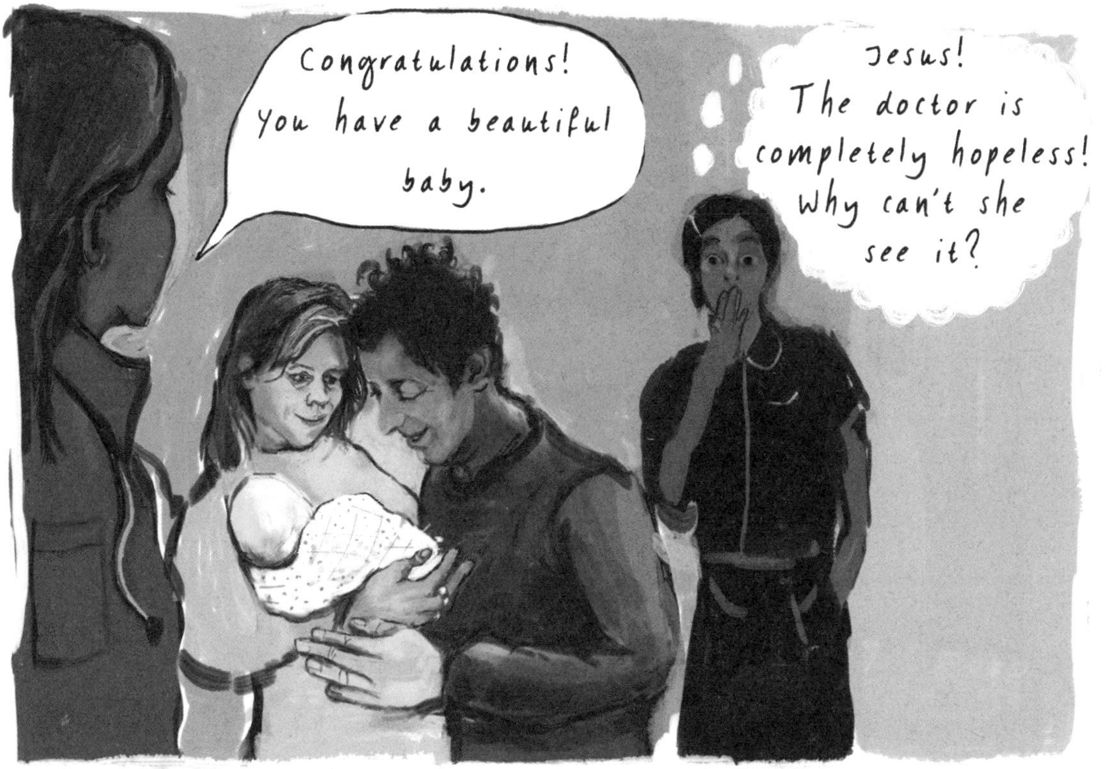
Congratulations! You have a beautiful baby.
Jesus! The doctor is completely hopeless! Why can't she see it?

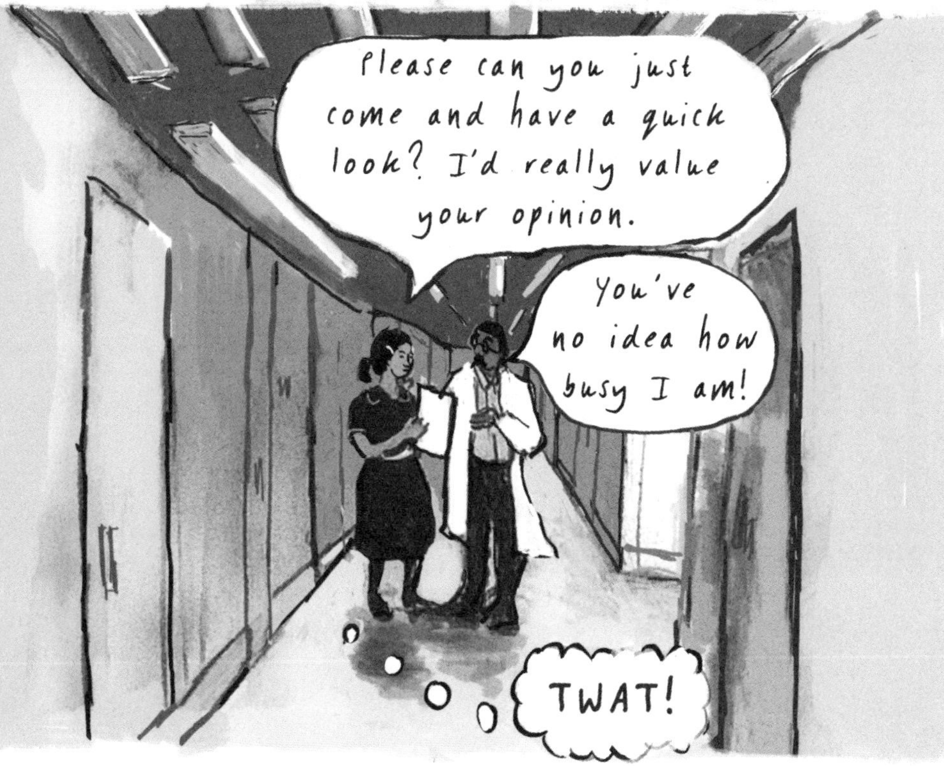
Please can you just come and have a quick look? I'd really value your opinion.
You've no idea how busy I am!
TWAT!

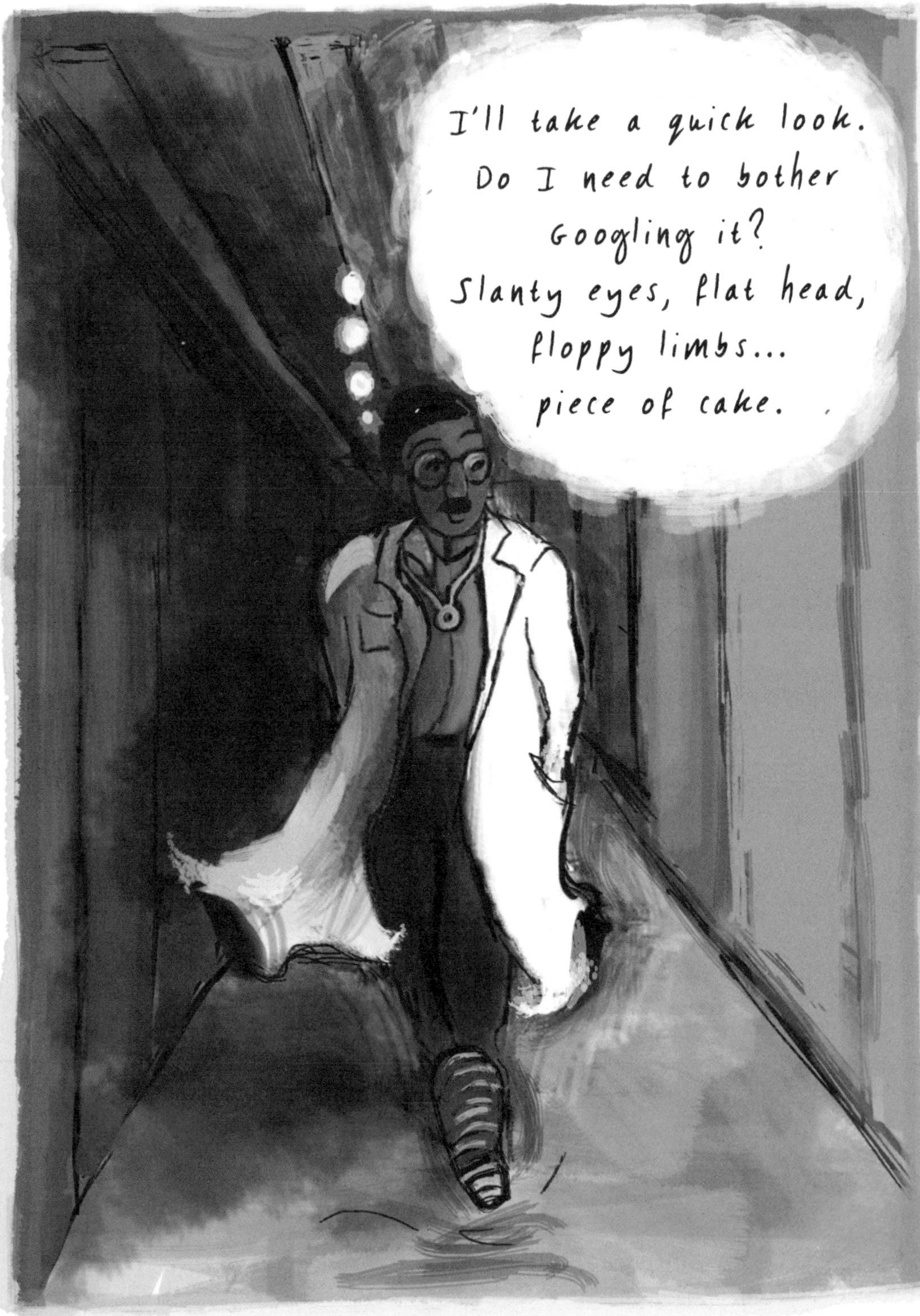
I'll take a quick look.
Do I need to bother
Googling it?
Slanty eyes, flat head,
floppy limbs...
piece of cake.

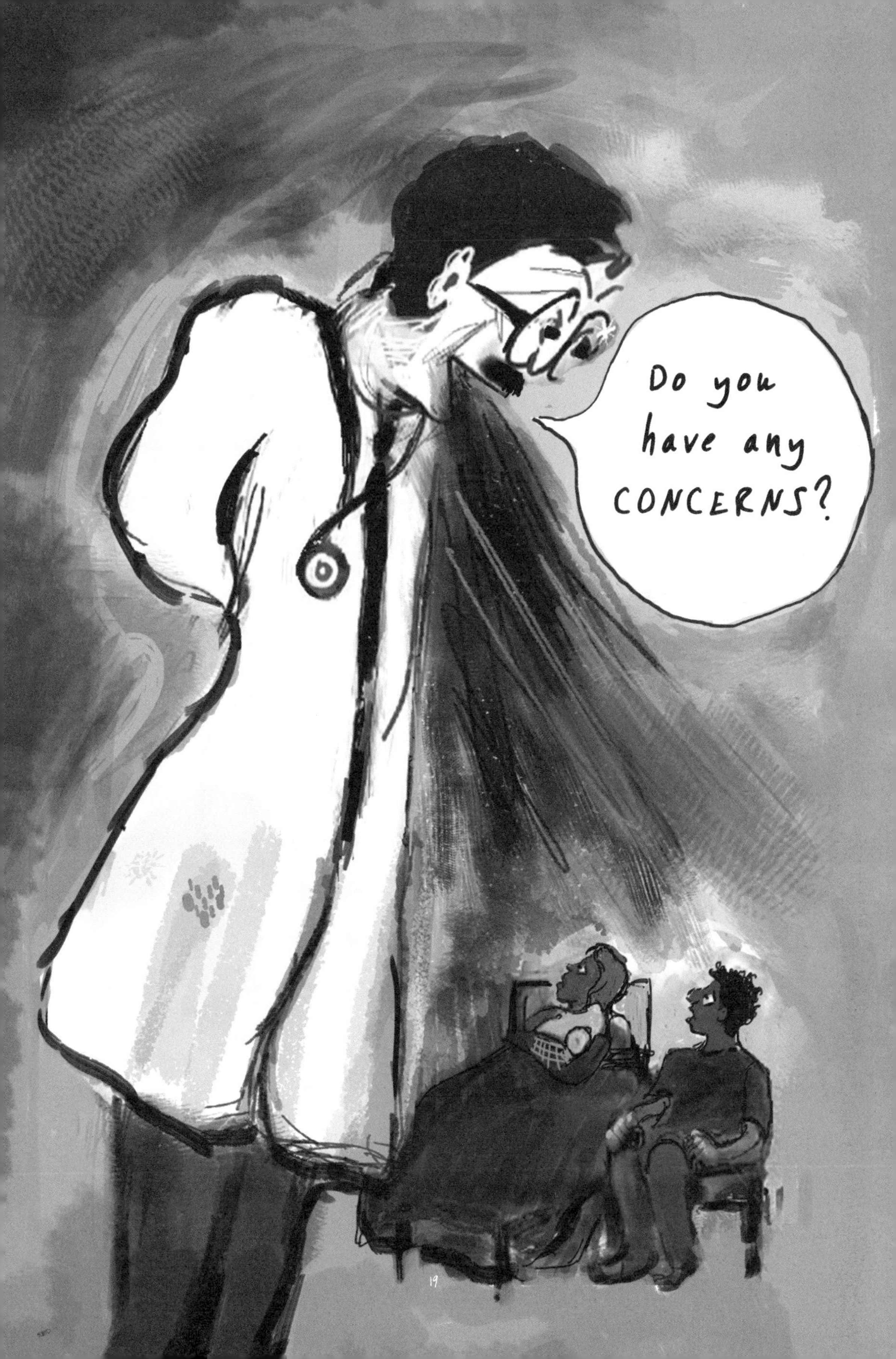
Do you have any CONCERNS?

Do you have any concerns?

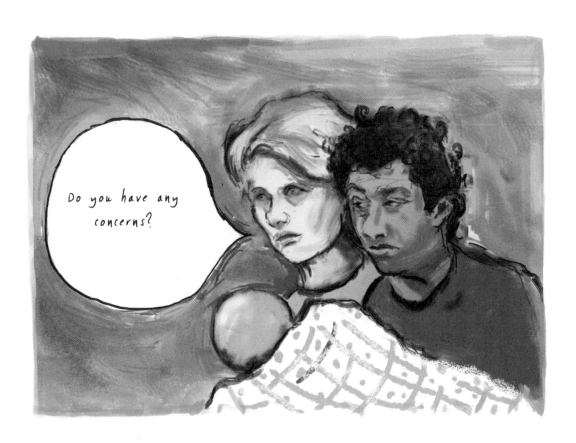

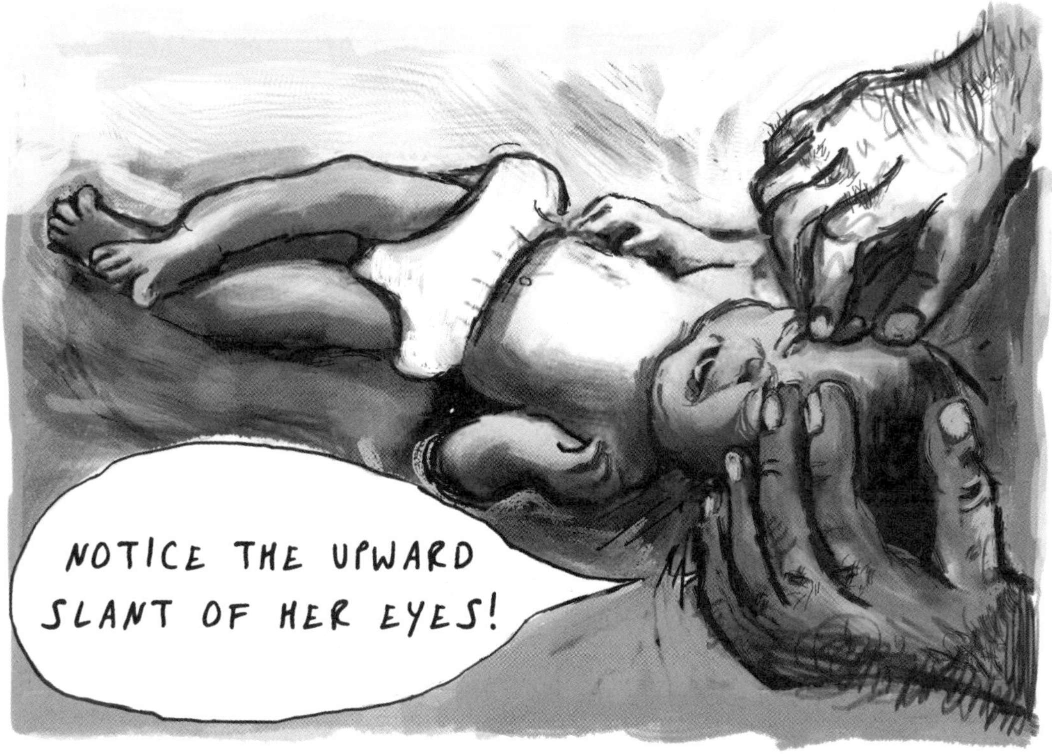
NOTICE THE UPWARD SLANT OF HER EYES!

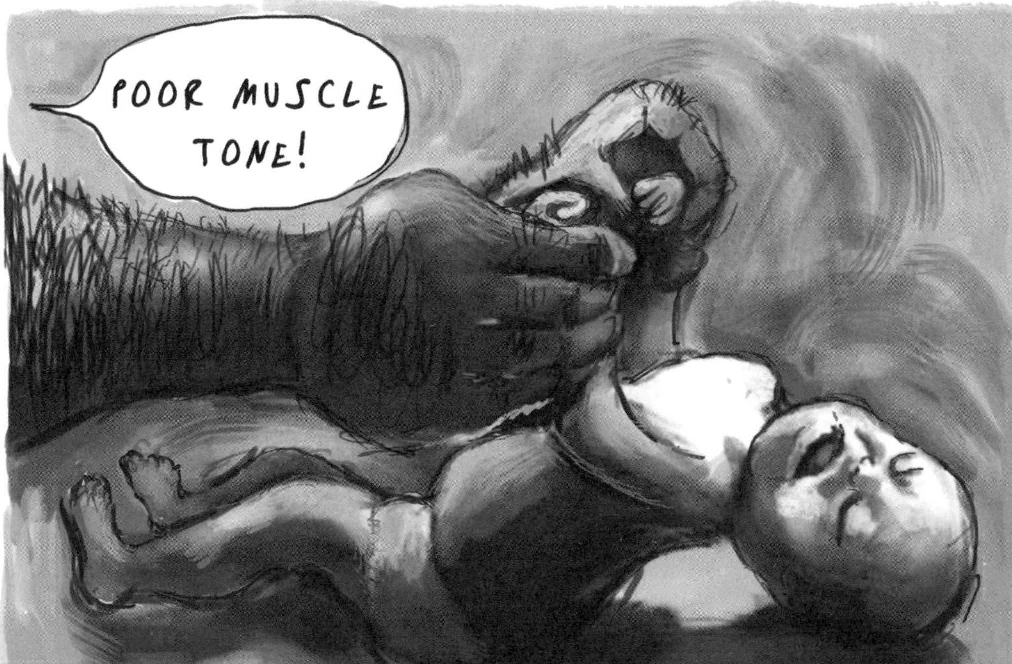
POOR MUSCLE TONE!

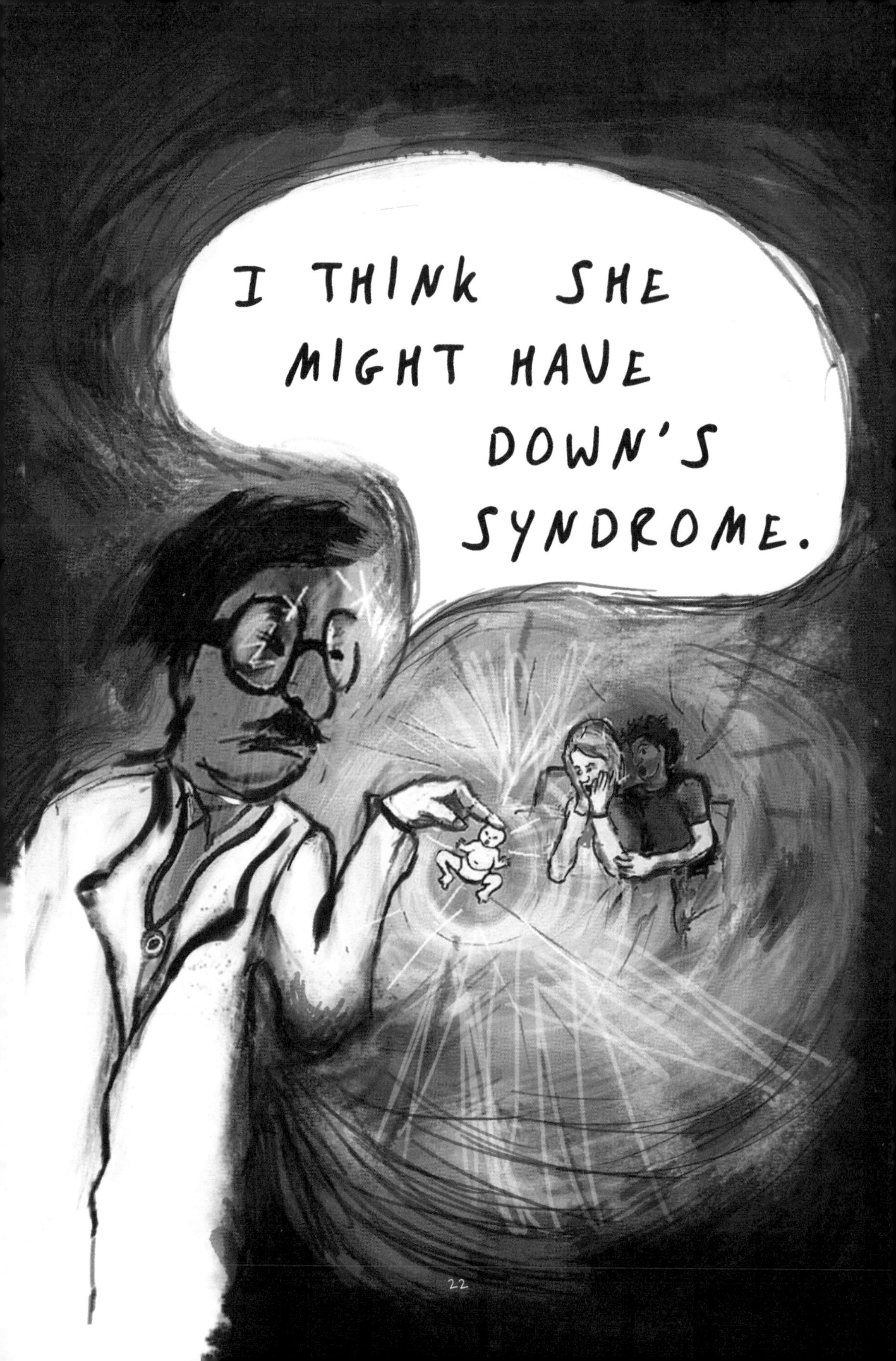
I THINK SHE MIGHT HAVE DOWN'S SYNDROME.

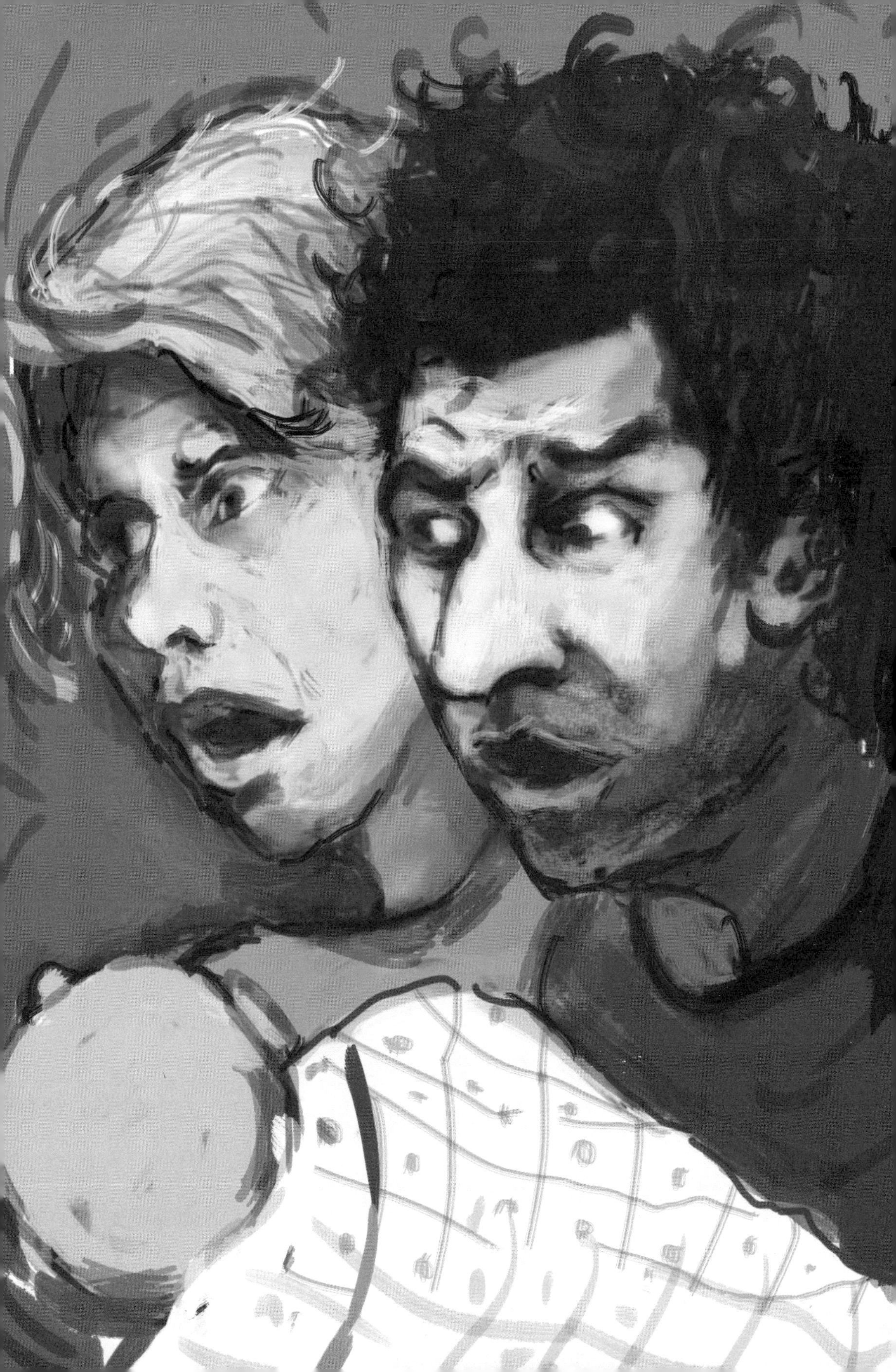

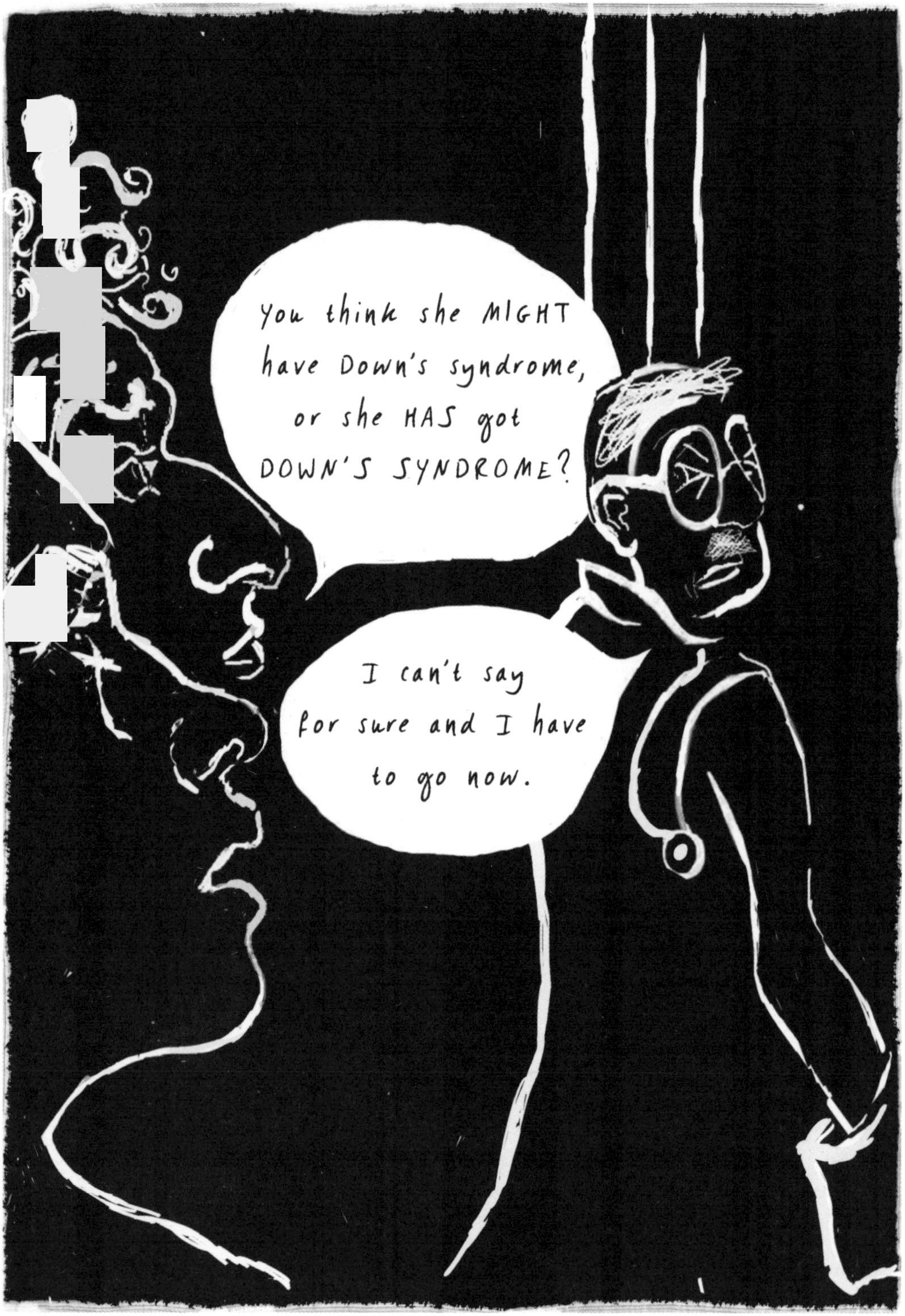
You think she MIGHT have Down's syndrome, or she HAS got DOWN'S SYNDROME?
I can't say for sure and I have to go now.

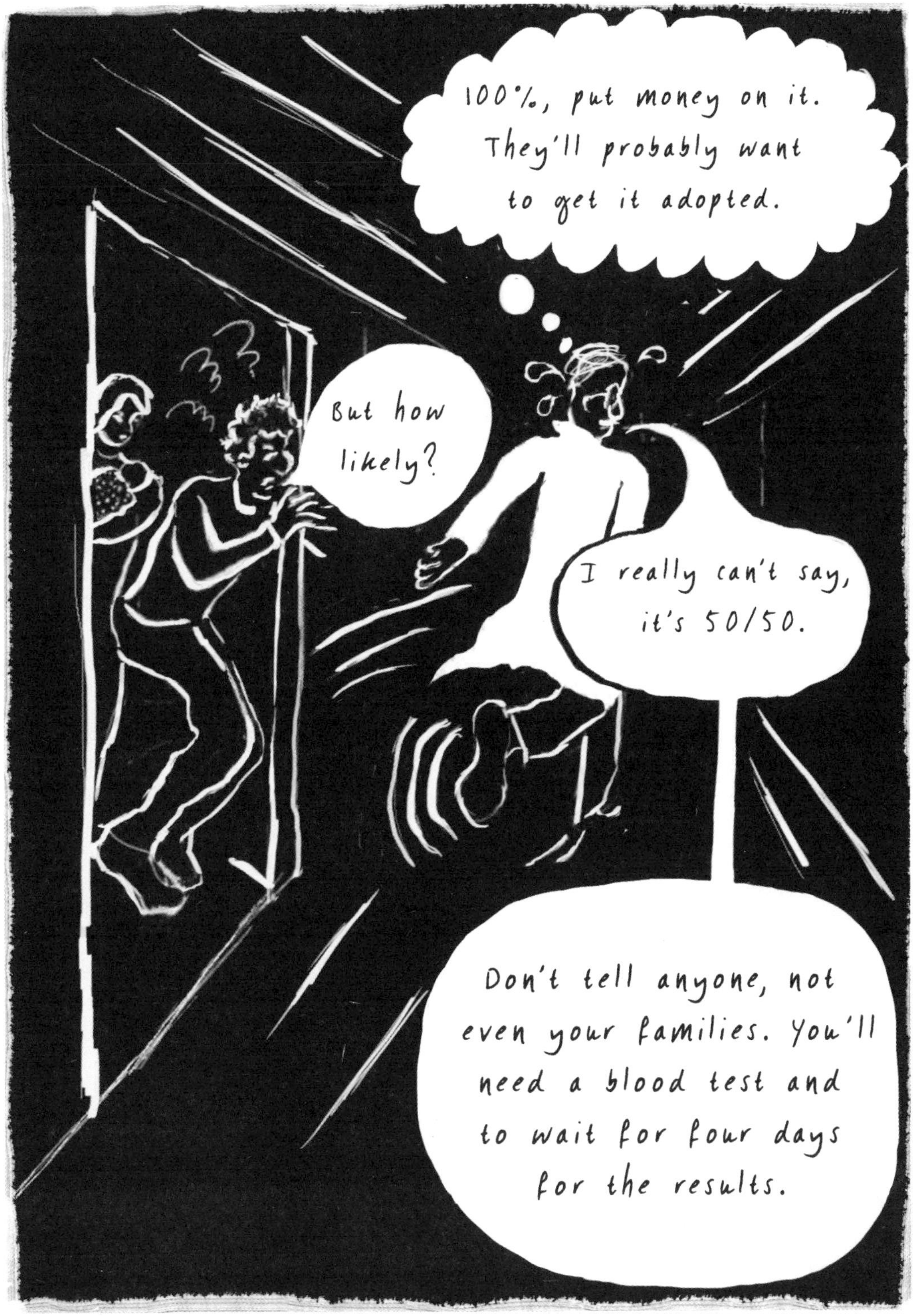
100%, put money on it. They'll probably want to get it adopted.
But how likely?
I really can't say, it's 50/50.
Don't tell anyone, not even your families. You'll need a blood test and to wait for four days for the results.

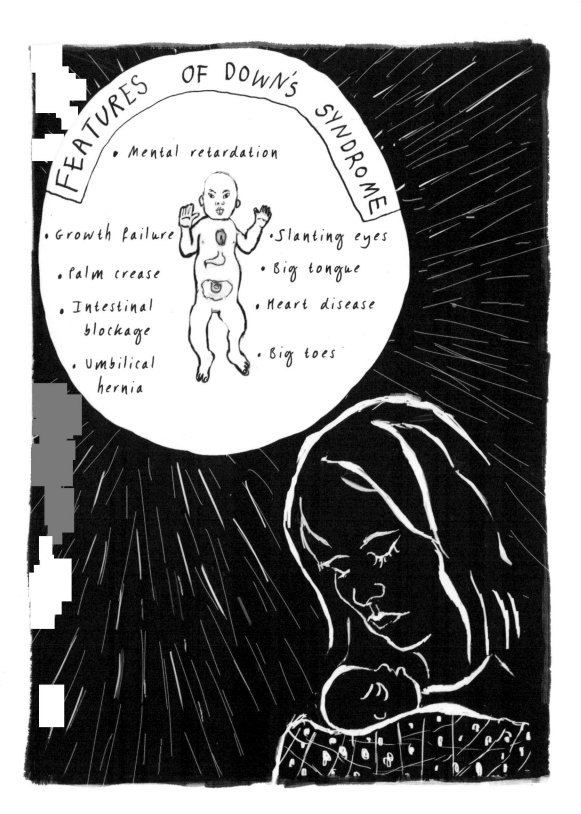

FEATURES OF DOWN'S SYNDROME

- Mental retardation
- Growth failure
- Palm crease
- Intestinal blockage
- Umbilical hernia
- Slanting eyes
- Big tongue
- Heart disease
- Big toes

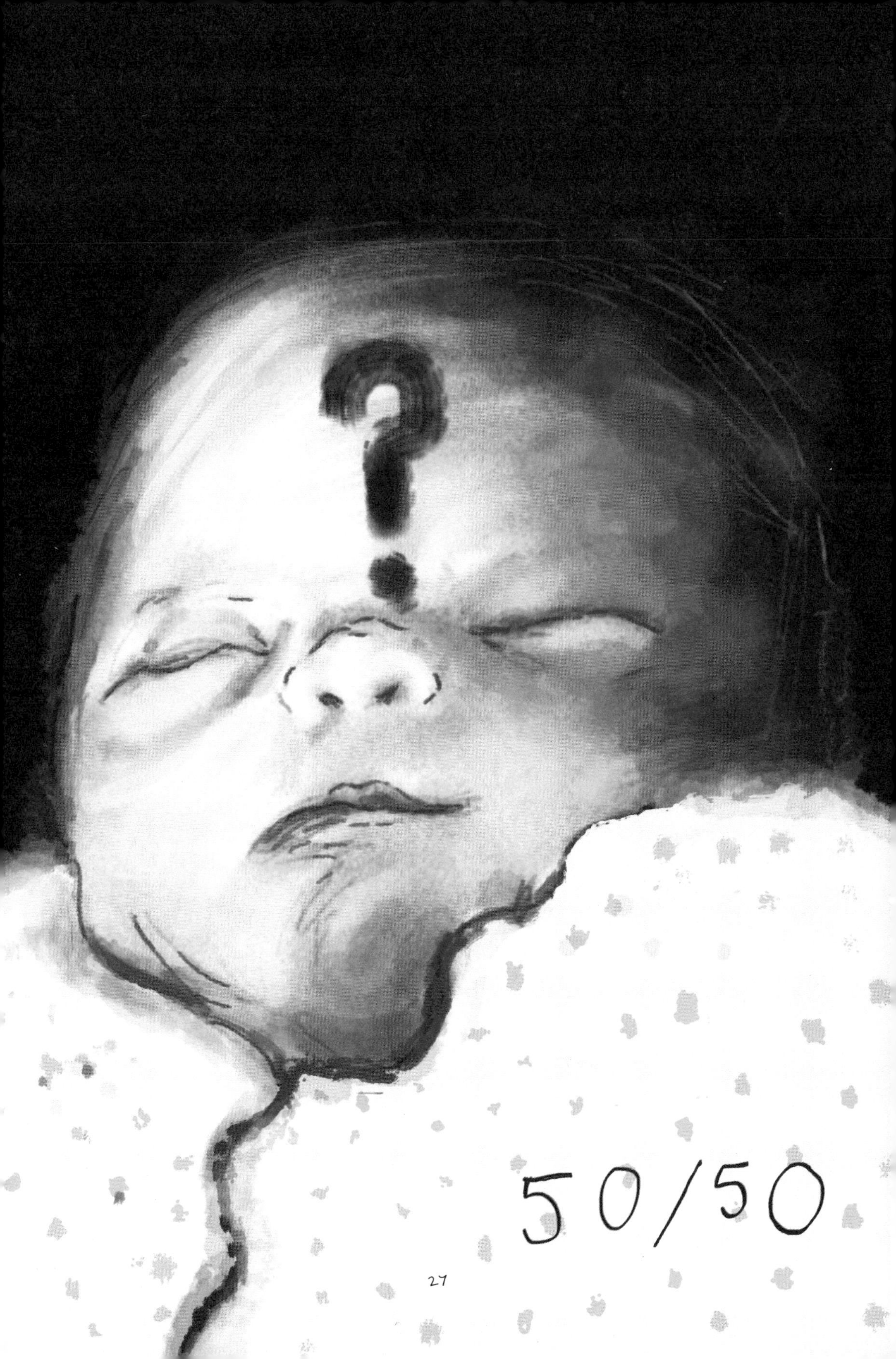
50/50

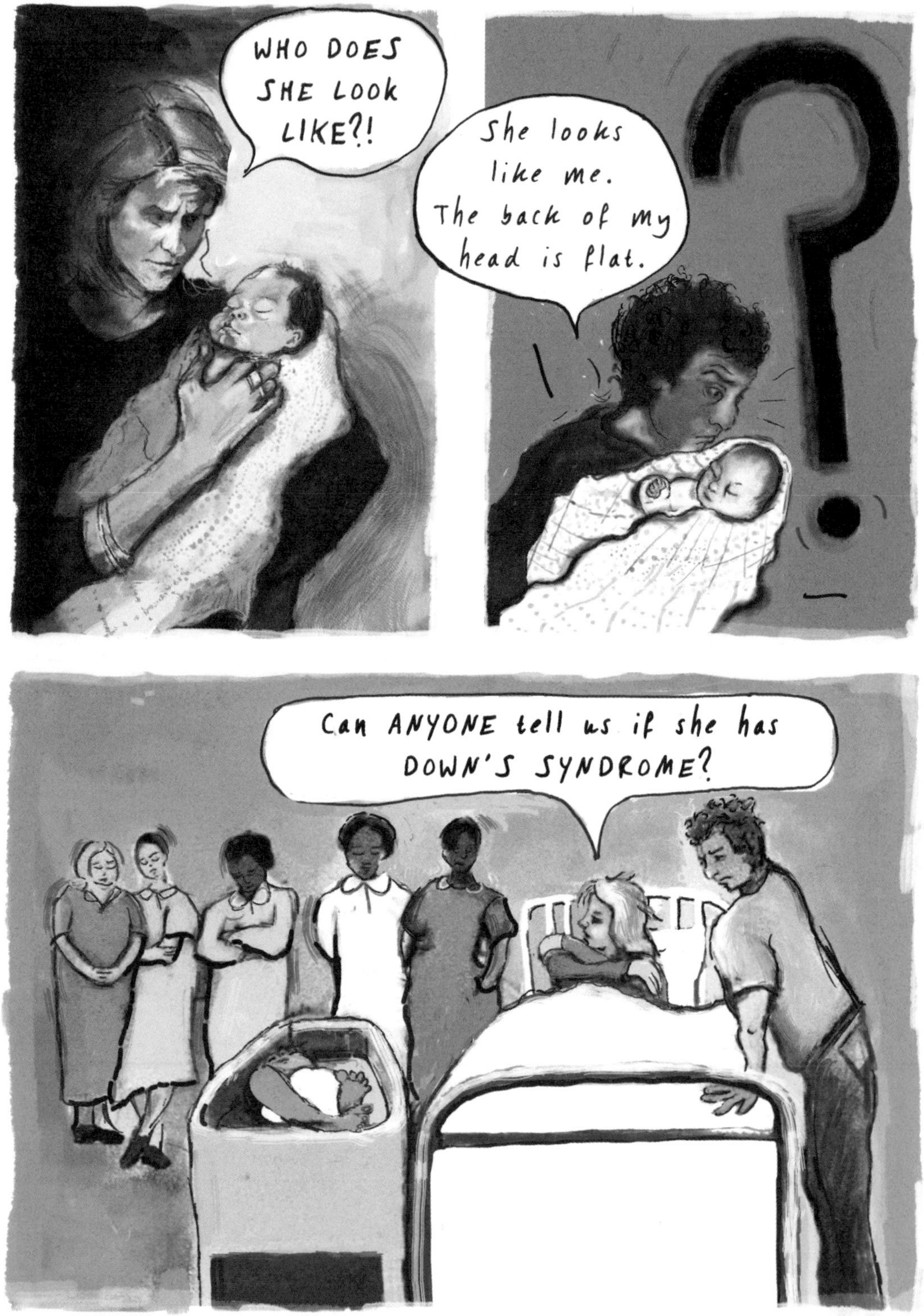
WHO DOES SHE LOOK LIKE?!
She looks like me. The back of my head is flat.
Can ANYONE tell us if she has DOWN'S SYNDROME?

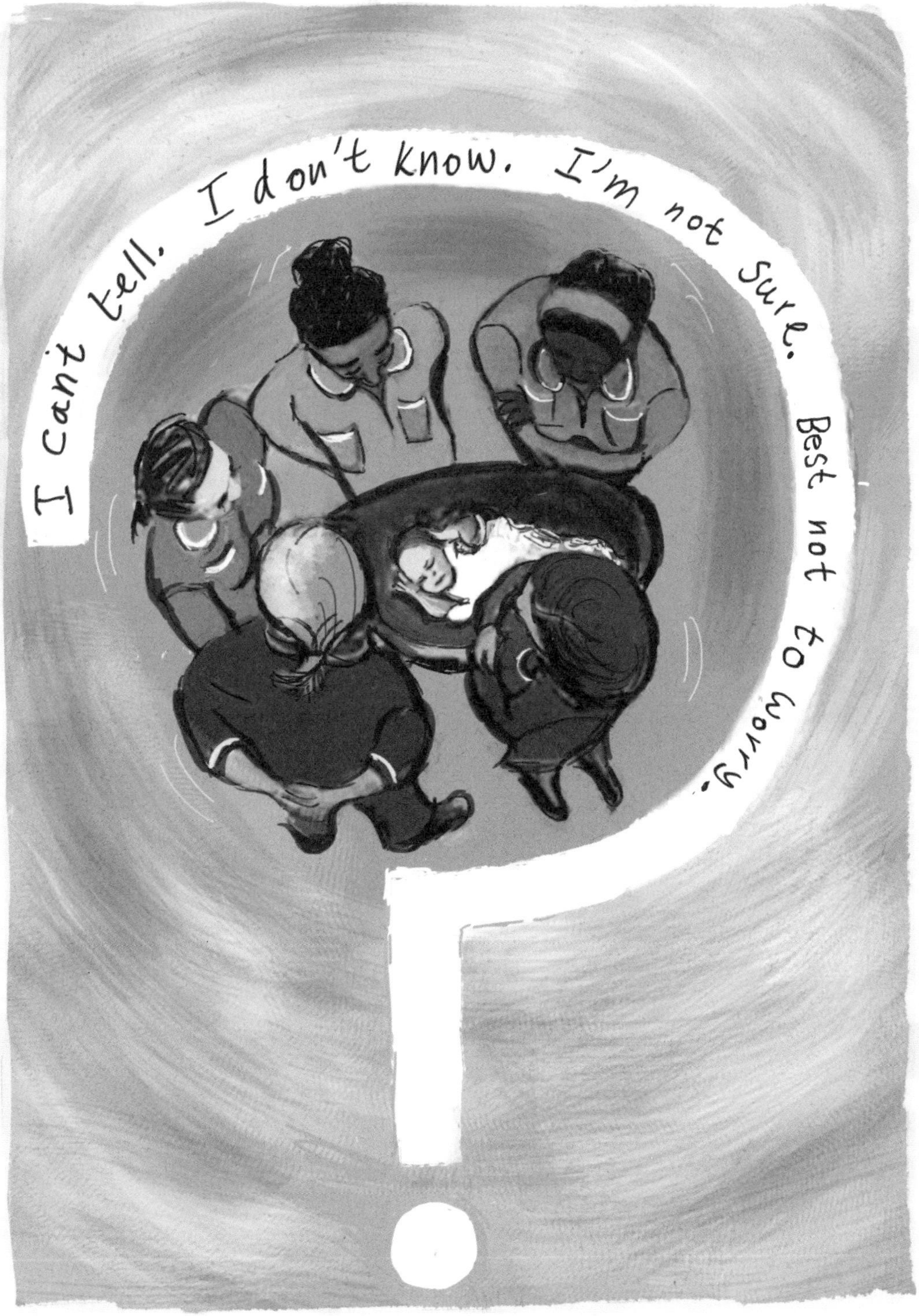
I can't tell. I don't know. I'm not sure. Best not to worry.

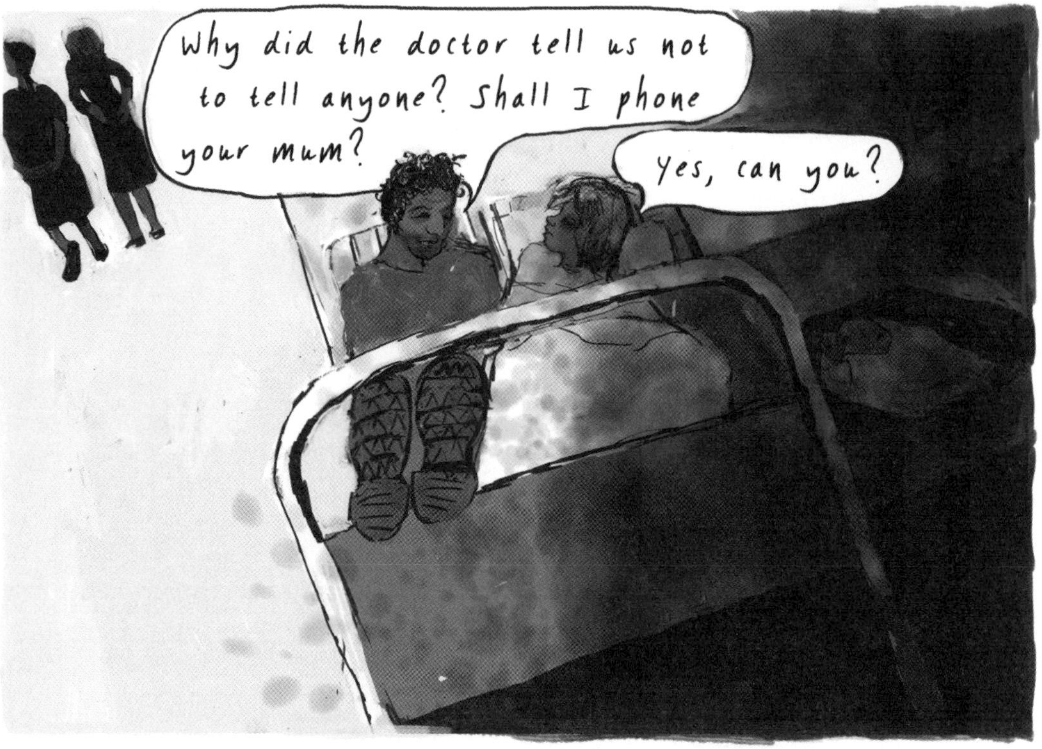
Why did the doctor tell us not to tell anyone? Shall I phone your mum?
Yes, can you?

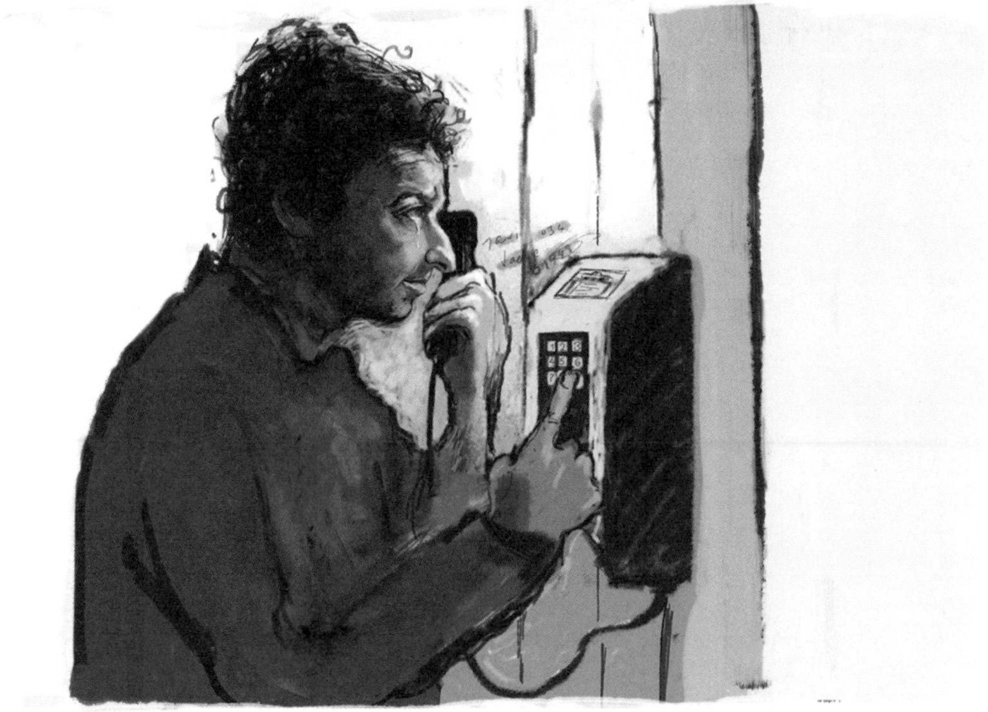

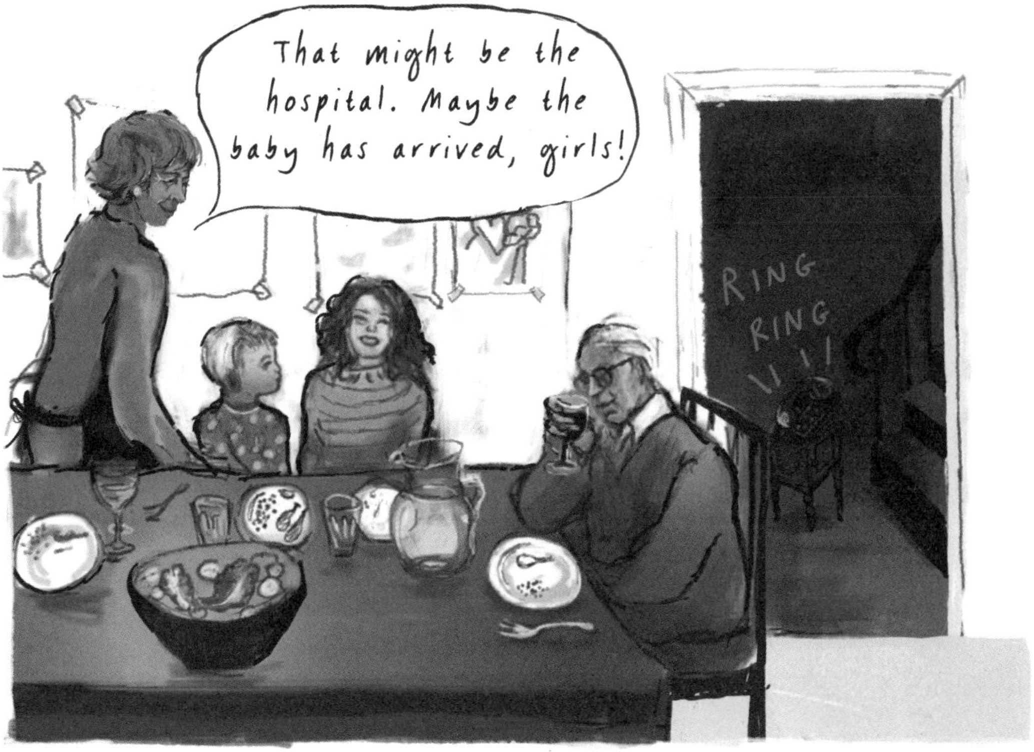
That might be the hospital. Maybe the baby has arrived, girls!
RING RING !!!

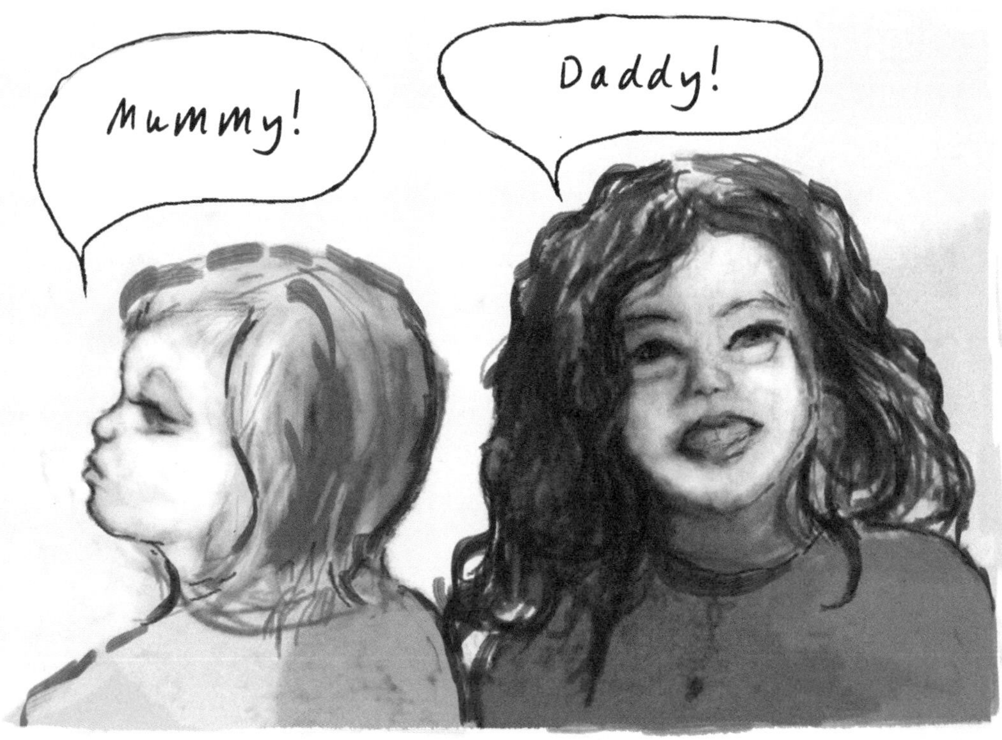
Mummy!
Daddy!

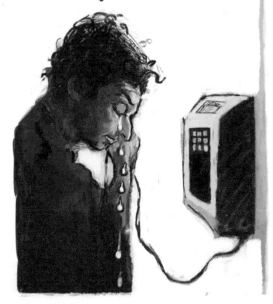

You need to sit down. We've got bad news.

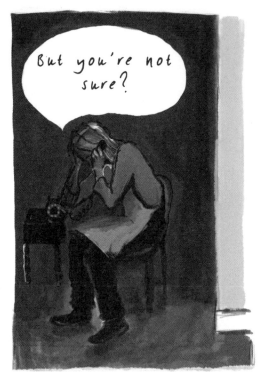

But you're not sure?

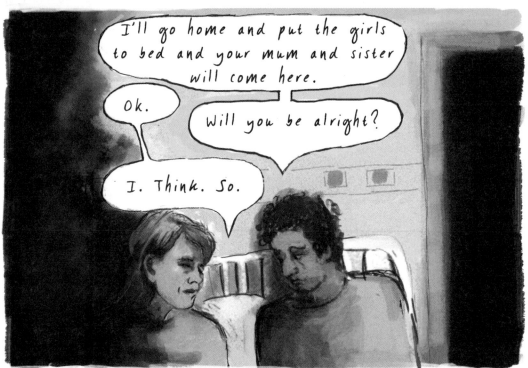

I'll go home and put the girls to bed and your mum and sister will come here.

Ok.

Will you be alright?

I. Think. So.

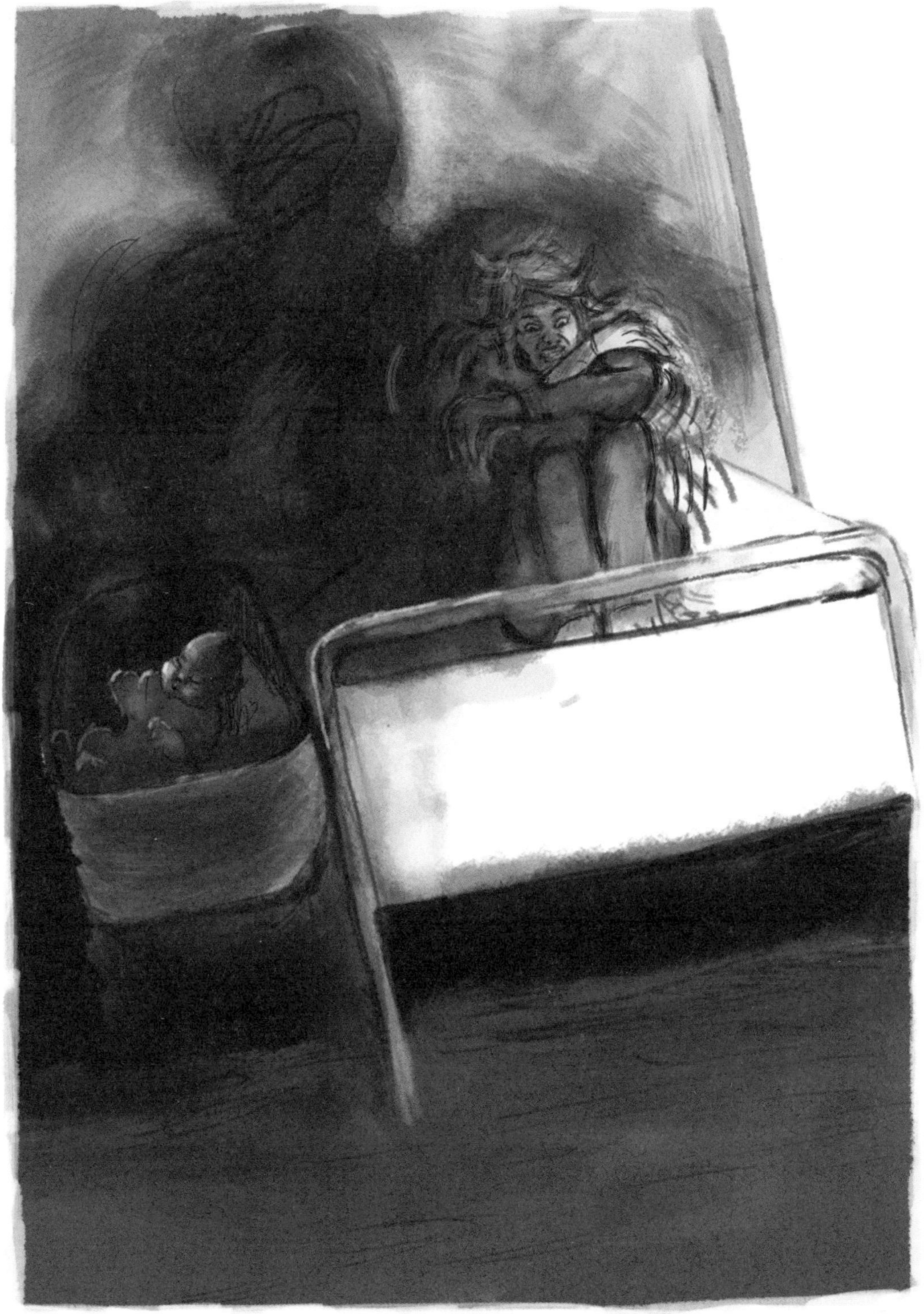

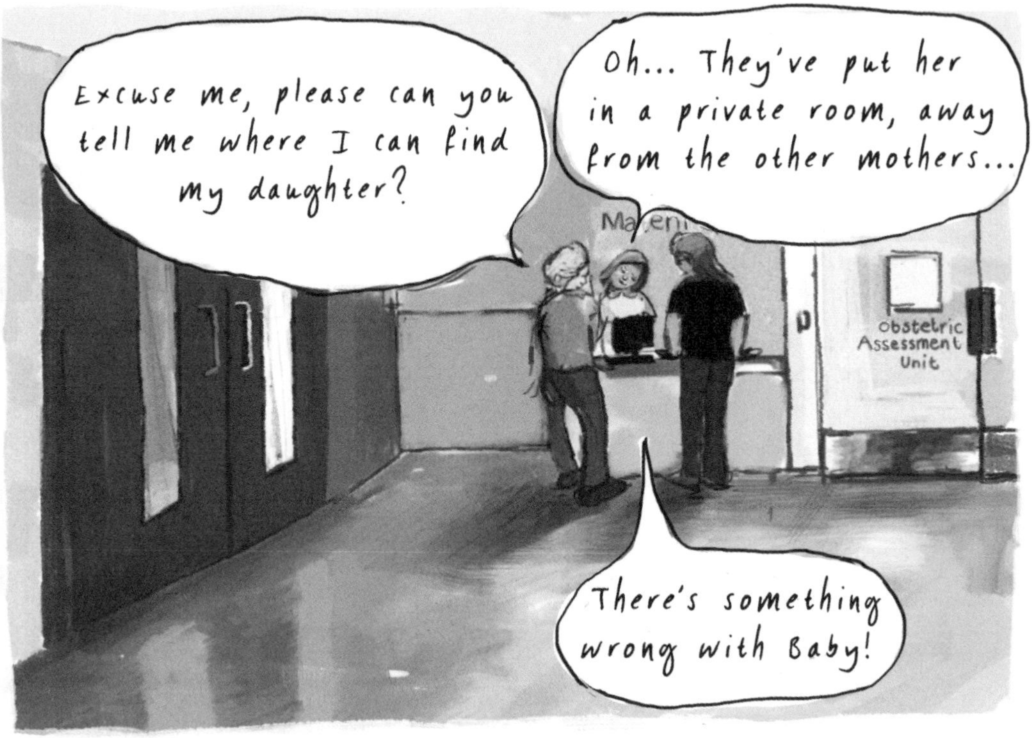
Excuse me, please can you tell me where I can find my daughter?
Oh... They've put her in a private room, away from the other mothers...
Maternity
Obstetric Assessment Unit
There's something wrong with Baby!

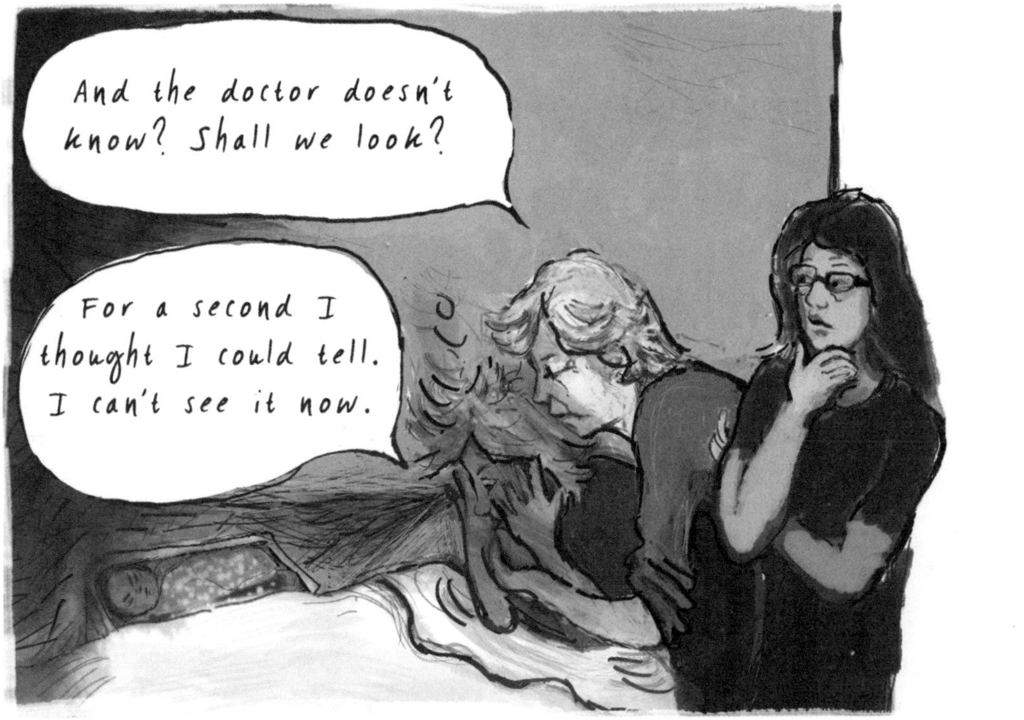
And the doctor doesn't know? Shall we look?
For a second I thought I could tell. I can't see it now.

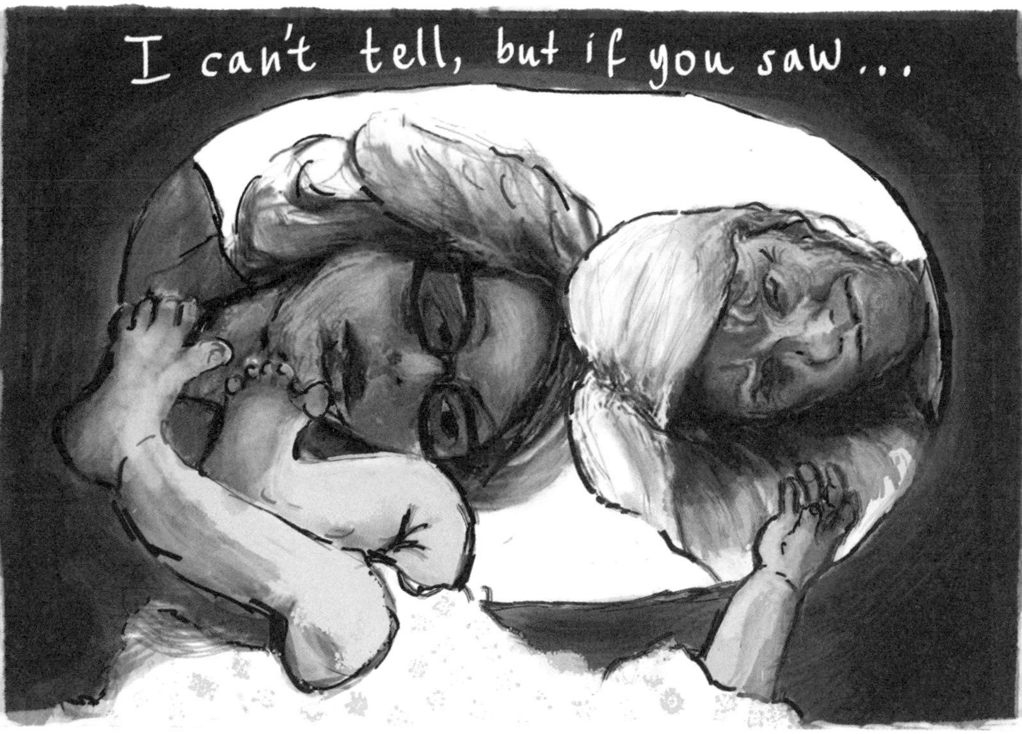
I can't tell, but if you saw...

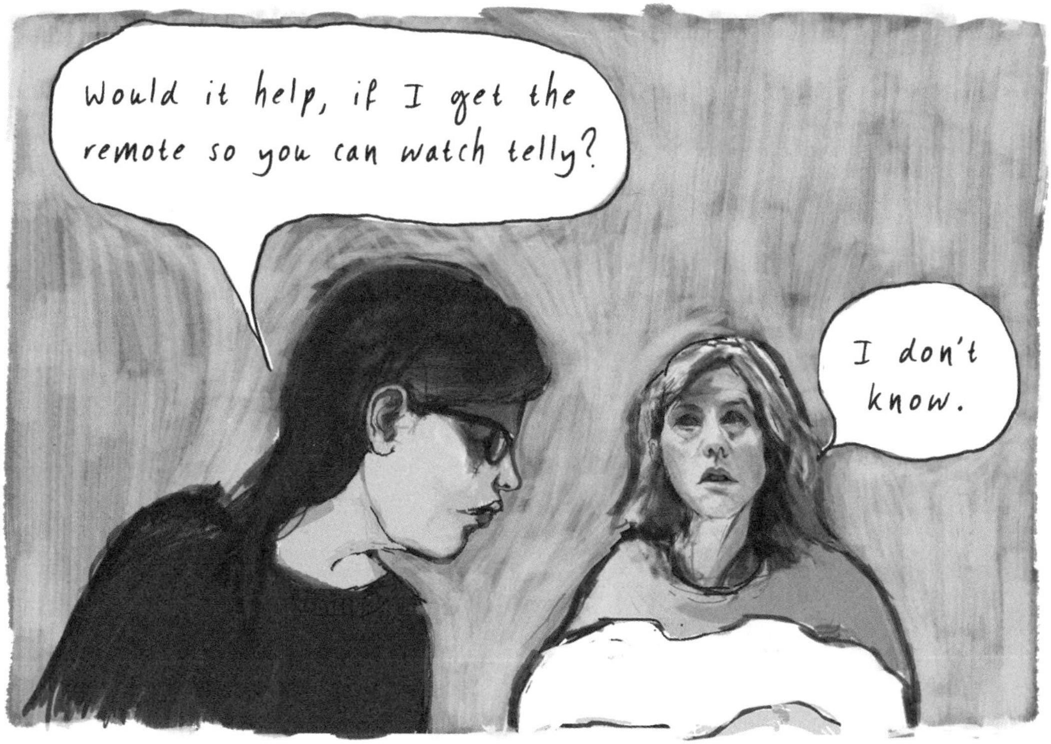
Would it help, if I get the remote so you can watch telly?
I don't know.

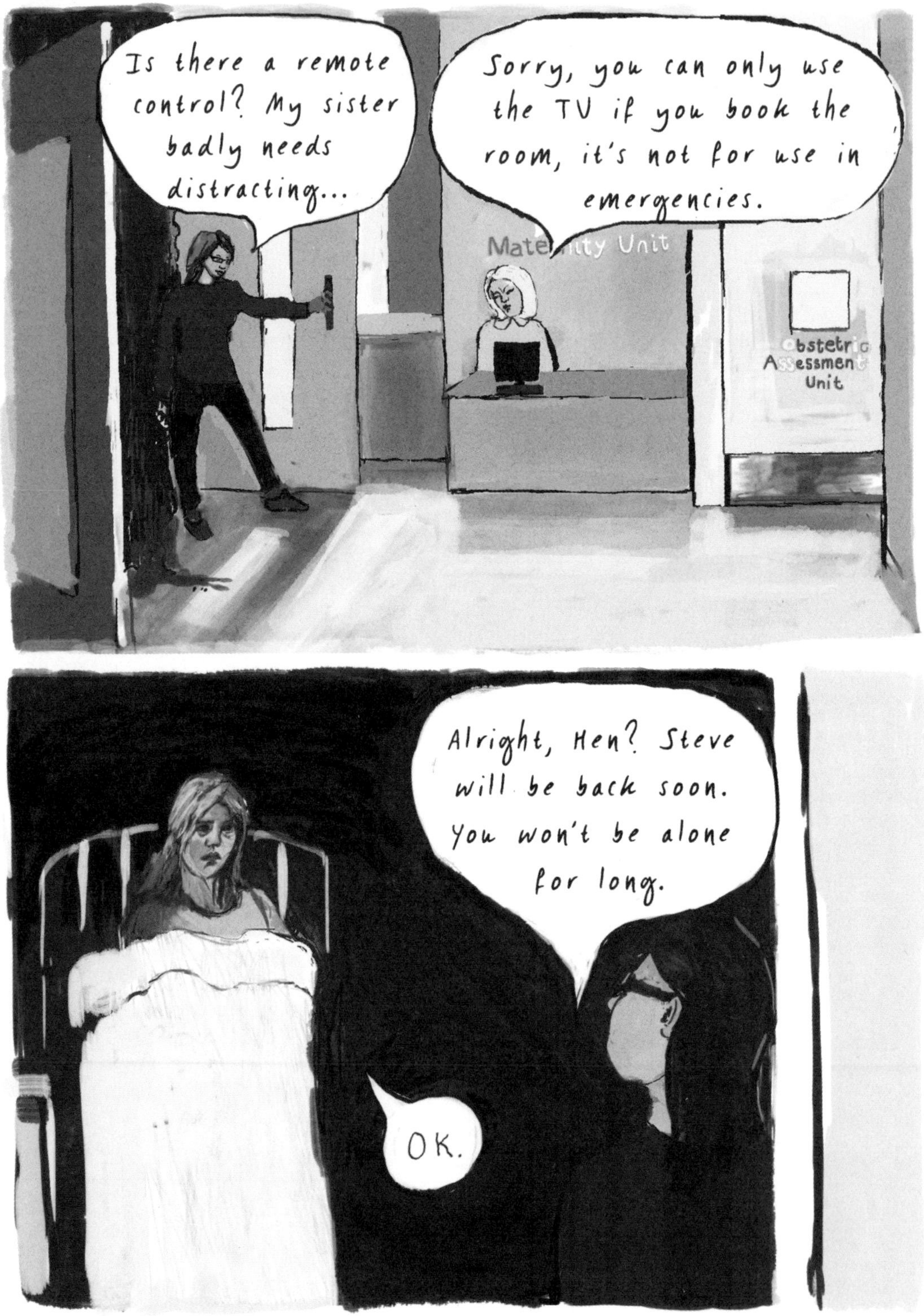
Is there a remote control? My sister badly needs distracting...
Sorry, you can only use the TV if you book the room, it's not for use in emergencies.
Alright, Hen? Steve will be back soon. You won't be alone for long.
OK.

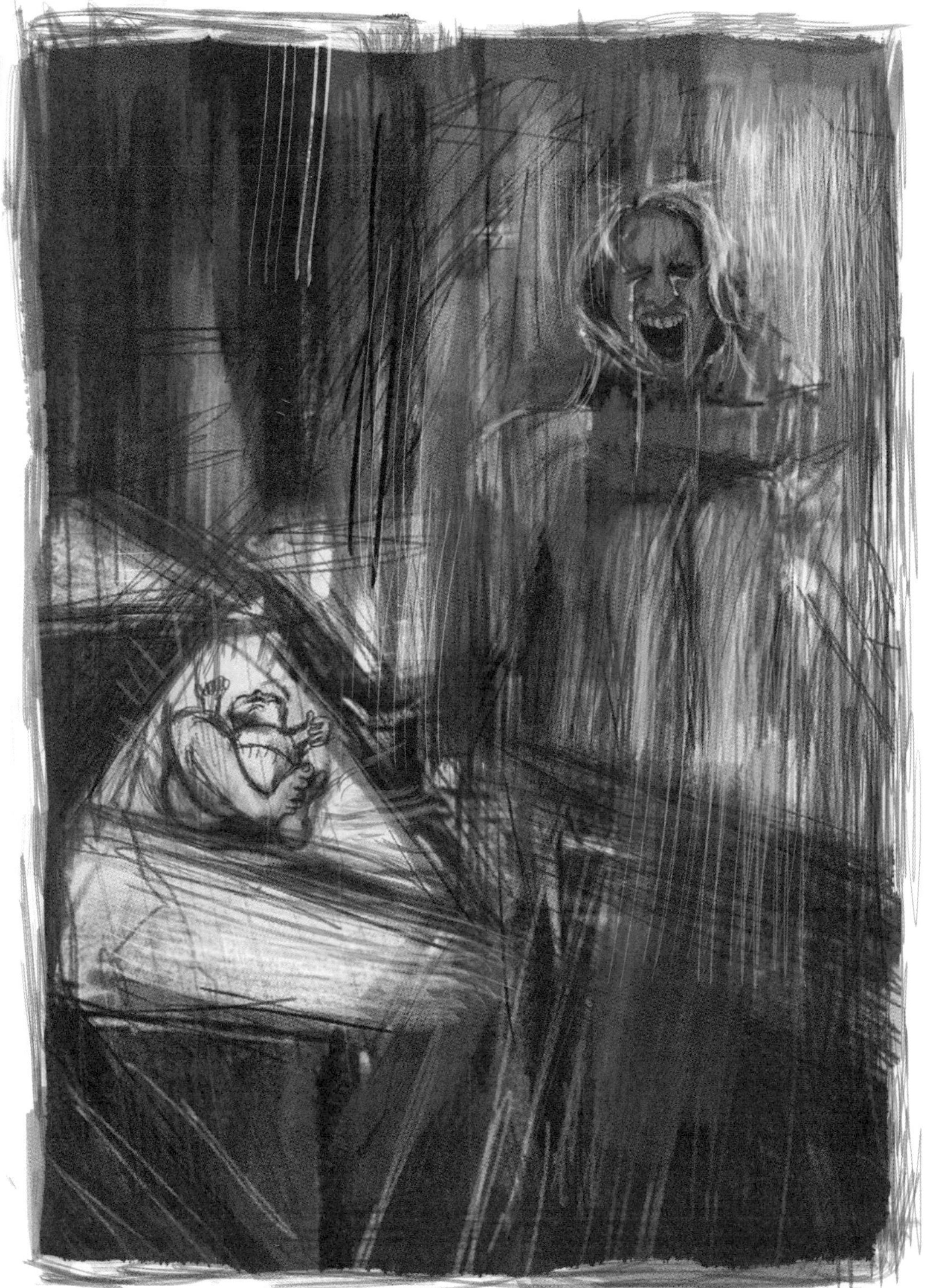

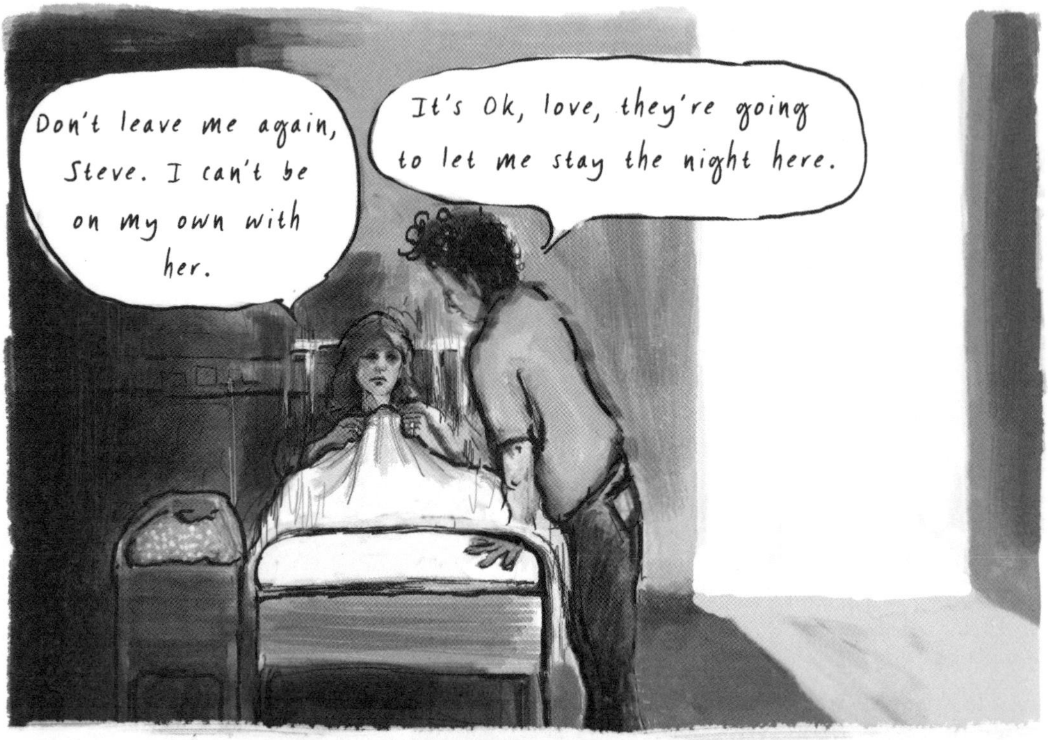
Don't leave me again, Steve. I can't be on my own with her.
It's Ok, love, they're going to let me stay the night here.

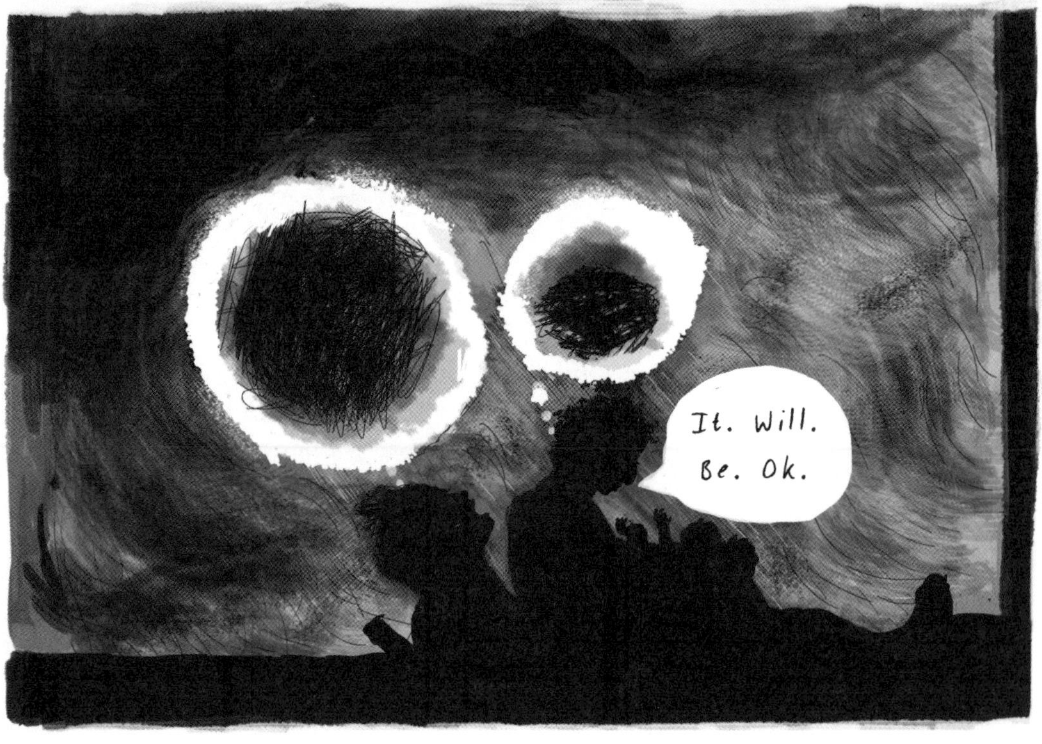
It. Will. Be. Ok.

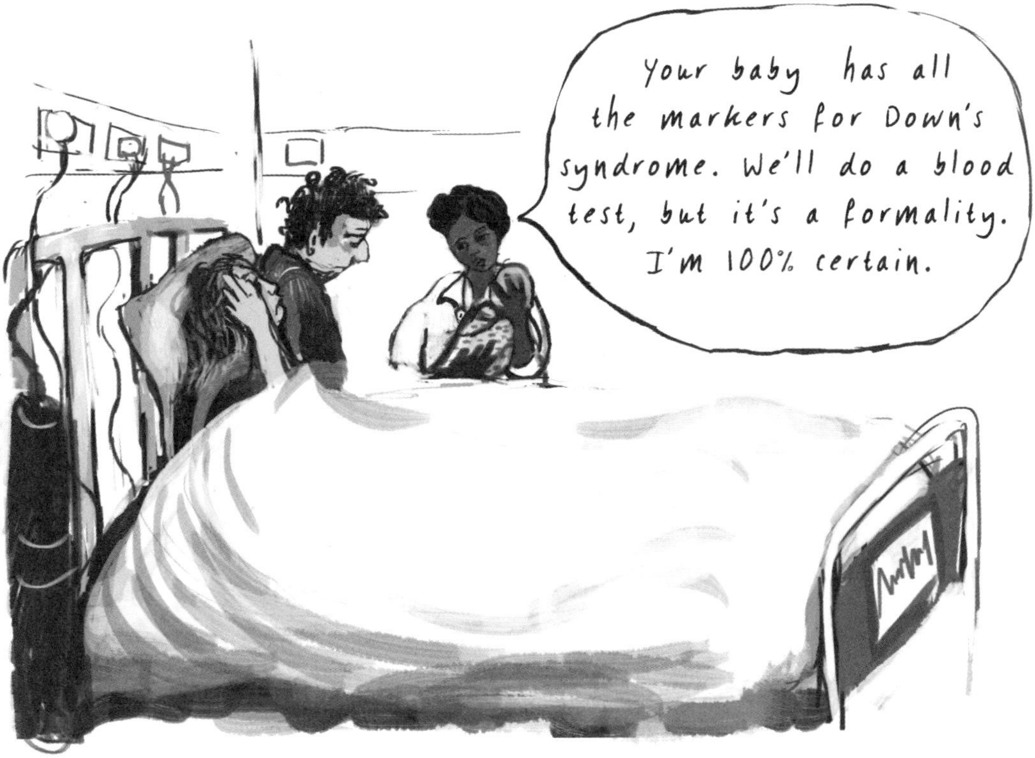
Your baby has all the markers for Down's syndrome. We'll do a blood test, but it's a formality. I'm 100% certain.

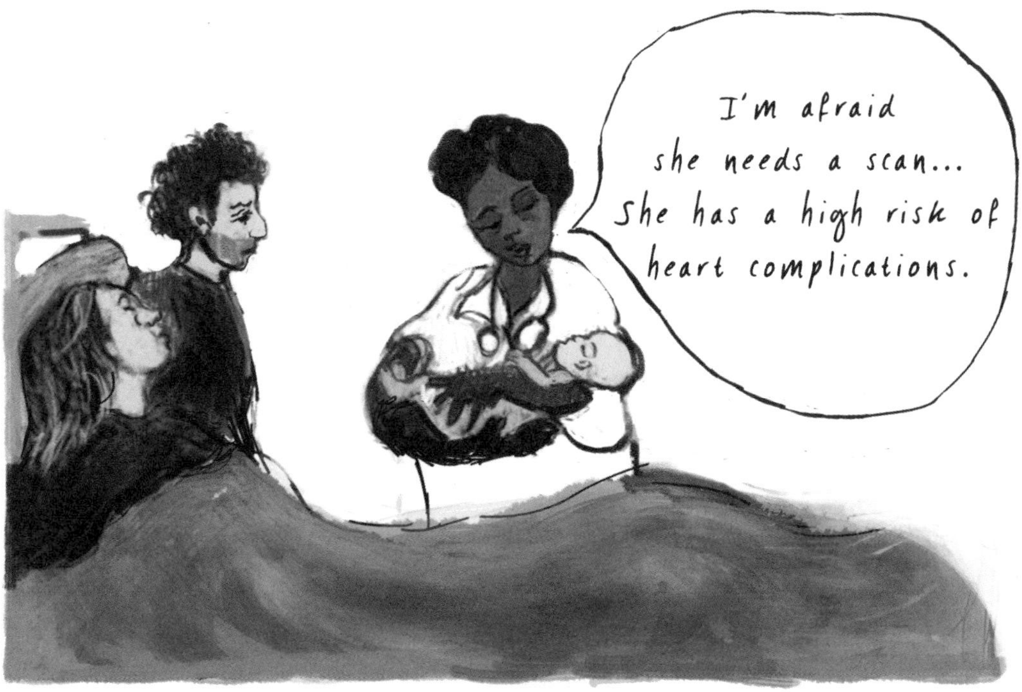
I'm afraid she needs a scan... She has a high risk of heart complications.

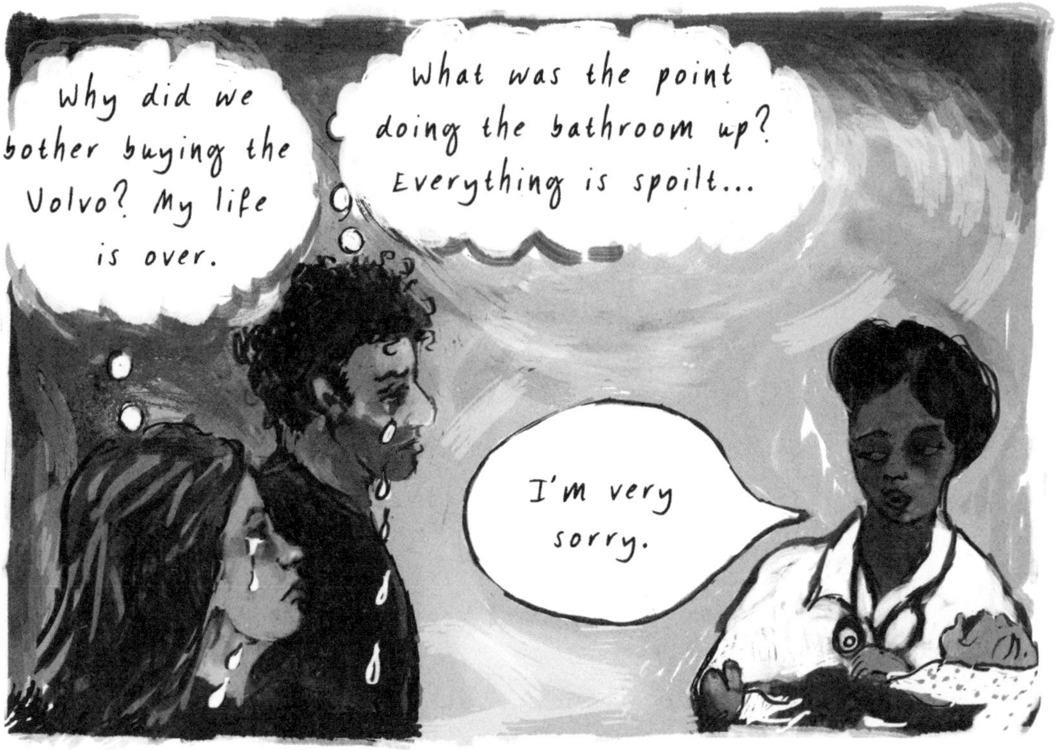
Why did we bother buying the Volvo? My life is over.
What was the point doing the bathroom up? Everything is spoilt...
I'm very sorry.

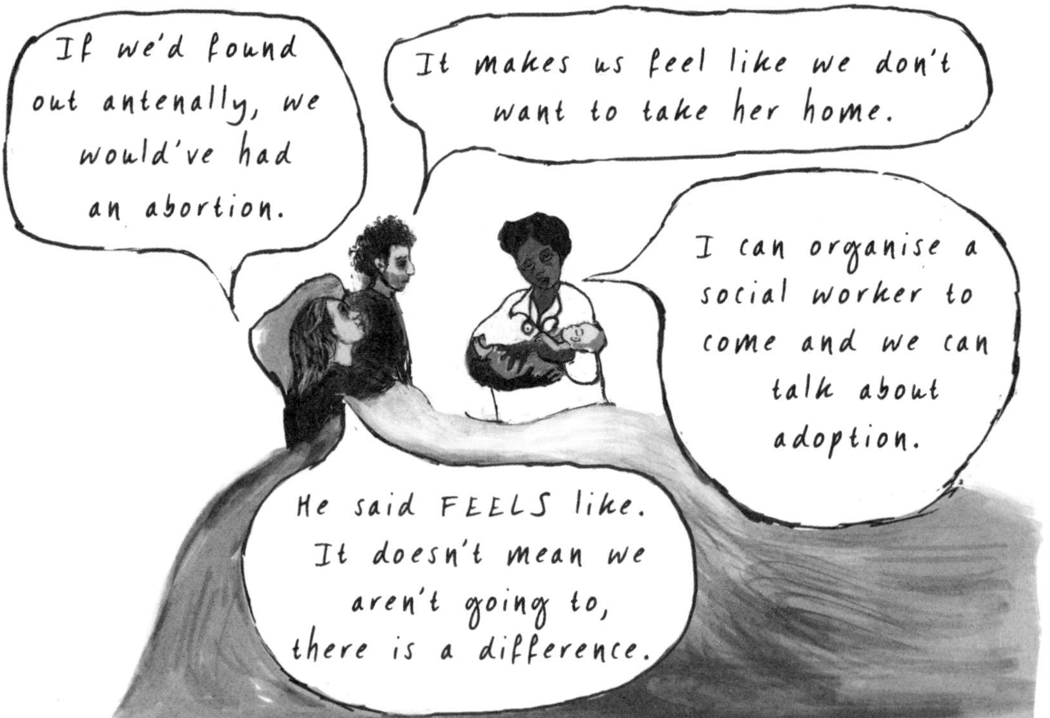
If we'd found out antenally, we would've had an abortion.
It makes us feel like we don't want to take her home.
I can organise a social worker to come and we can talk about adoption.
He said FEELS like. It doesn't mean we aren't going to, there is a difference.

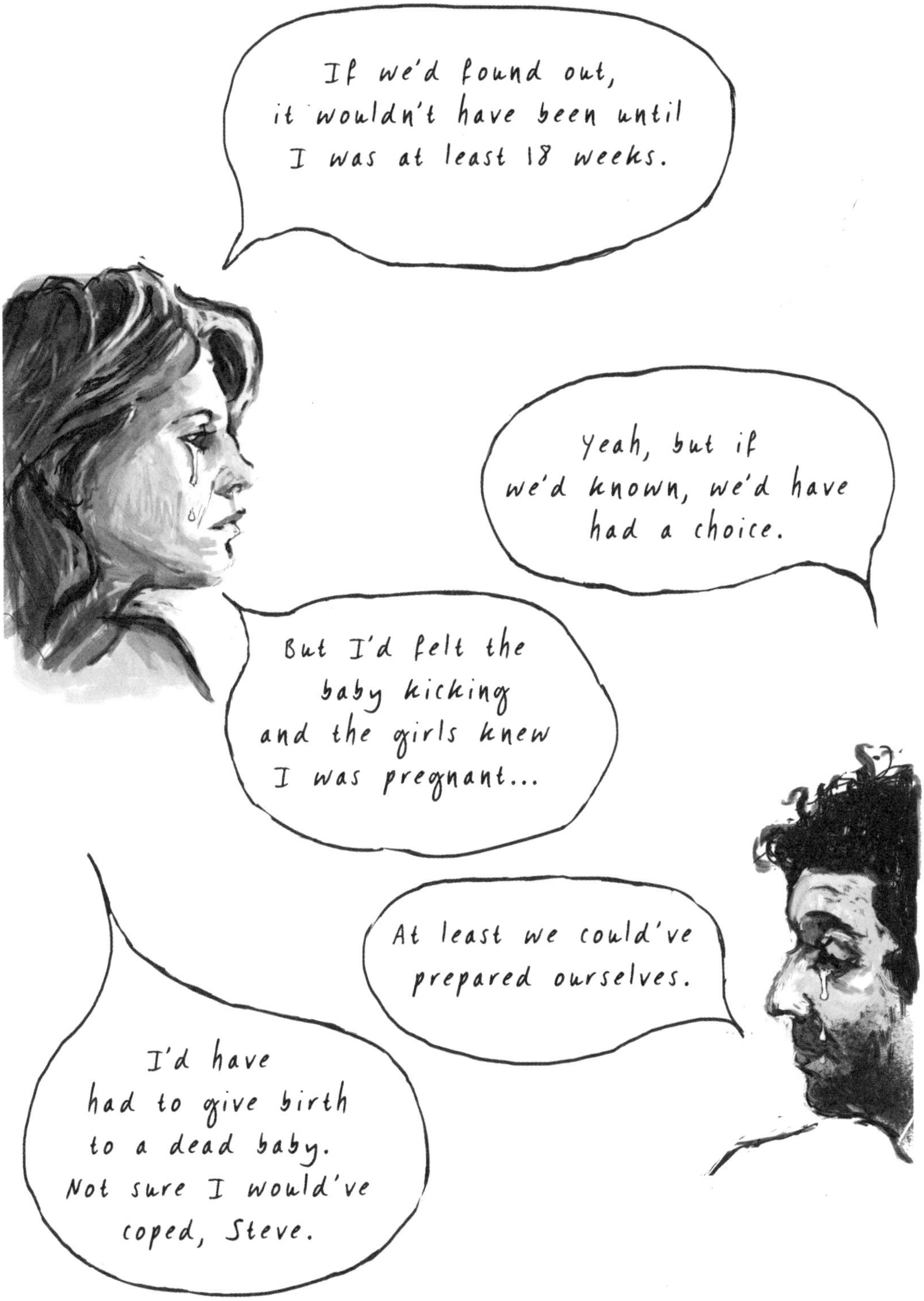

If we'd found out,
it wouldn't have been until
I was at least 18 weeks.

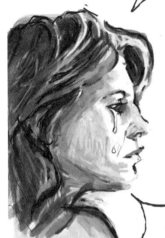

Yeah, but if
we'd known, we'd have
had a choice.

But I'd felt the
baby kicking
and the girls knew
I was pregnant...

At least we could've
prepared ourselves.

I'd have
had to give birth
to a dead baby.
Not sure I would've
coped, Steve.

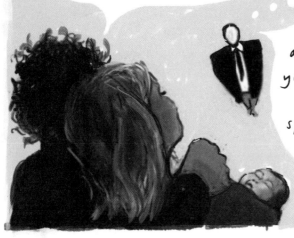

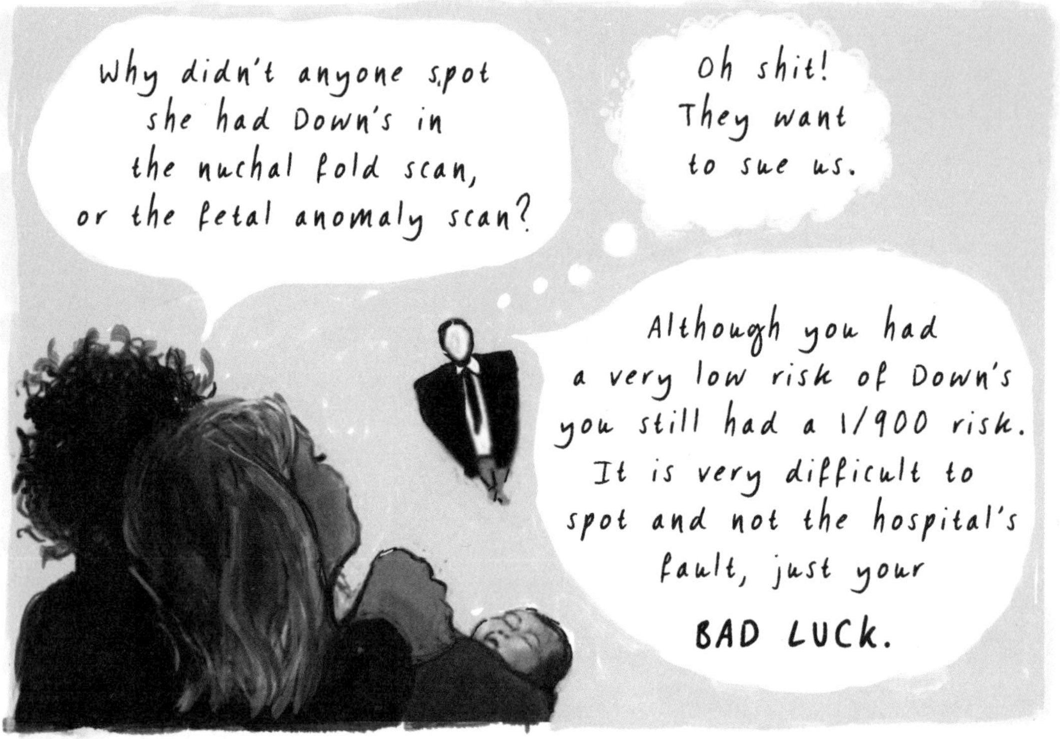

Why didn't anyone spot she had Down's in the nuchal fold scan, or the fetal anomaly scan?

Oh shit! They want to sue us.

Although you had a very low risk of Down's you still had a 1/900 risk. It is very difficult to spot and not the hospital's fault, just your **BAD LUCK.**

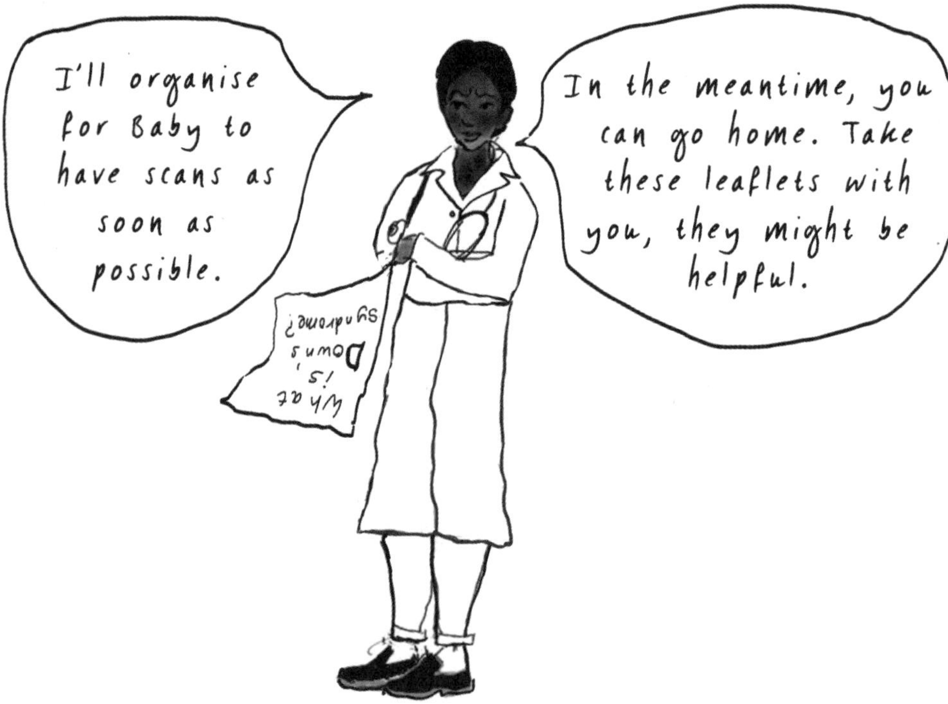

I'll organise for Baby to have scans as soon as possible.

In the meantime, you can go home. Take these leaflets with you, they might be helpful.

What is, Down's Syndrome?

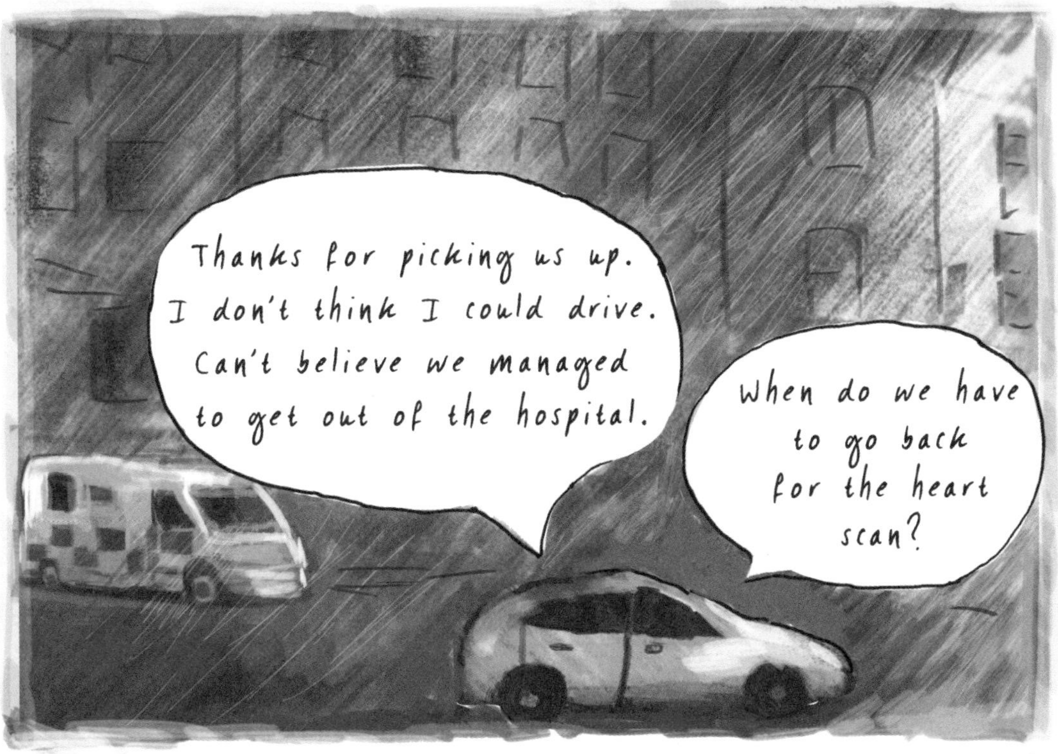
Thanks for picking us up. I don't think I could drive. Can't believe we managed to get out of the hospital.
When do we have to go back for the heart scan?

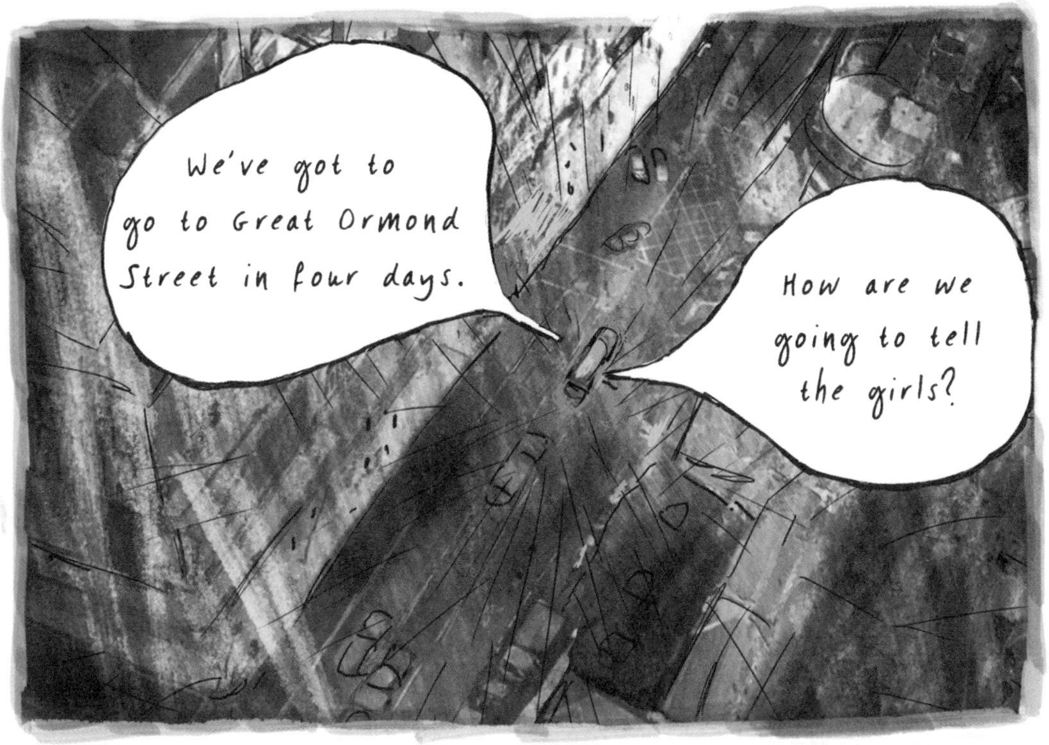
We've got to go to Great Ormond Street in four days.
How are we going to tell the girls?

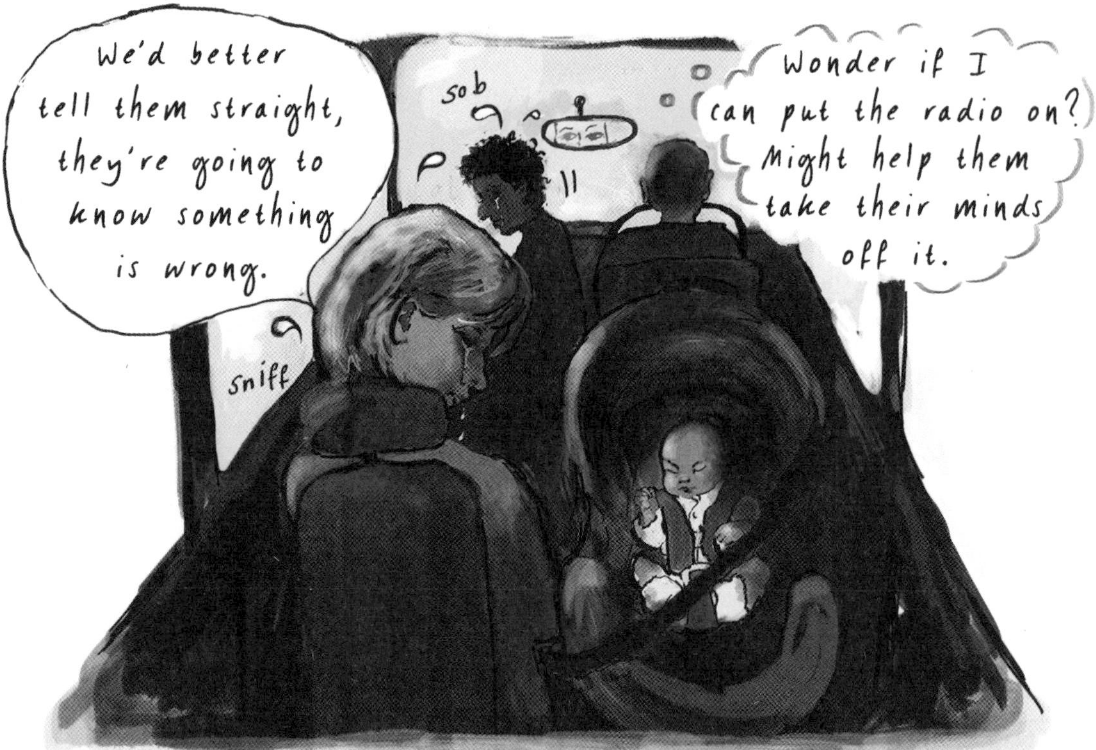
We'd better tell them straight, they're going to know something is wrong.
sob
sniff
Wonder if I can put the radio on? Might help them take their minds off it.

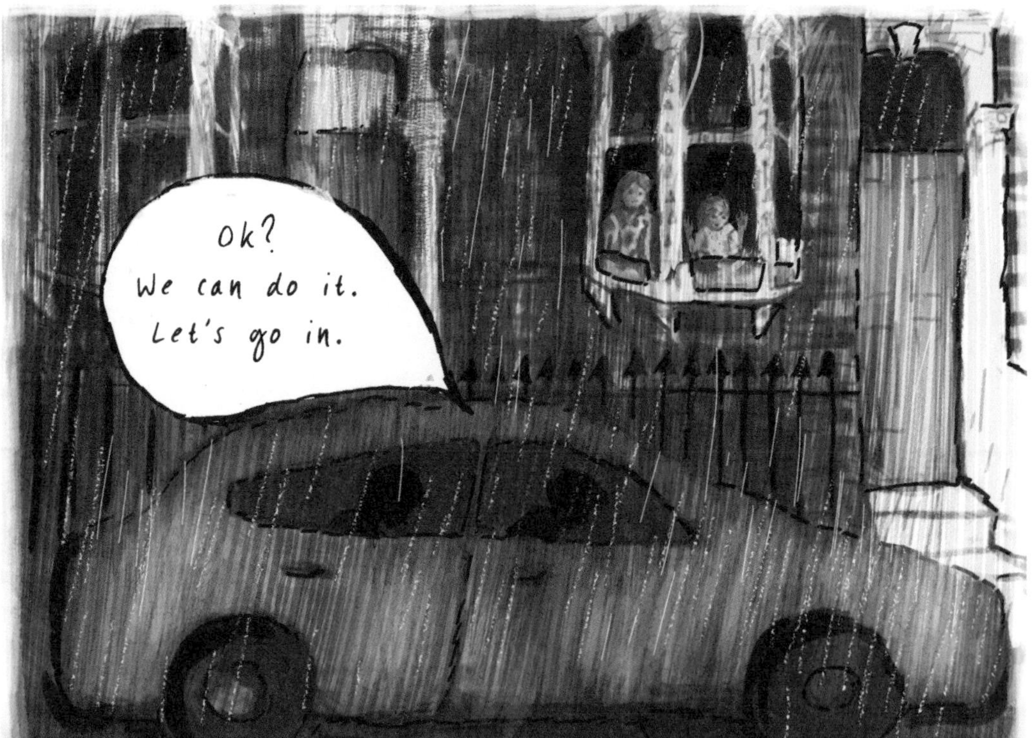
Ok? We can do it. Let's go in.

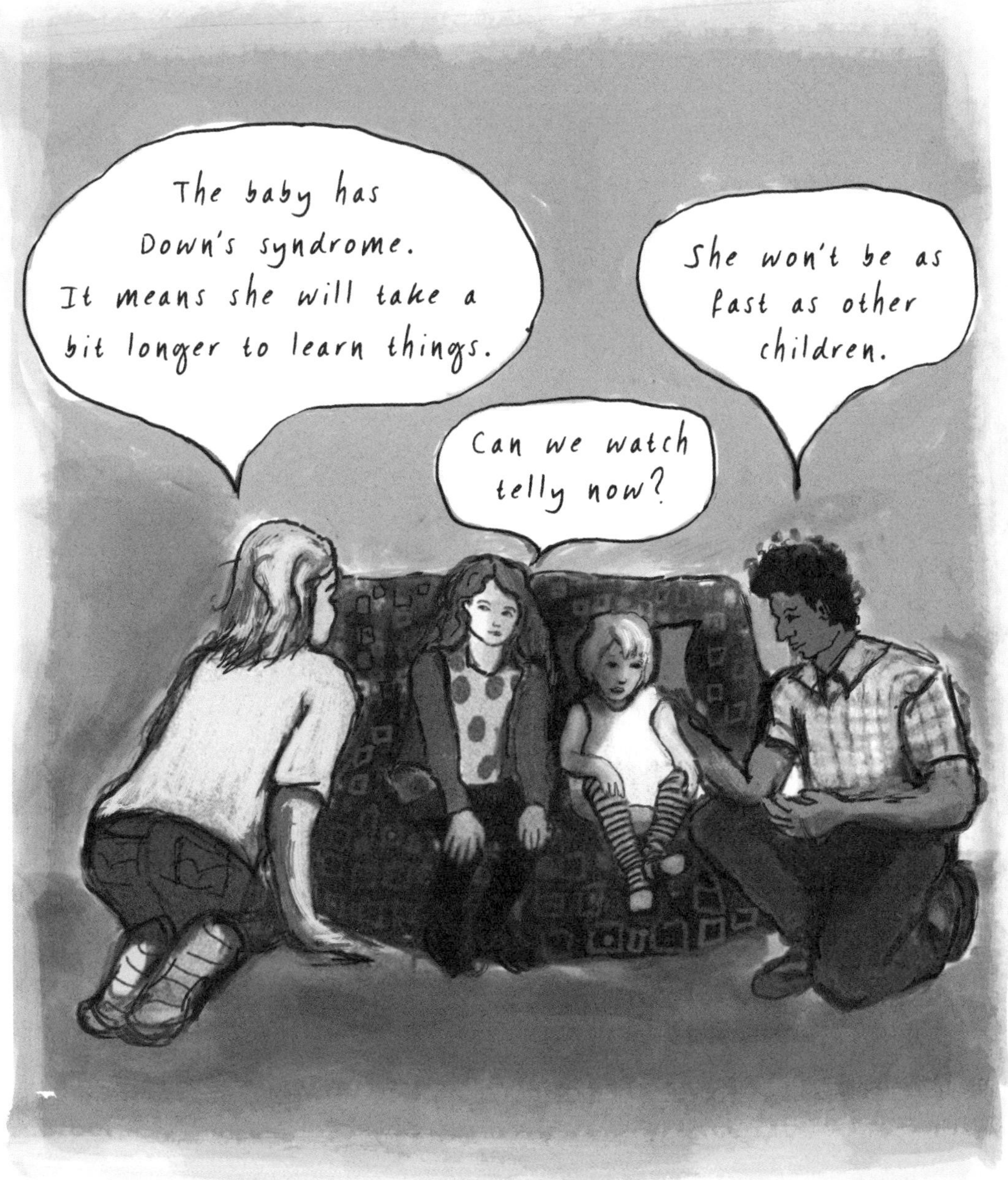
The baby has Down's syndrome. It means she will take a bit longer to learn things.
She won't be as fast as other children.
Can we watch telly now?

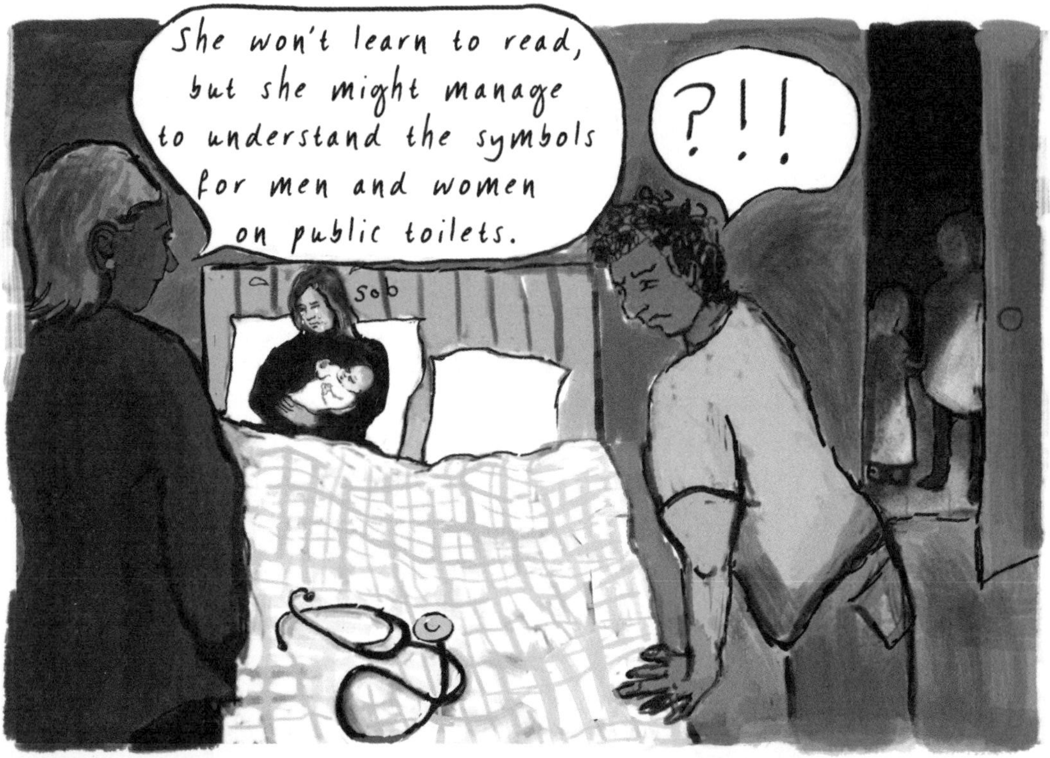
She won't learn to read, but she might manage to understand the symbols for men and women on public toilets.
?!!
sob

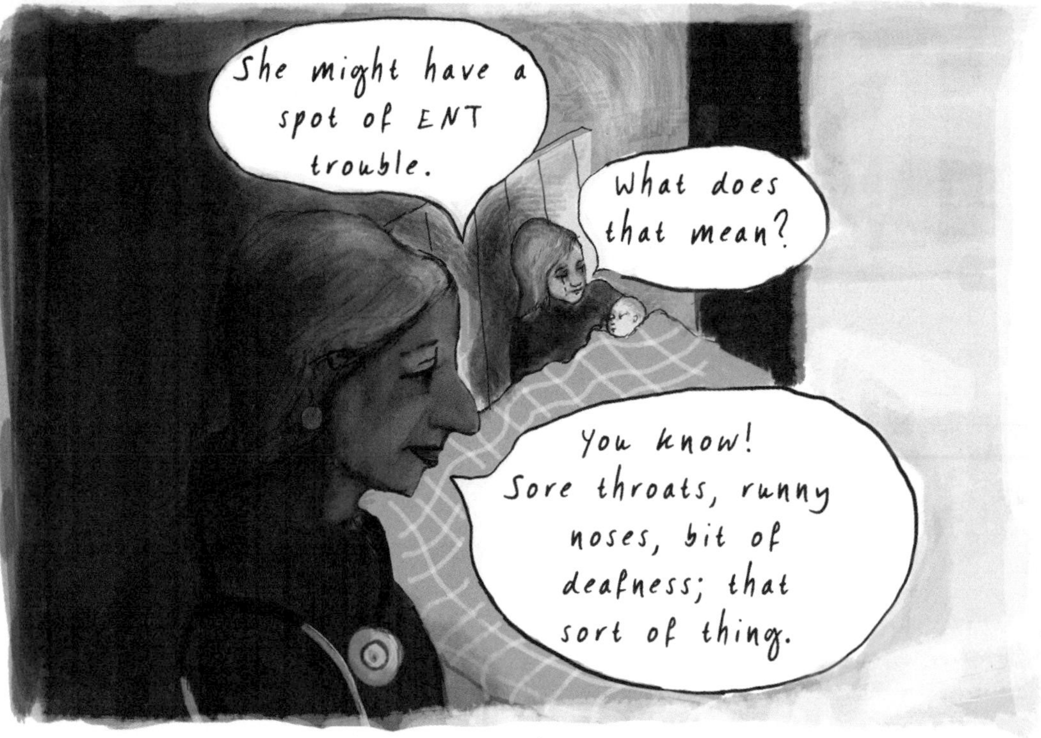
She might have a spot of ENT trouble.
What does that mean?
You know! Sore throats, runny noses, bit of deafness; that sort of thing.

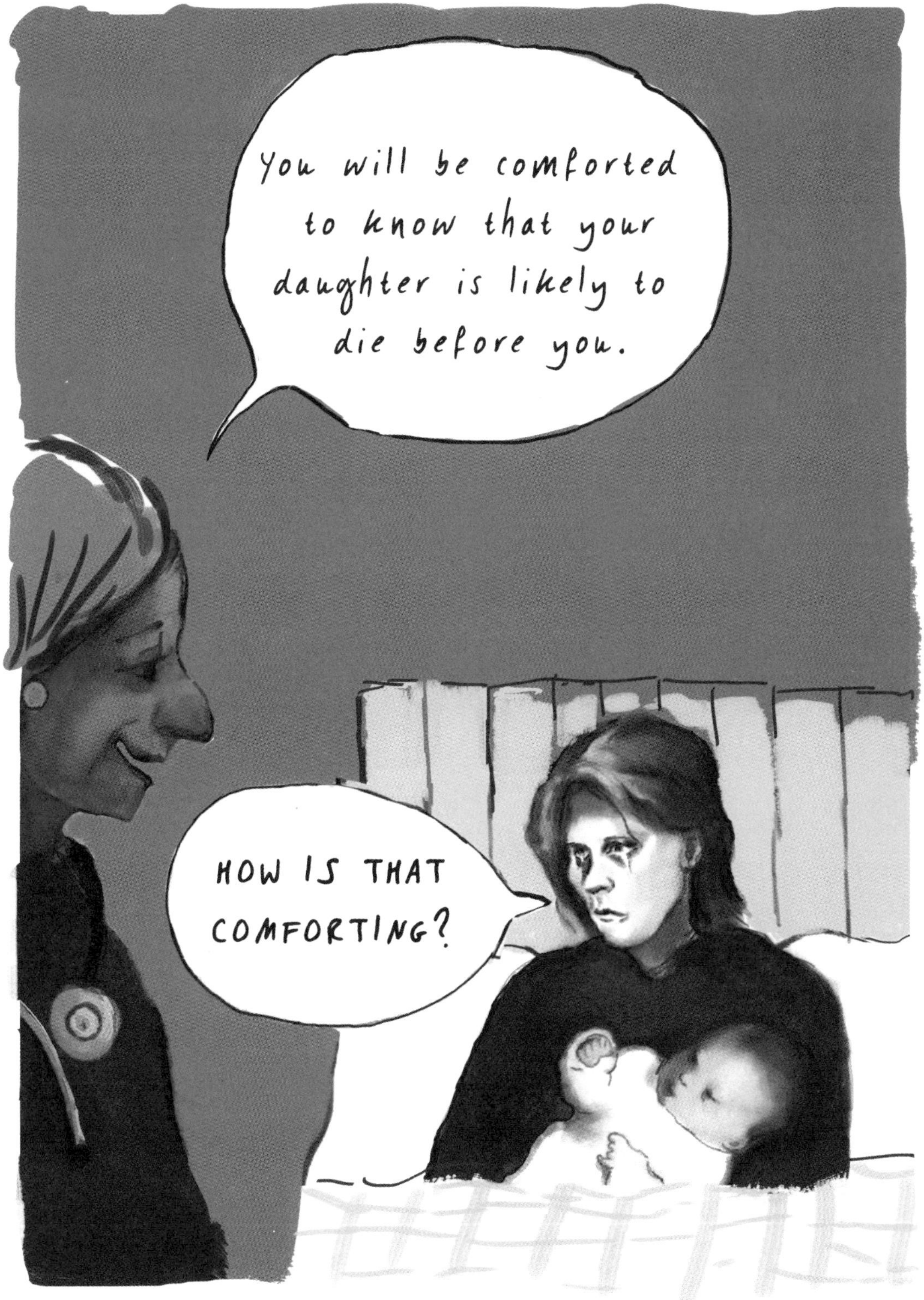
you will be comforted to know that your daughter is likely to die before you.
HOW IS THAT COMFORTING?

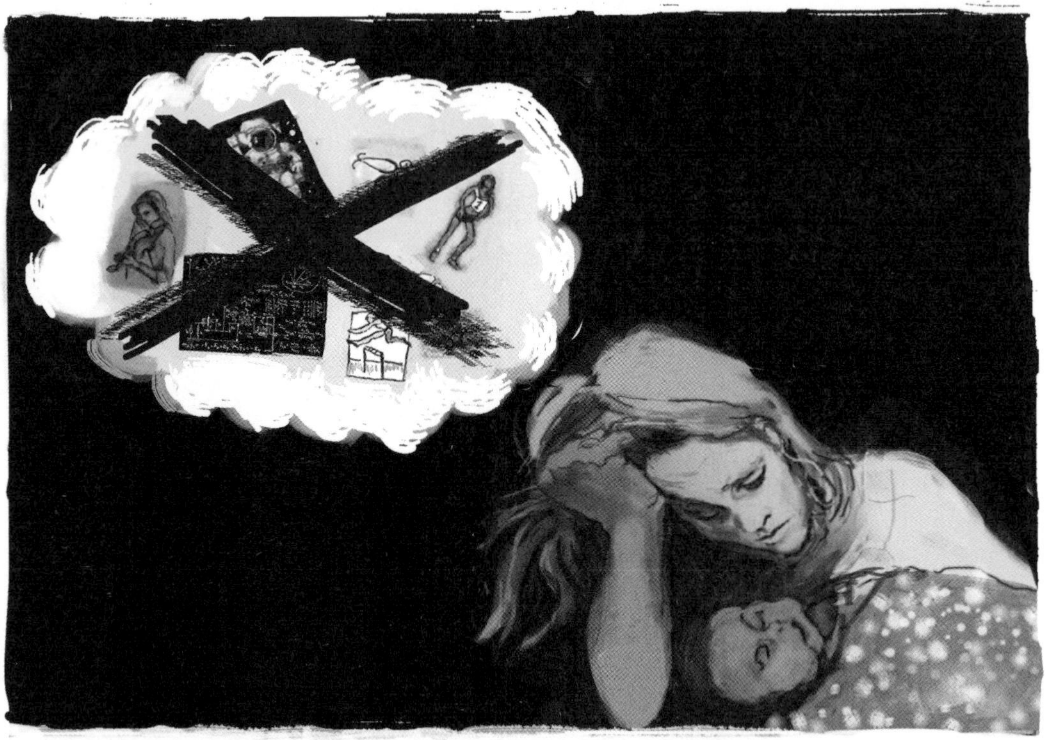

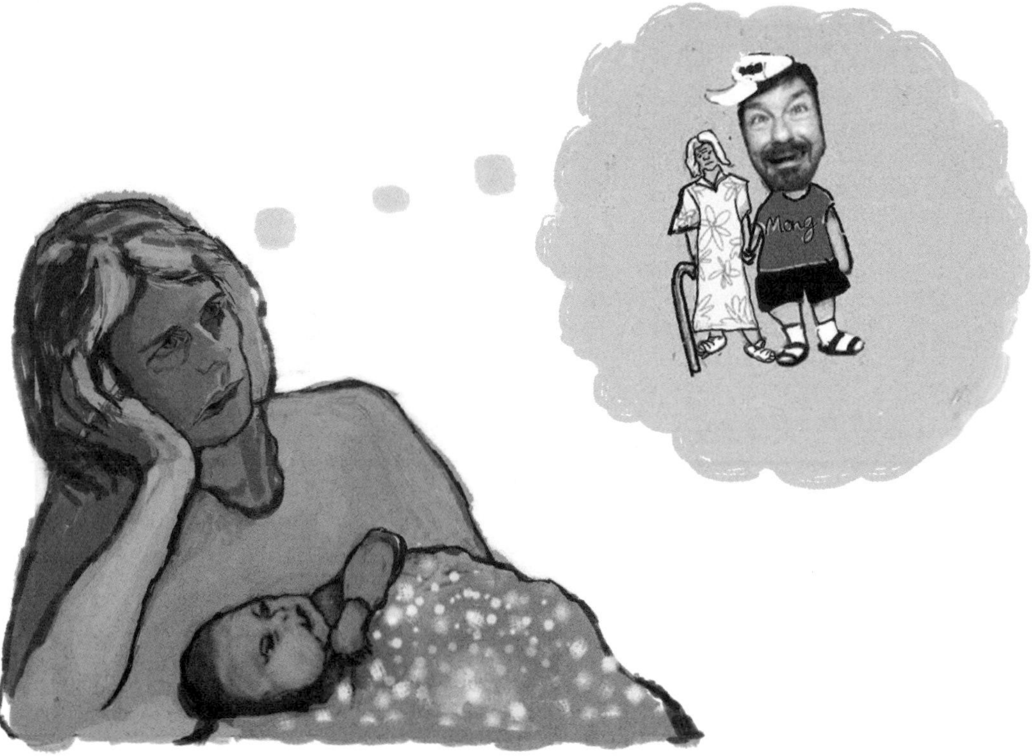
Mong

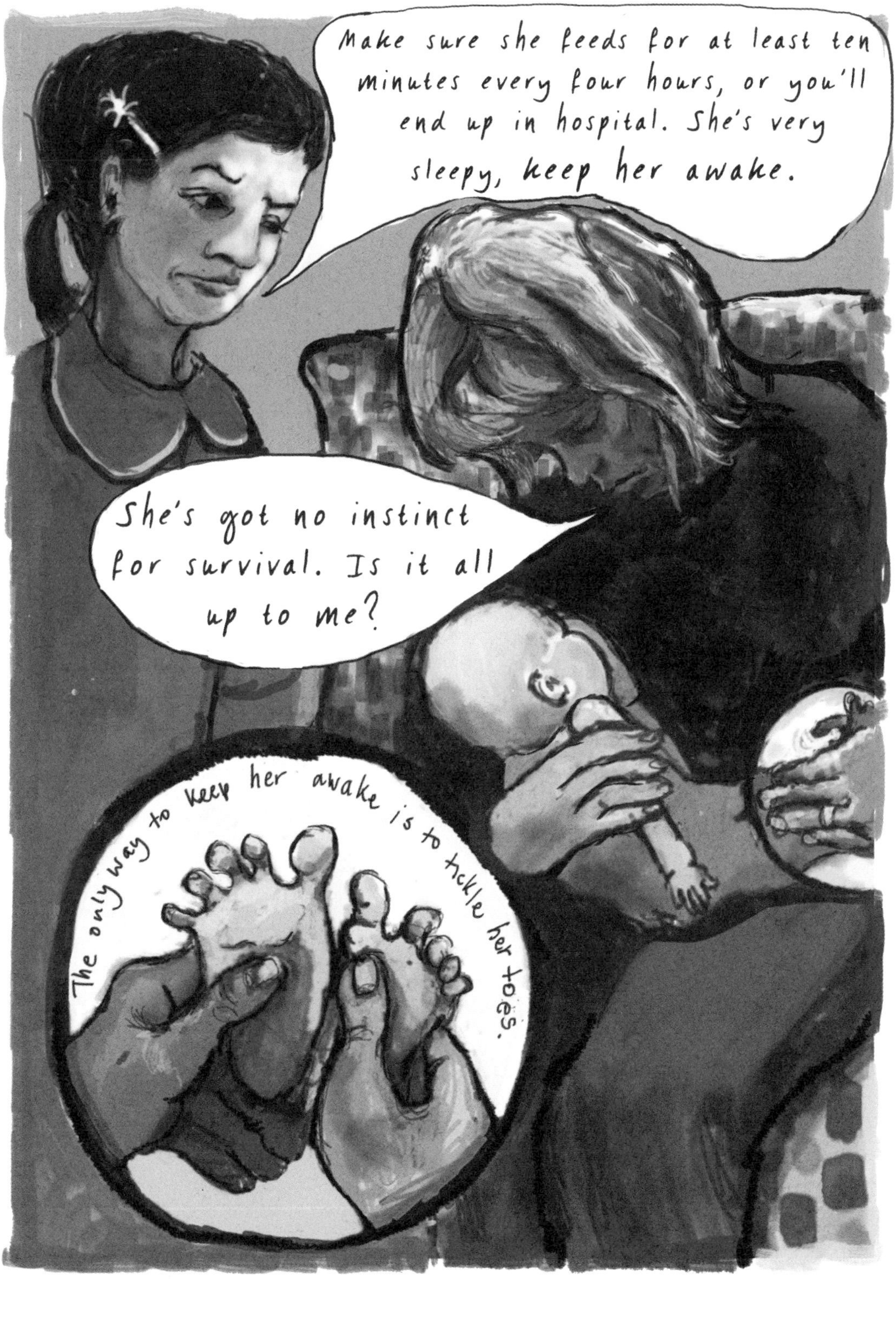
Make sure she feeds for at least ten minutes every four hours, or you'll end up in hospital. She's very sleepy, keep her awake.
She's got no instinct for survival. Is it all up to me?
The only way to keep her awake is to tickle her toes.

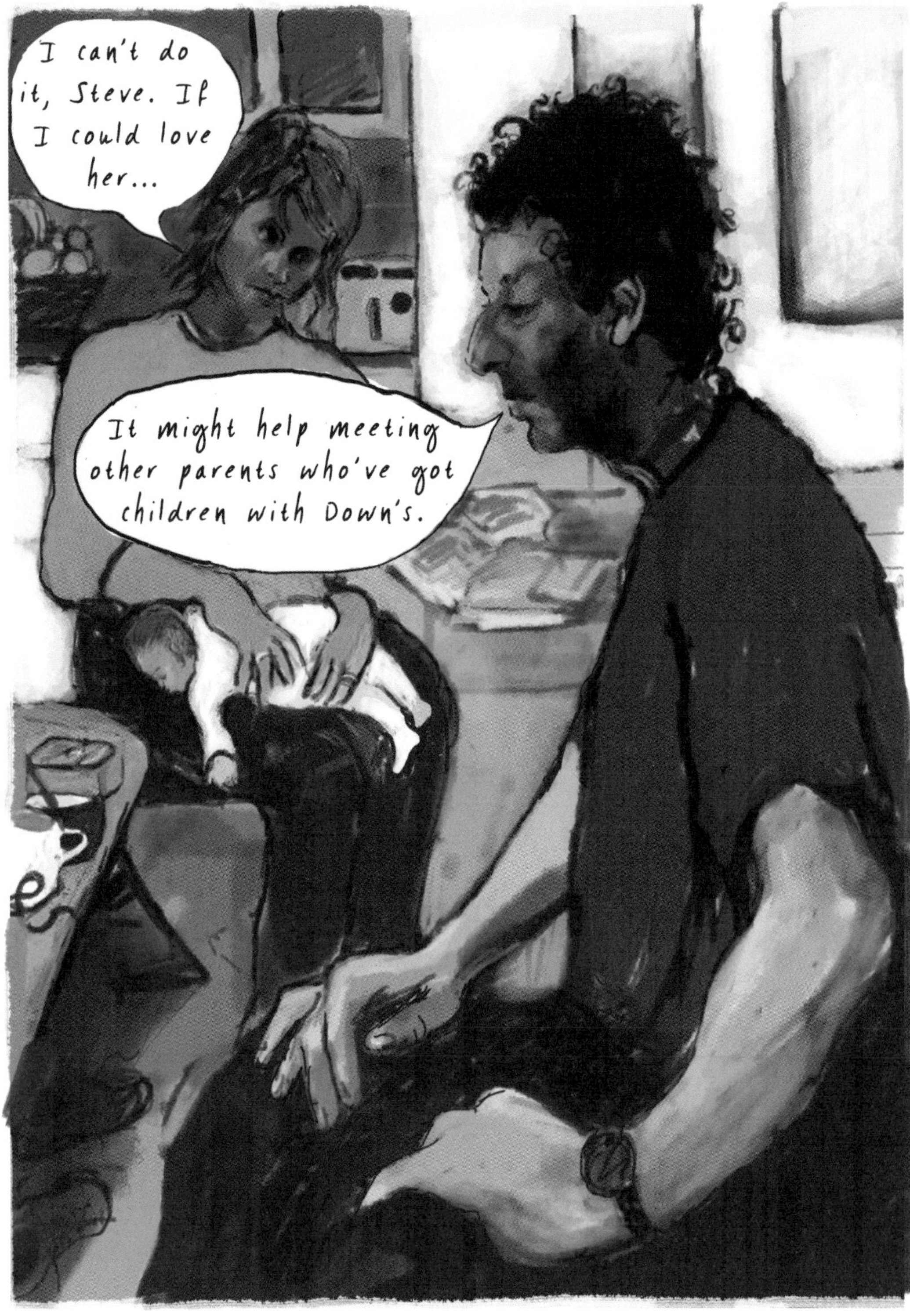
I can't do it, Steve. If I could love her...
It might help meeting other parents who've got children with Down's.

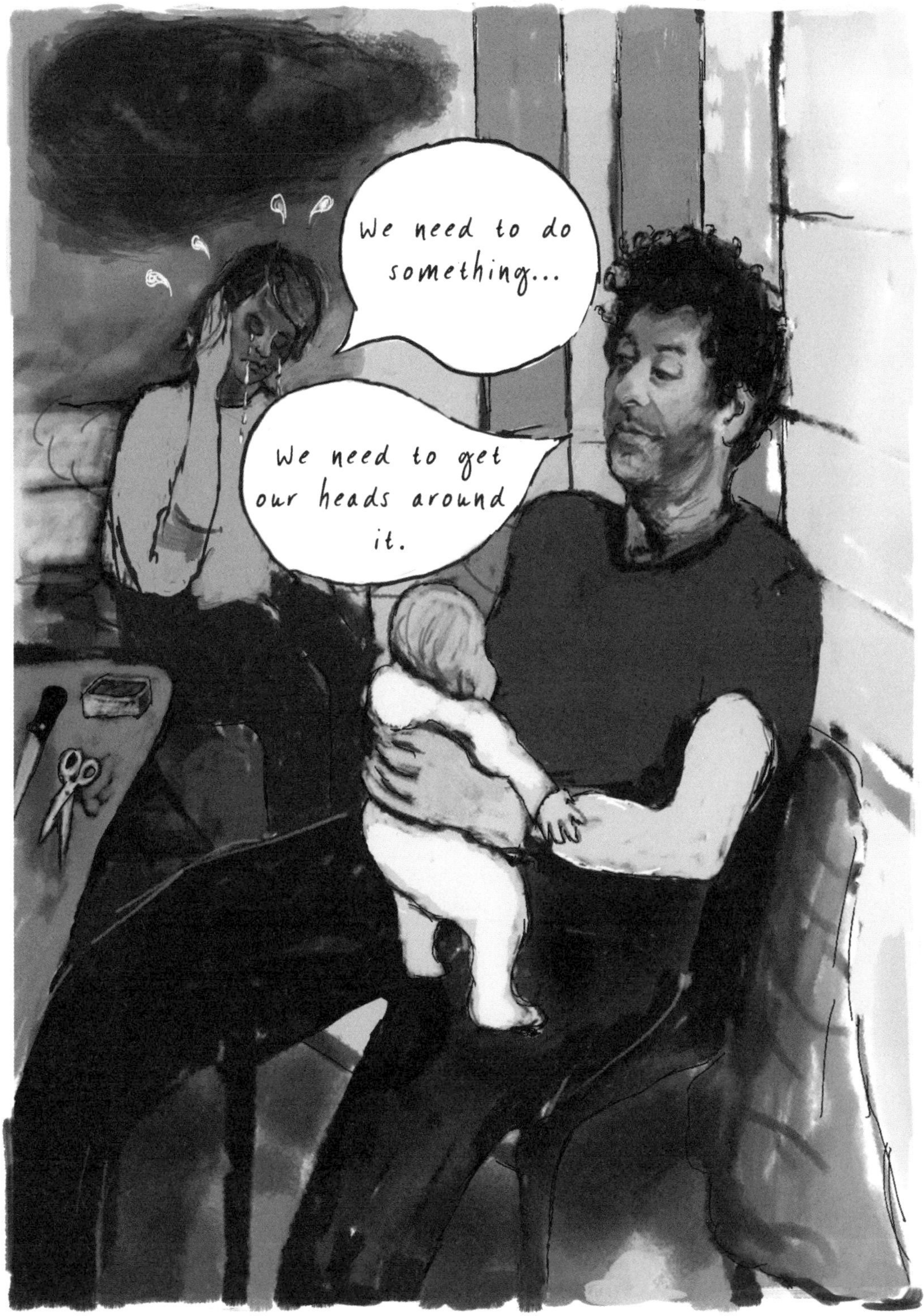
We need to do something...
We need to get our heads around it.

Nothing will help.

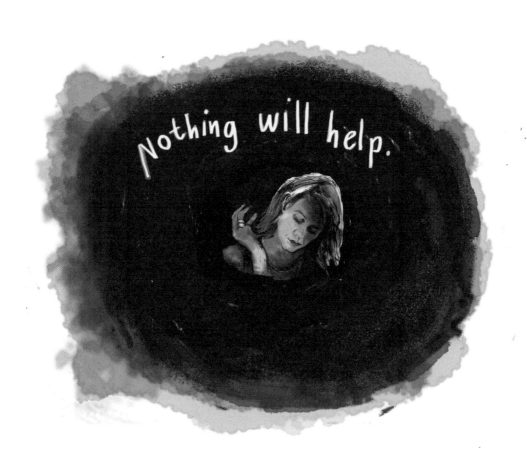

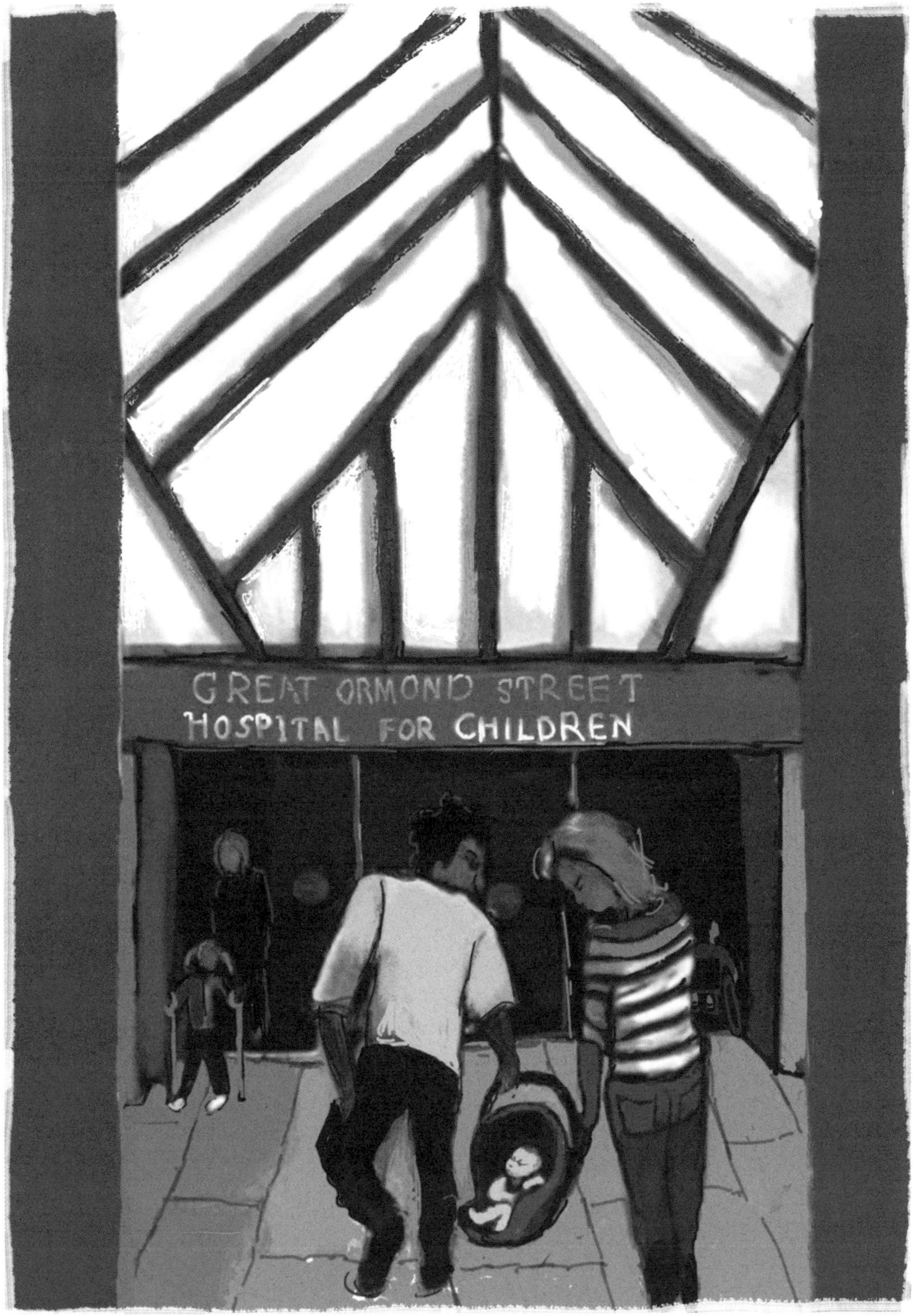
GREAT ORMOND STREET
HOSPITAL FOR CHILDREN

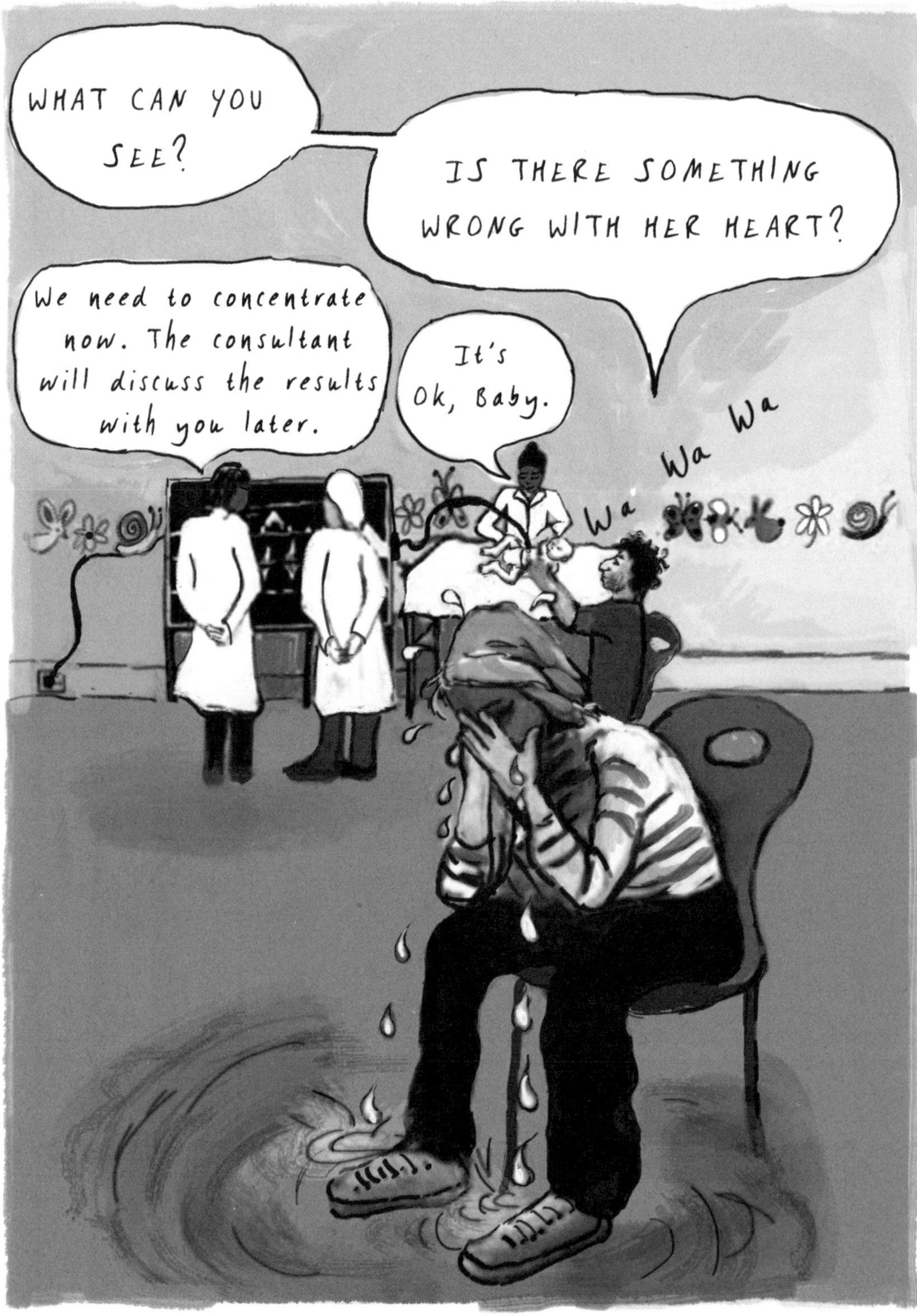
WHAT CAN YOU SEE?
IS THERE SOMETHING WRONG WITH HER HEART?
We need to concentrate now. The consultant will discuss the results with you later.
It's Ok, Baby.
Wa Wa Wa

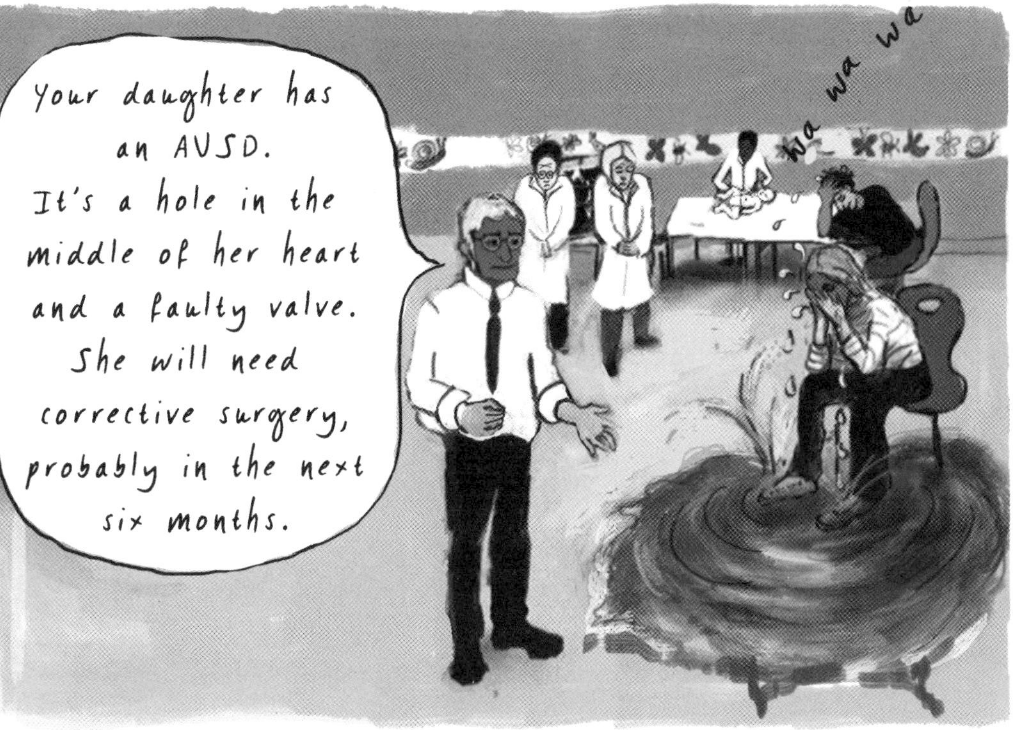
Your daughter has an AVSD. It's a hole in the middle of her heart and a faulty valve. She will need corrective surgery, probably in the next six months.
wa wa wa

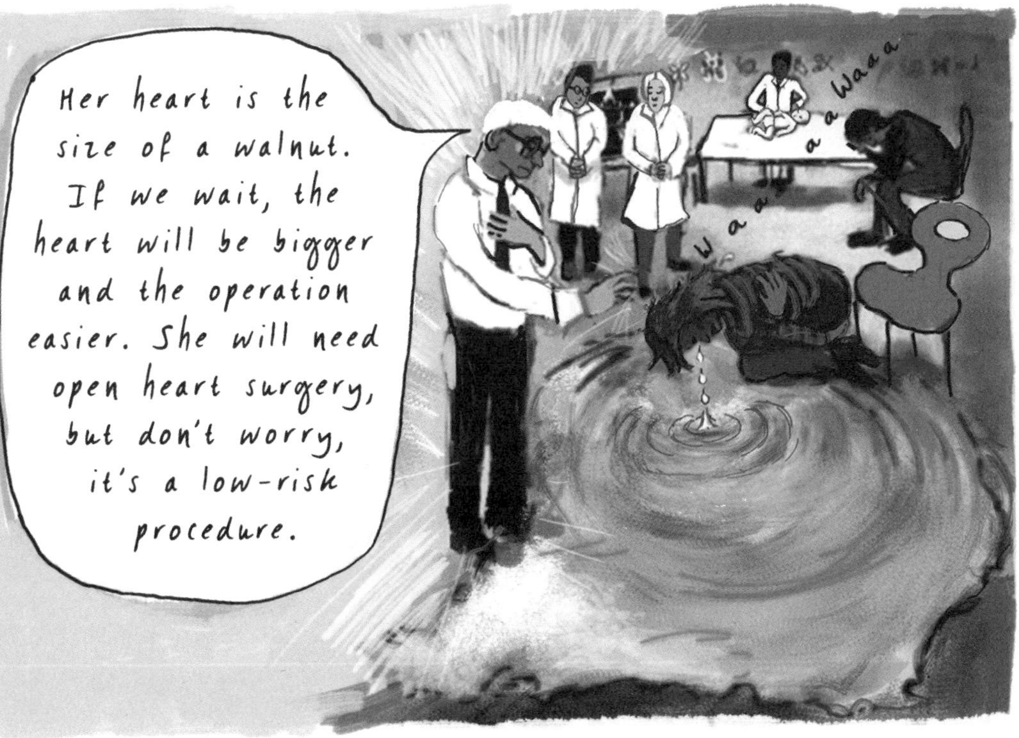
Her heart is the size of a walnut. If we wait, the heart will be bigger and the operation easier. She will need open heart surgery, but don't worry, it's a low-risk procedure.
Waaaa Waaa

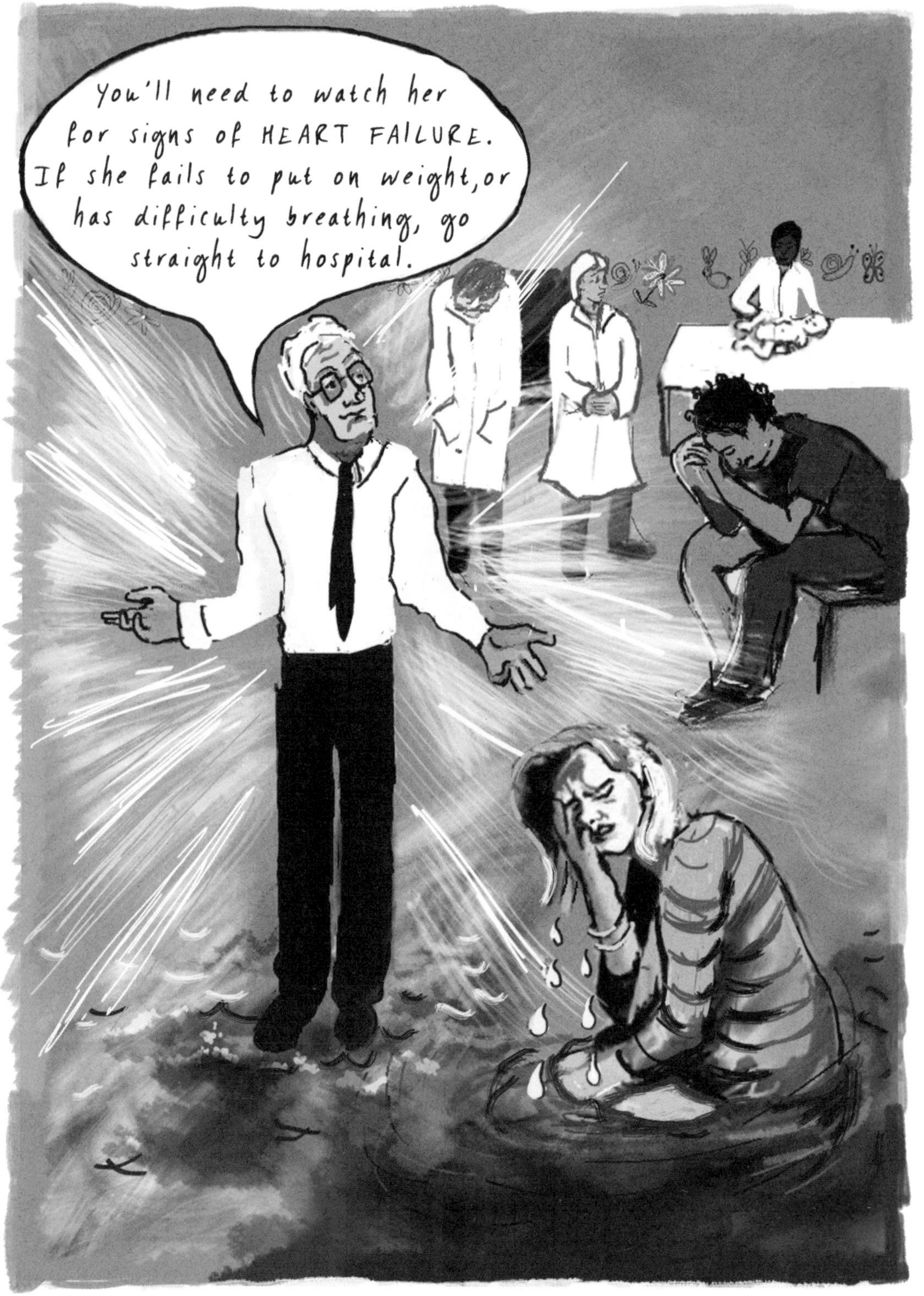
You'll need to watch her for signs of HEART FAILURE. If she fails to put on weight, or has difficulty breathing, go straight to hospital.

But how can I watch her ALL THE TIME when I've got two other children to look after?

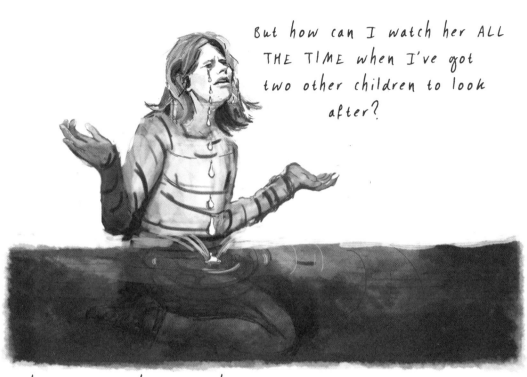

Why couldn't they see she had a heart condition when I was pregnant? I had so many scans and they looked in such detail...

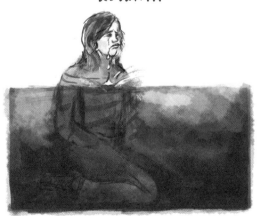

...and they were so confident that everything was fine. Are your scanning machines much more sophisticated here?

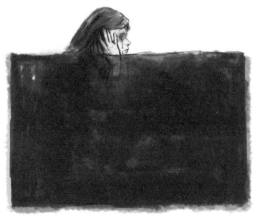

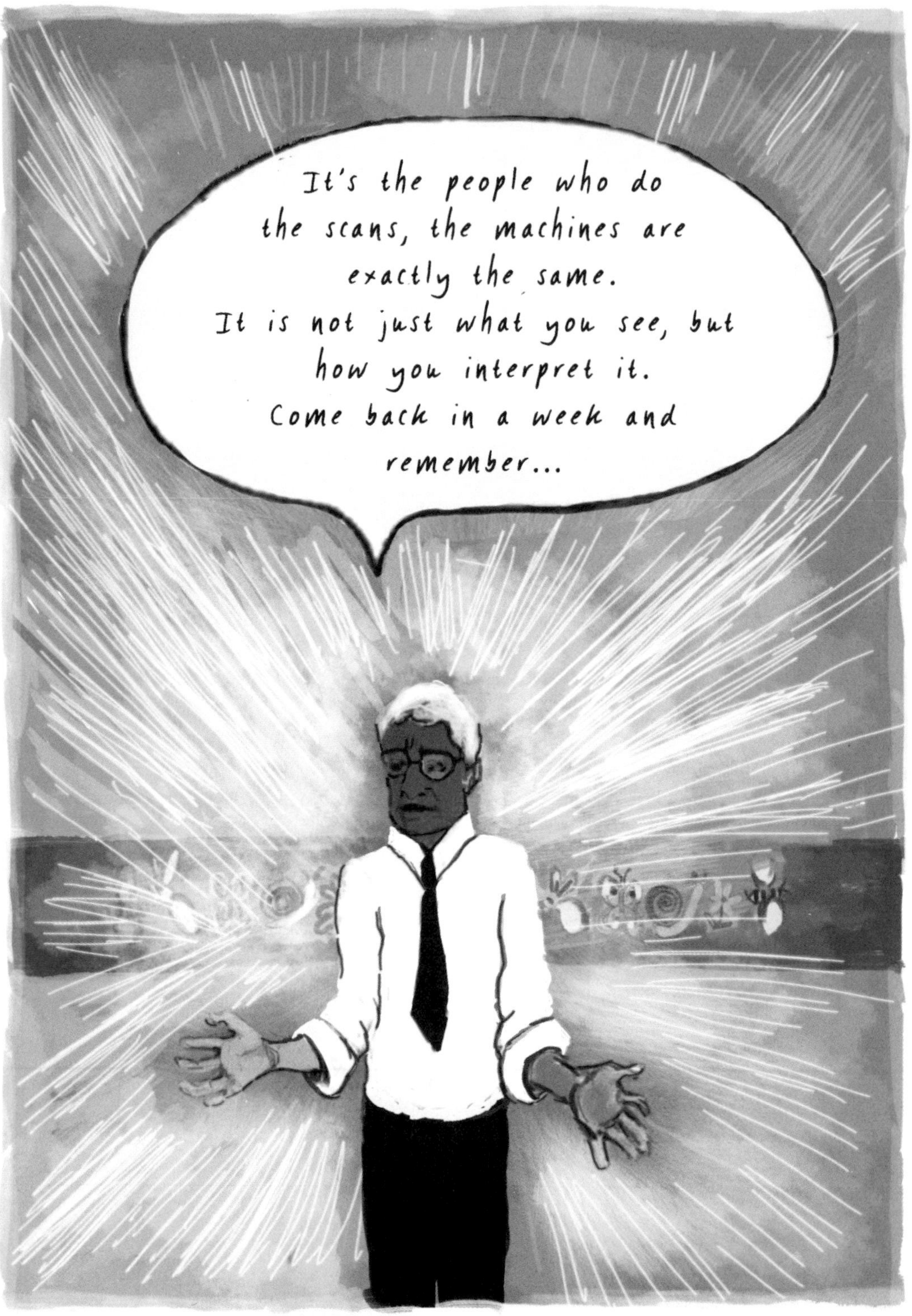
It's the people who do the scans, the machines are exactly the same. It is not just what you see, but how you interpret it. Come back in a week and remember...

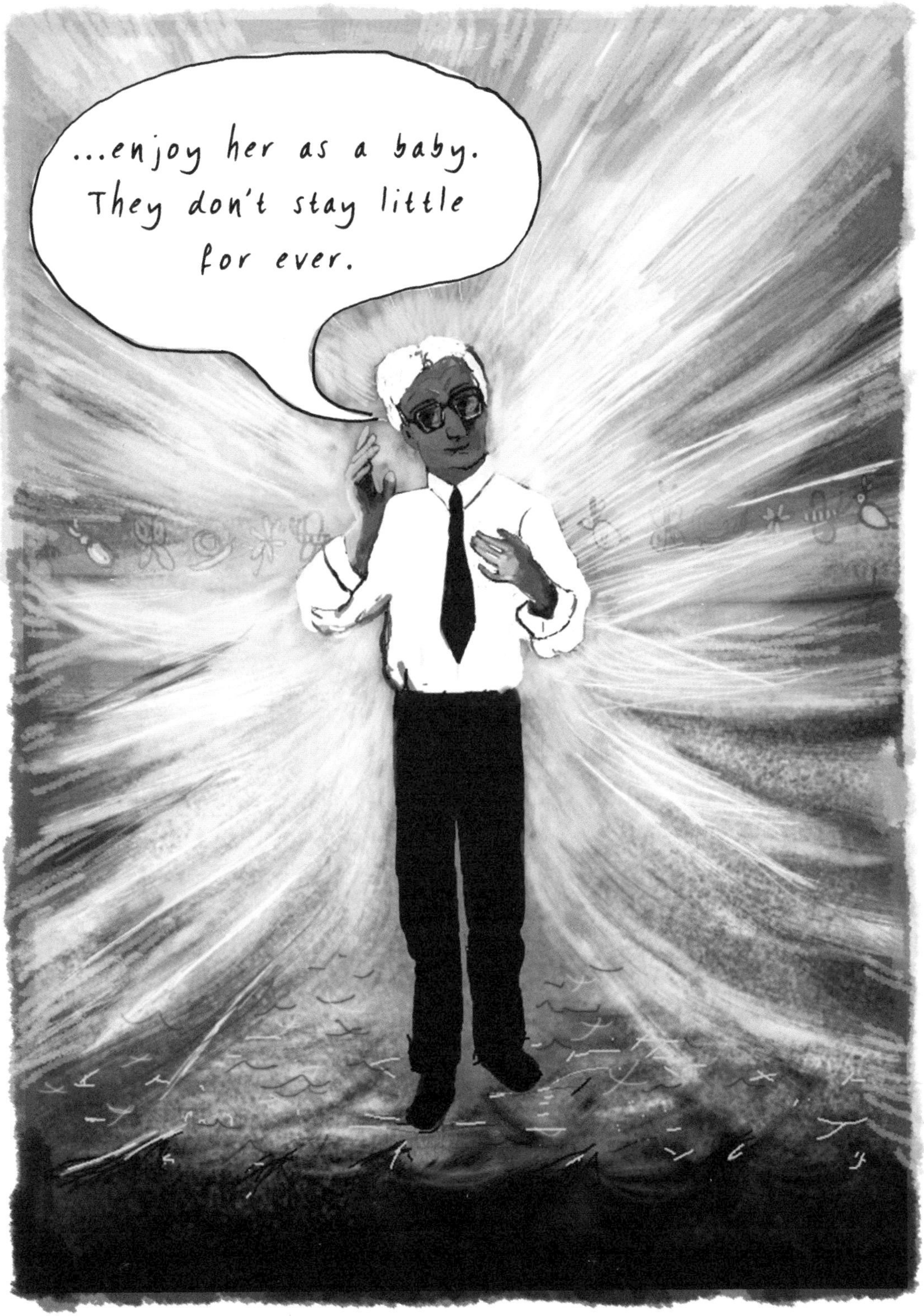
...enjoy her as a baby. They don't stay little for ever.

What does that mean?
Is he saying she'll die, so we
need to make the most of her now,
or that she is going to be a
hideous nightmare when she grows
up and we'll regret not loving
her enough as a baby?

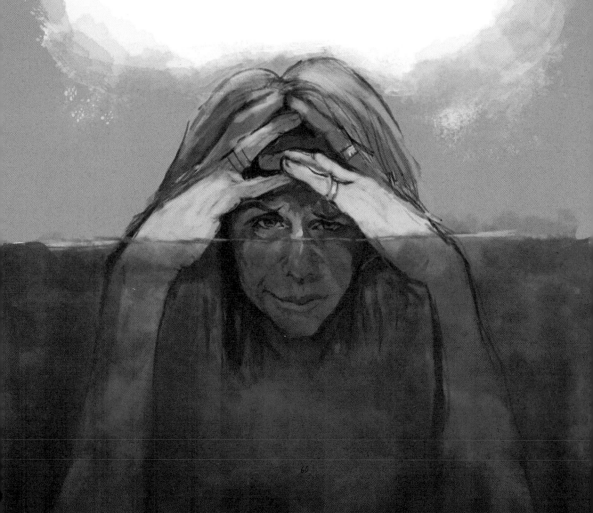

OPERATION

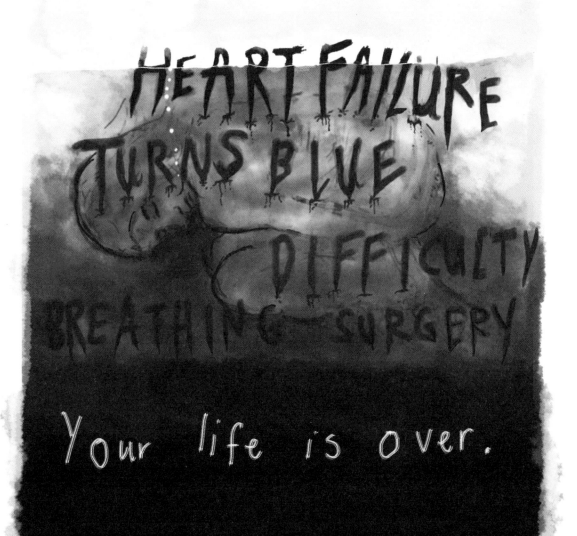

HEART FAILURE
TURNS BLUE
DIFFICULTY
BREATHING SURGERY

Your life is over.

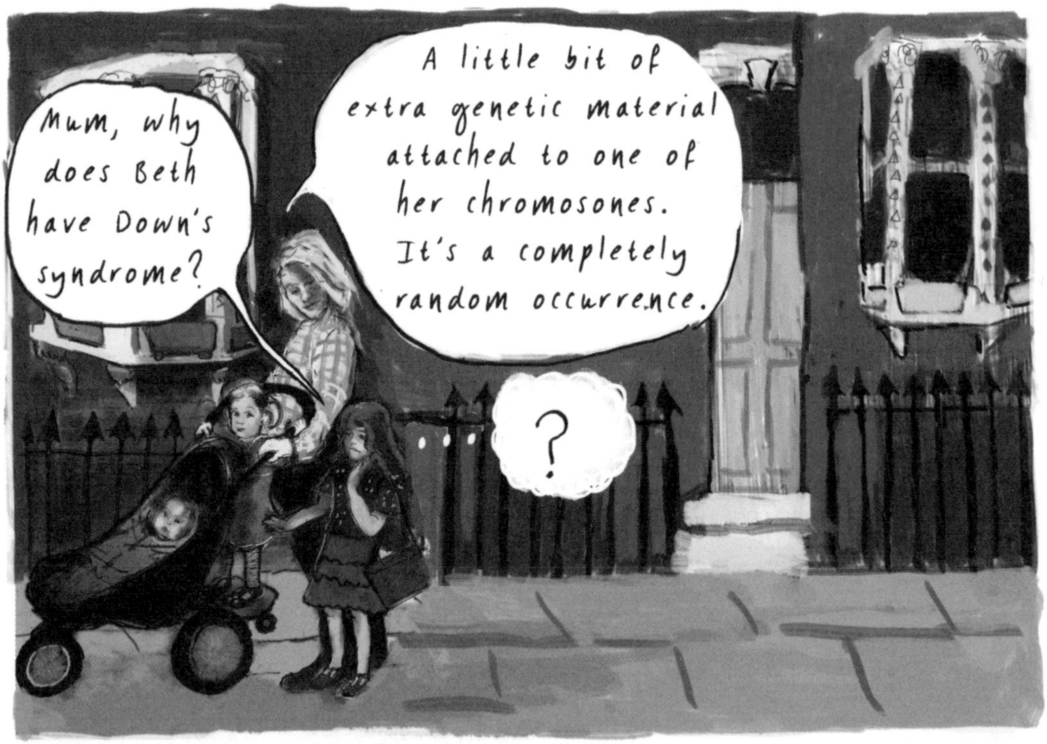
Mum, why does Beth have Down's syndrome?
A little bit of extra genetic material attached to one of her chromosones. It's a completely random occurrence.
?

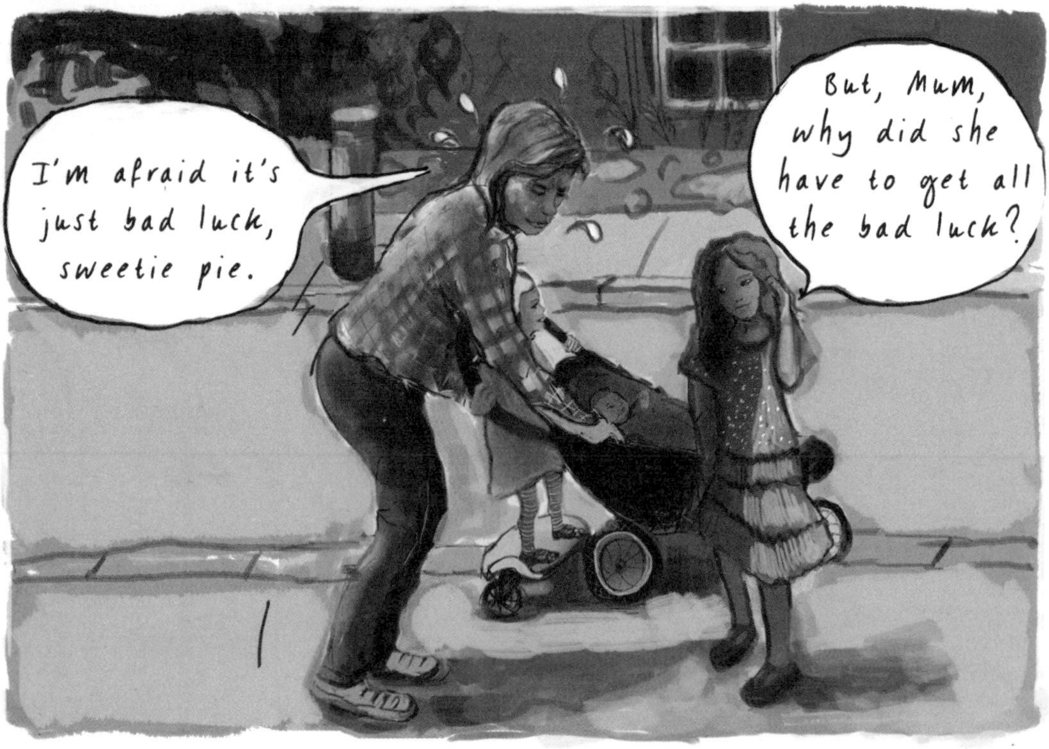
I'm afraid it's just bad luck, sweetie pie.
But, Mum, why did she have to get all the bad luck?

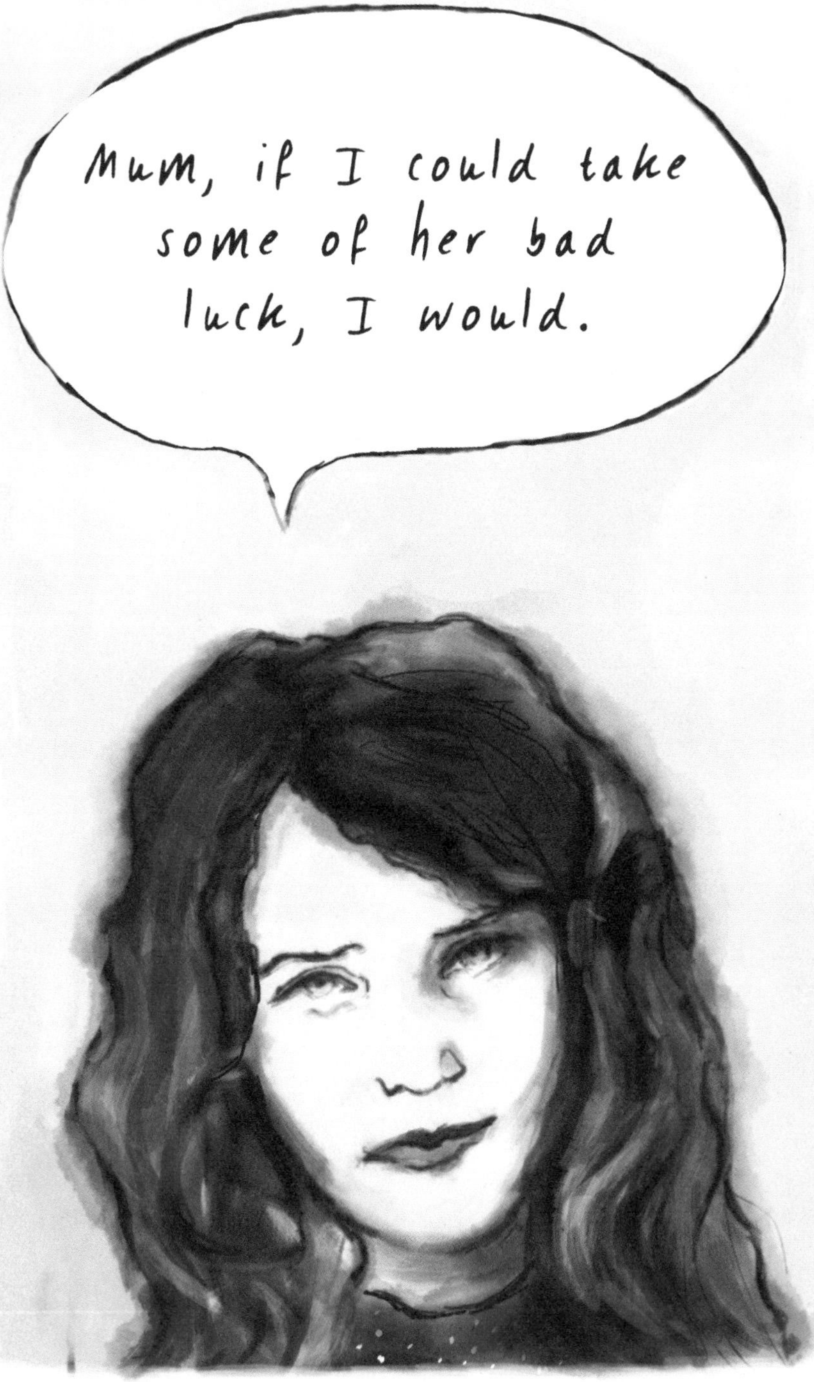
Mum, if I could take some of her bad luck, I would.

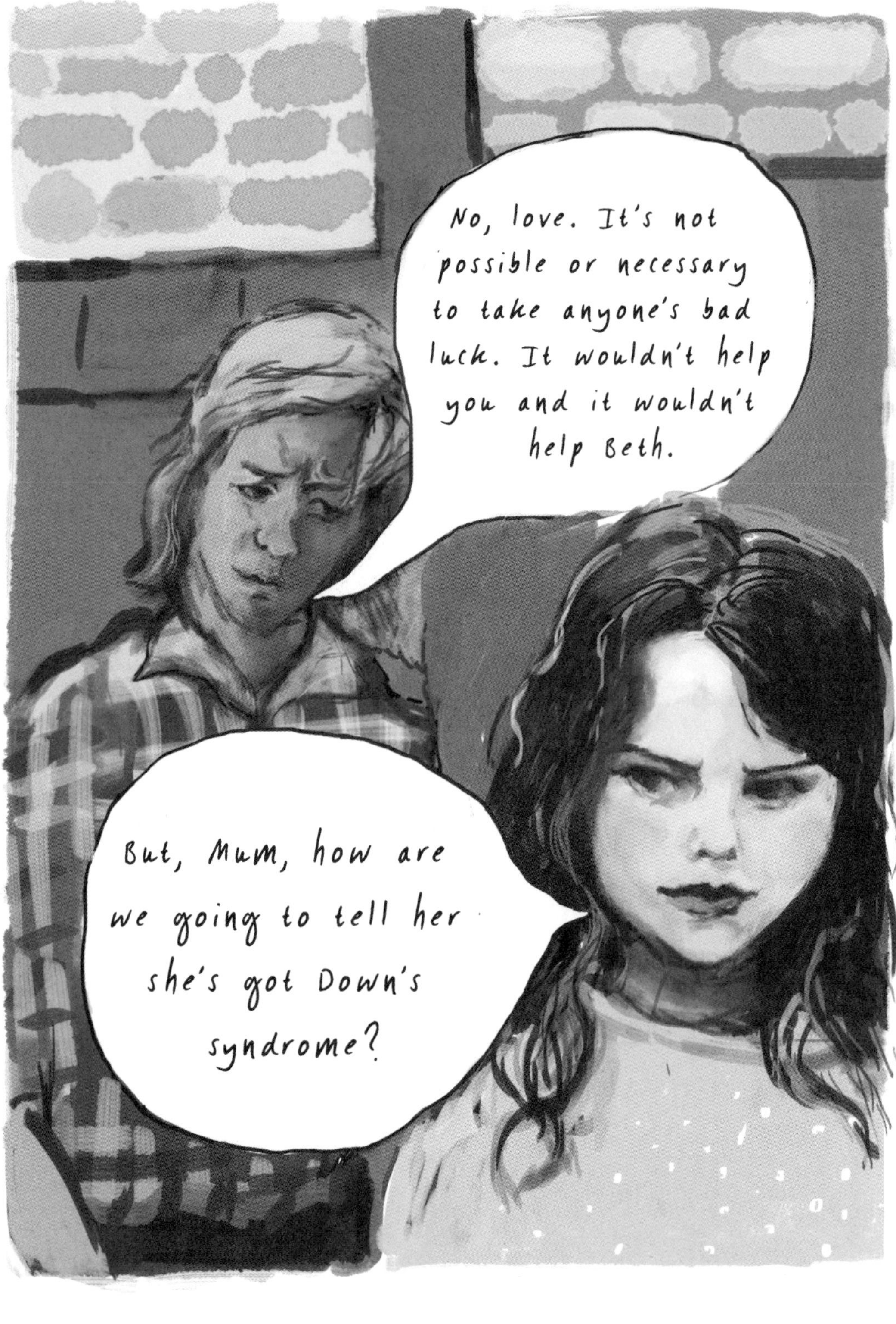
No, love. It's not possible or necessary to take anyone's bad luck. It wouldn't help you and it wouldn't help Beth.
But, Mum, how are we going to tell her she's got Down's syndrome?

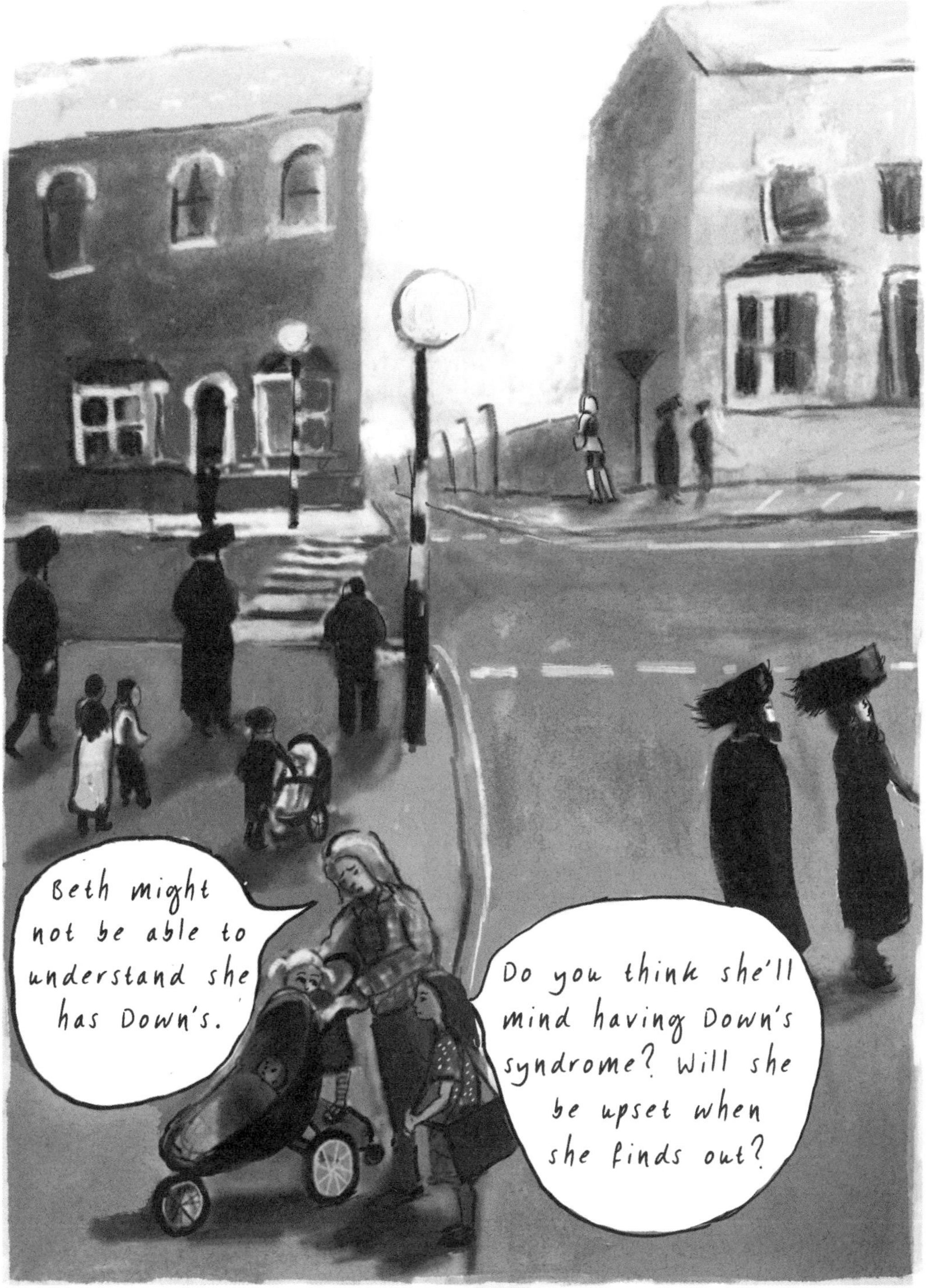
Beth might not be able to understand she has Down's.
Do you think she'll mind having Down's syndrome? Will she be upset when she finds out?

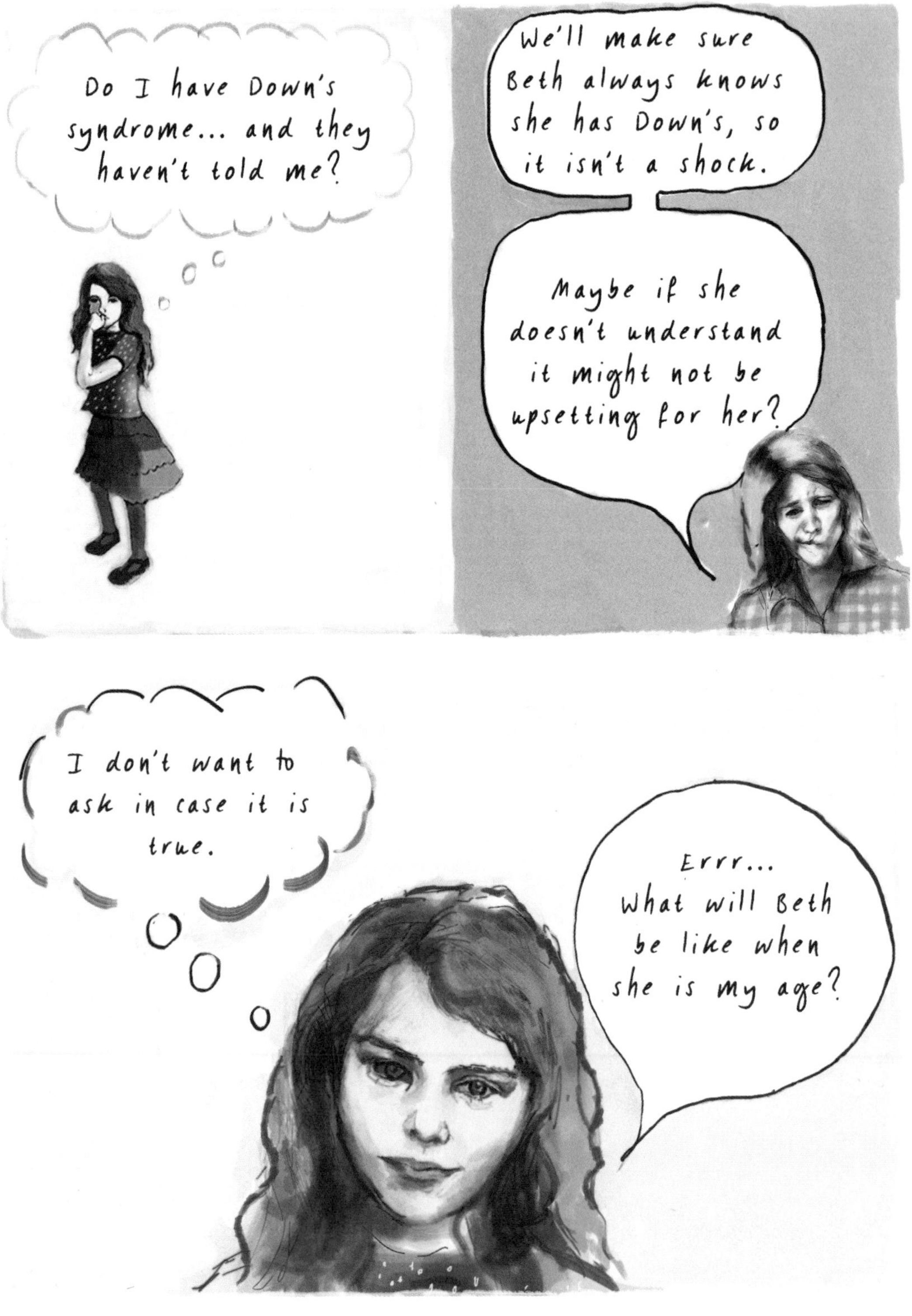

Do I have Down's syndrome... and they haven't told me?

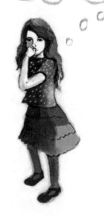

We'll make sure Beth always knows she has Down's, so it isn't a shock.

Maybe if she doesn't understand it might not be upsetting for her?

I don't want to ask in case it is true.

Errr... What will Beth be like when she is my age?

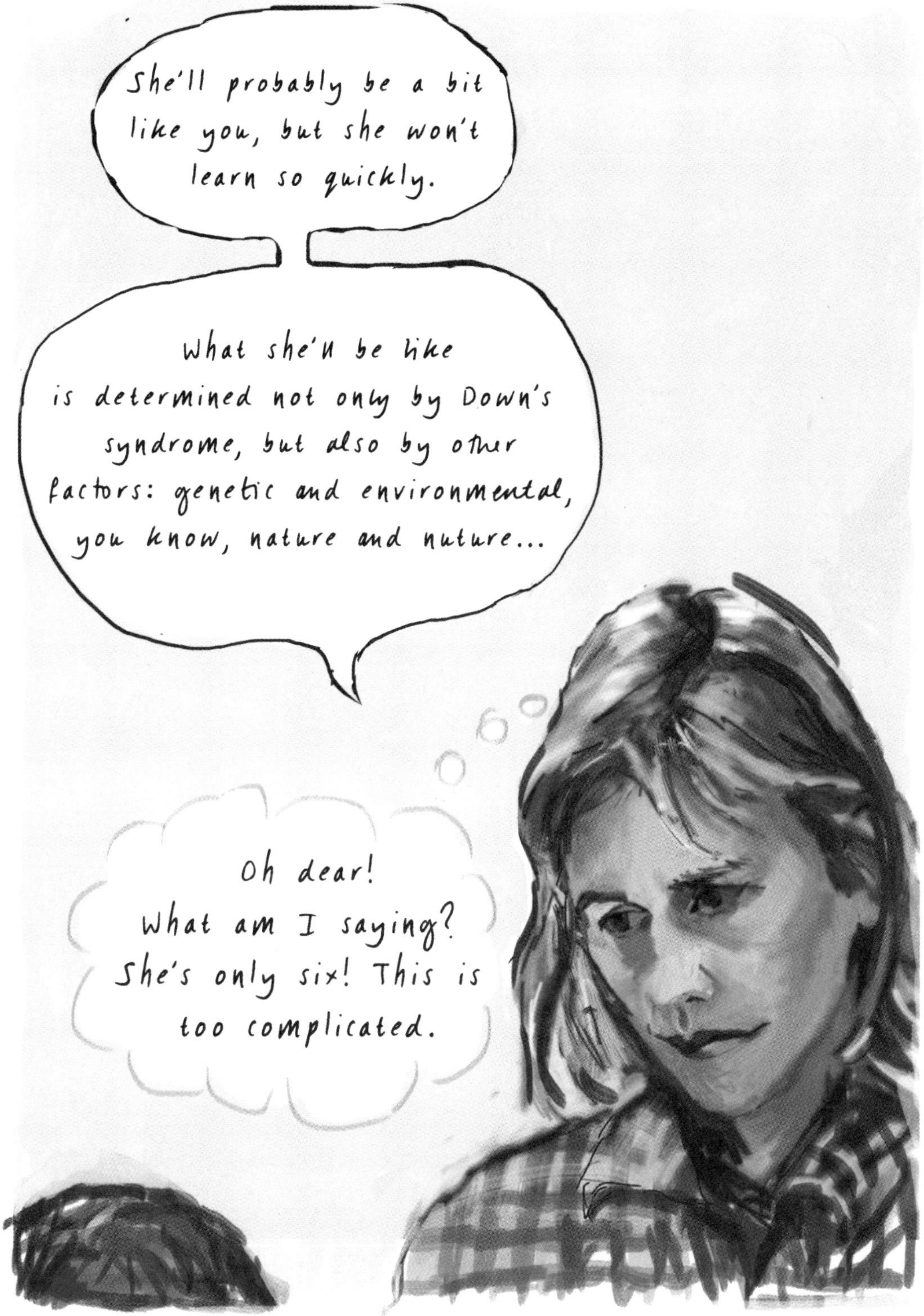

She'll probably be a bit like you, but she won't learn so quickly.

What she'll be like is determined not only by Down's syndrome, but also by other factors: genetic and environmental, you know, nature and nuture...

Oh dear! What am I saying? She's only six! This is too complicated.

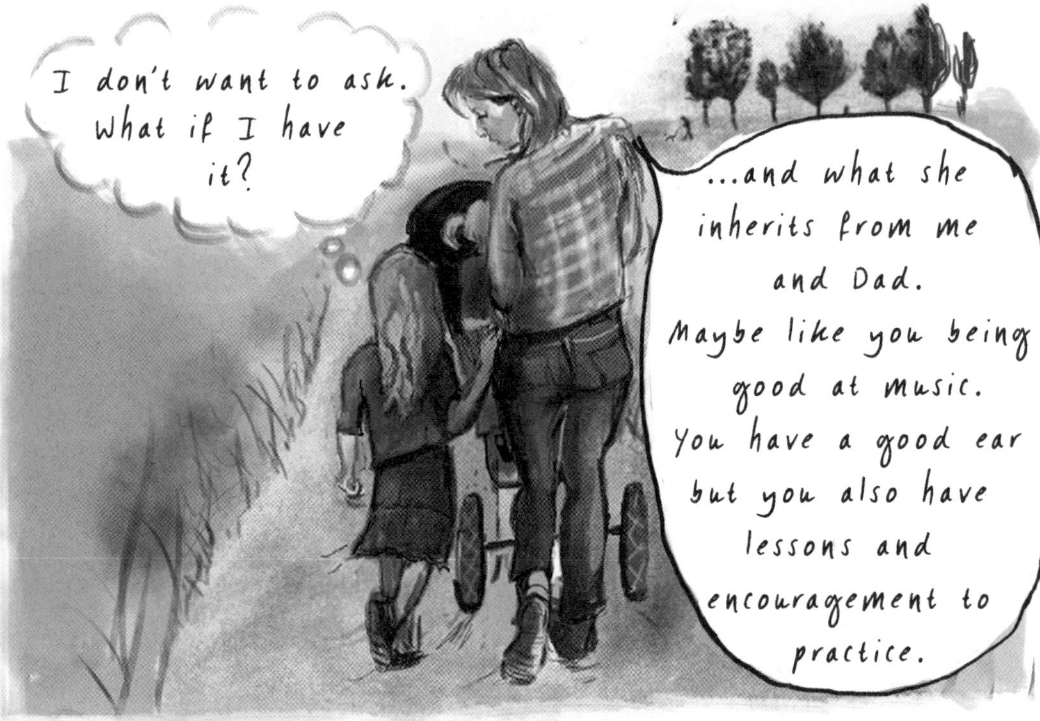
I don't want to ask. What if I have it?
...and what she inherits from me and Dad. Maybe like you being good at music. You have a good ear but you also have lessons and encouragement to practice.

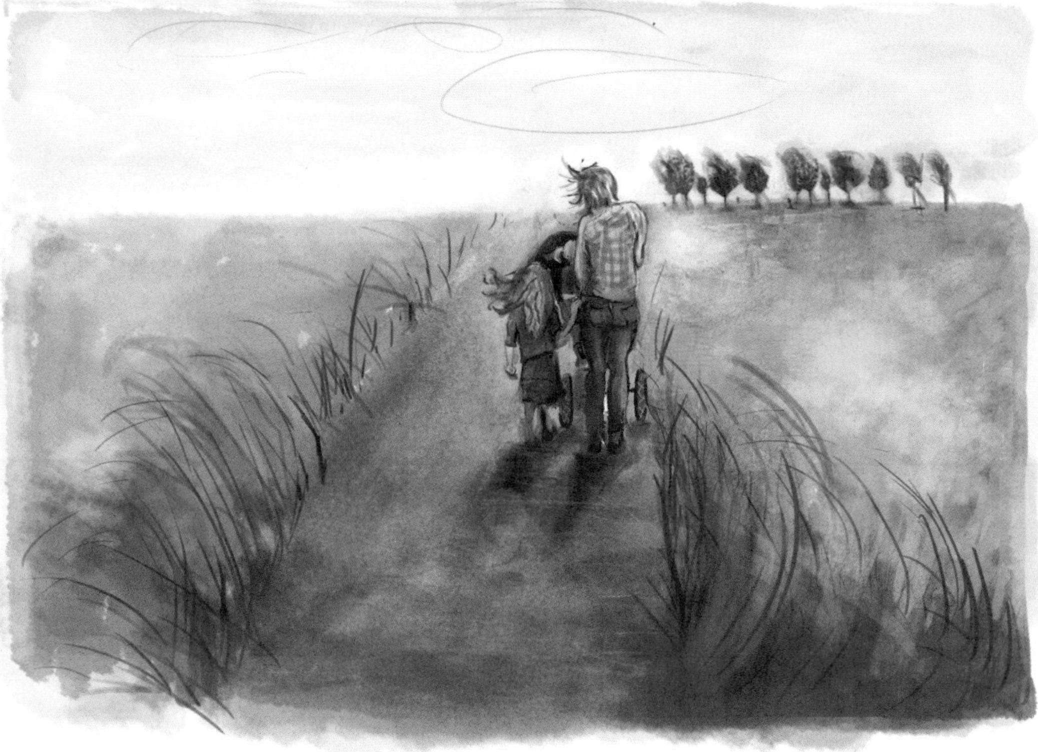

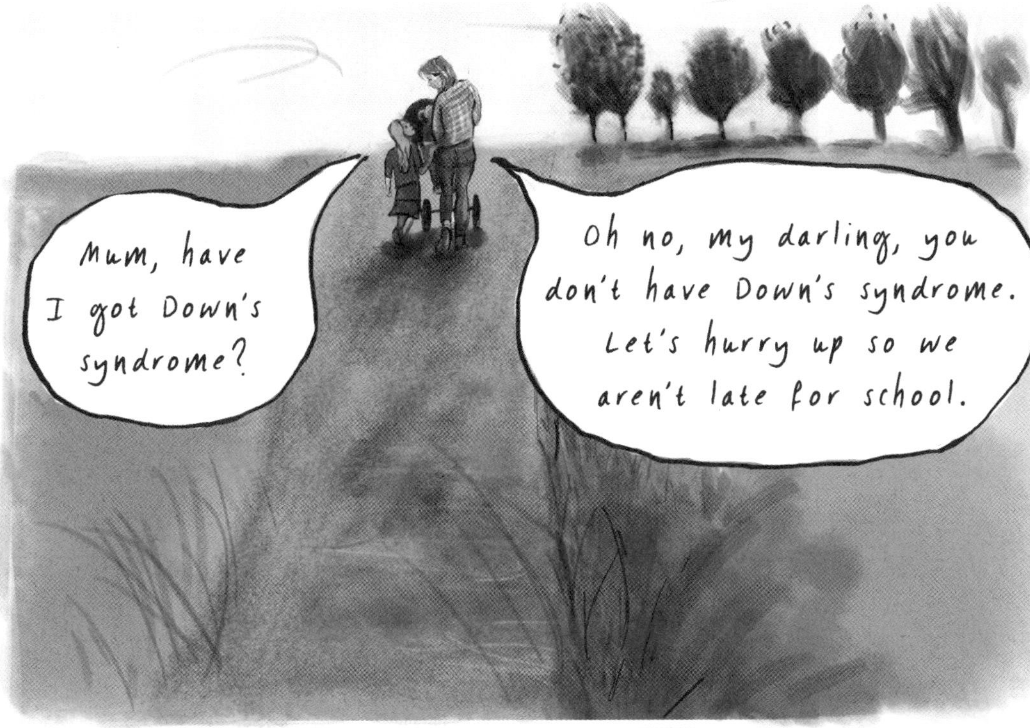
Mum, have I got Down's syndrome?
Oh no, my darling, you don't have Down's syndrome. Let's hurry up so we aren't late for school.

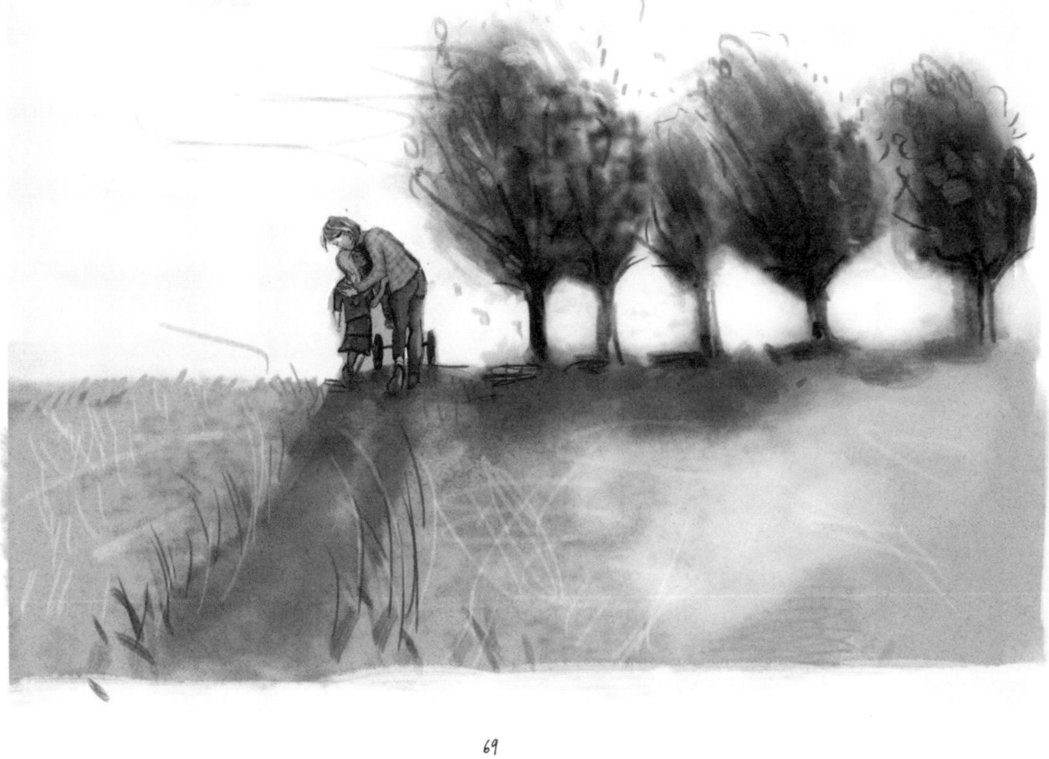

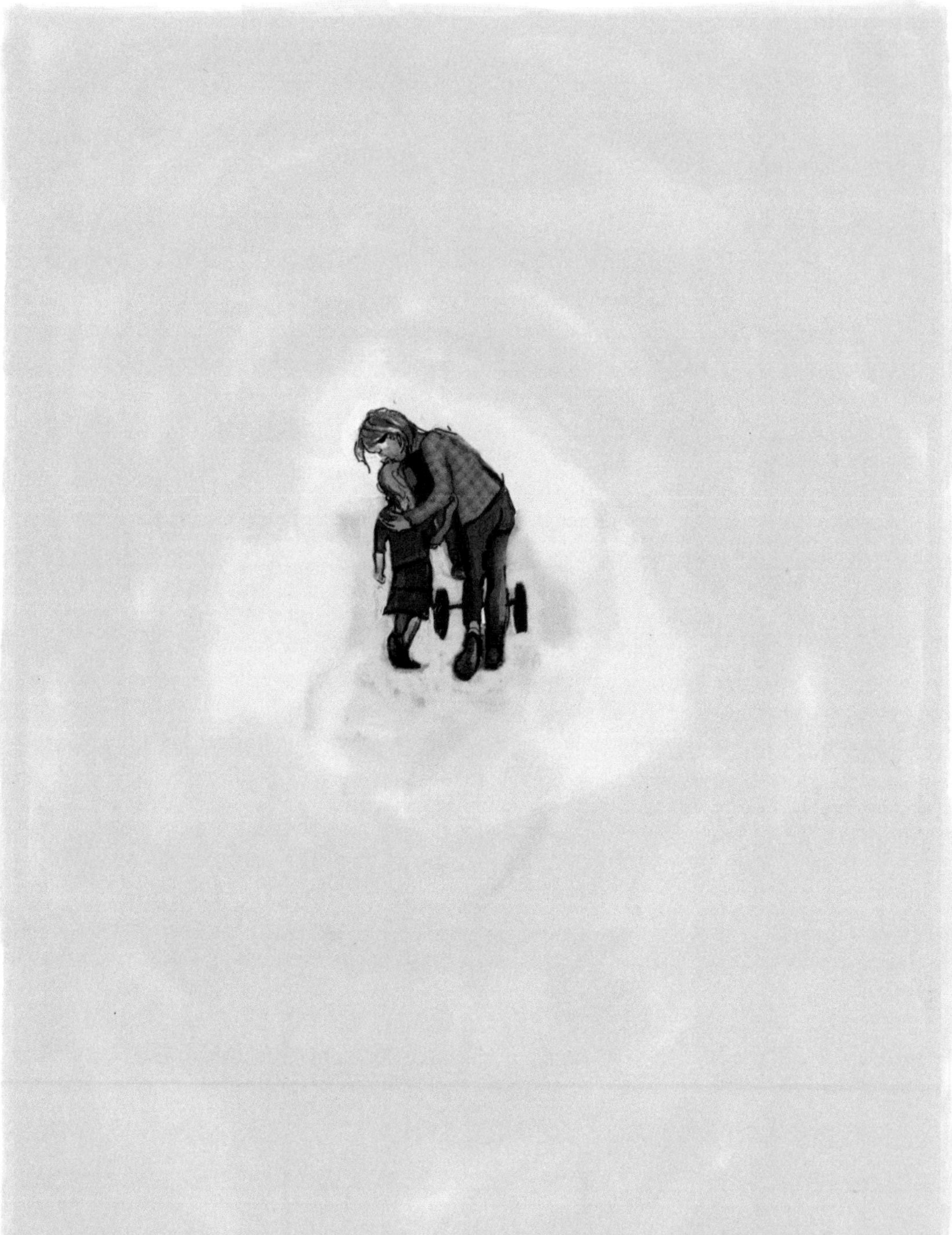

Part Two

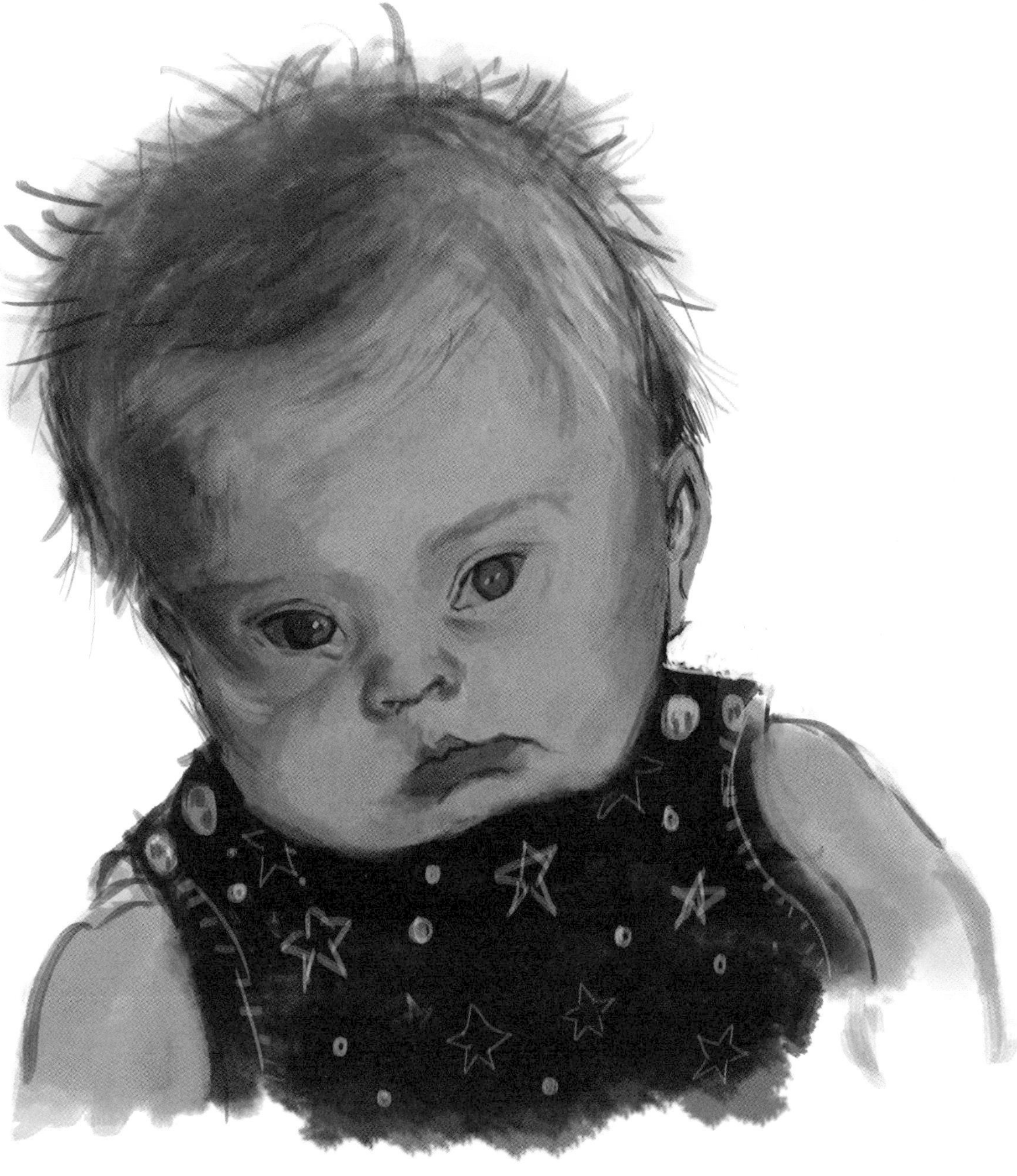

April 2001

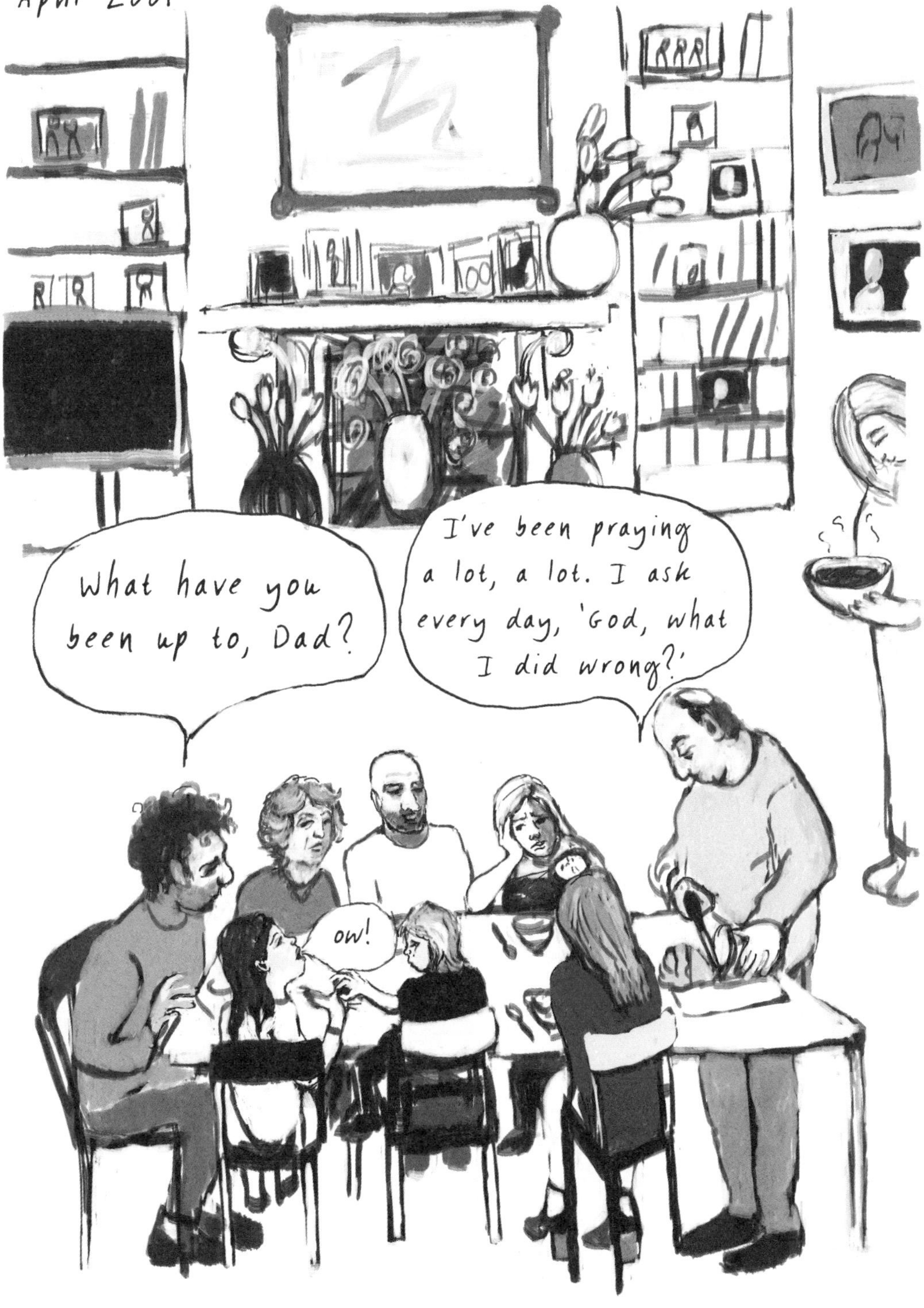
What have you been up to, Dad?
I've been praying a lot, a lot. I ask every day, 'God, what I did wrong?'
ow!

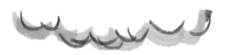

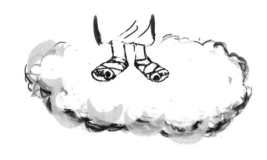

Why, God?
Why visit us with
this disability
business?

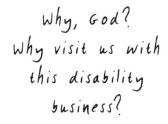

This Down's syndrome
nonsense?

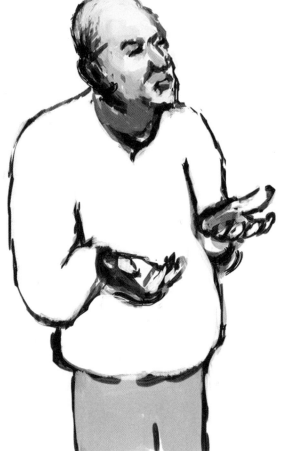

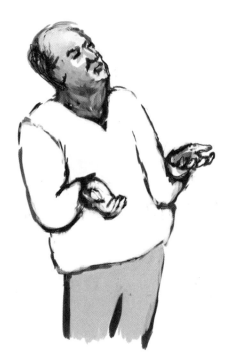

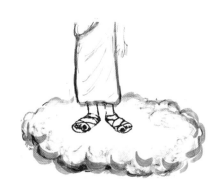

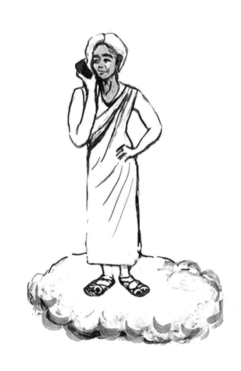

They can't put her
in a home?

Why, God? Everything I do
I do for my
family.

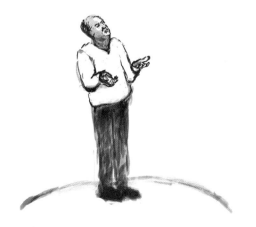

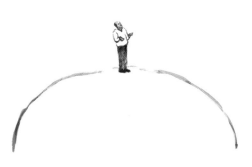

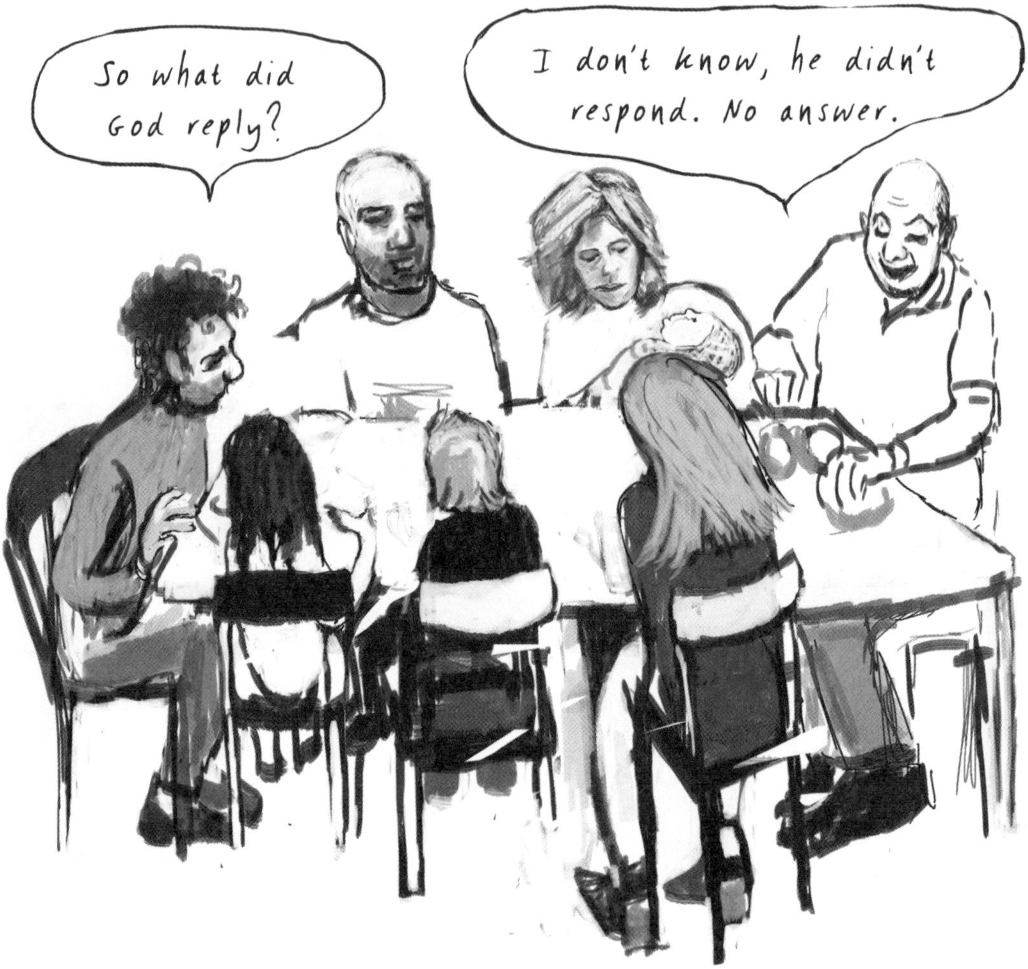
So what did God reply?
I don't know, he didn't respond. No answer.

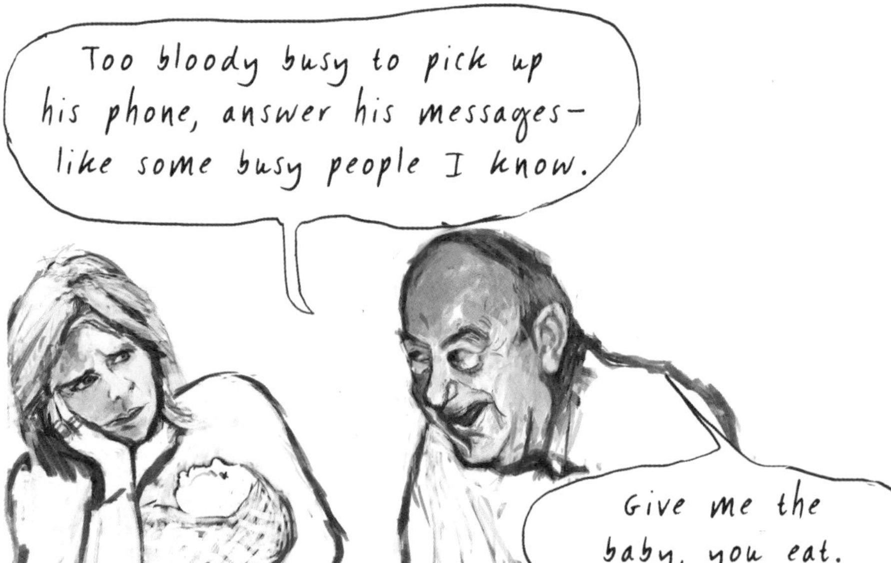
Too bloody busy to pick up his phone, answer his messages- like some busy people I know.
Give me the baby, you eat.

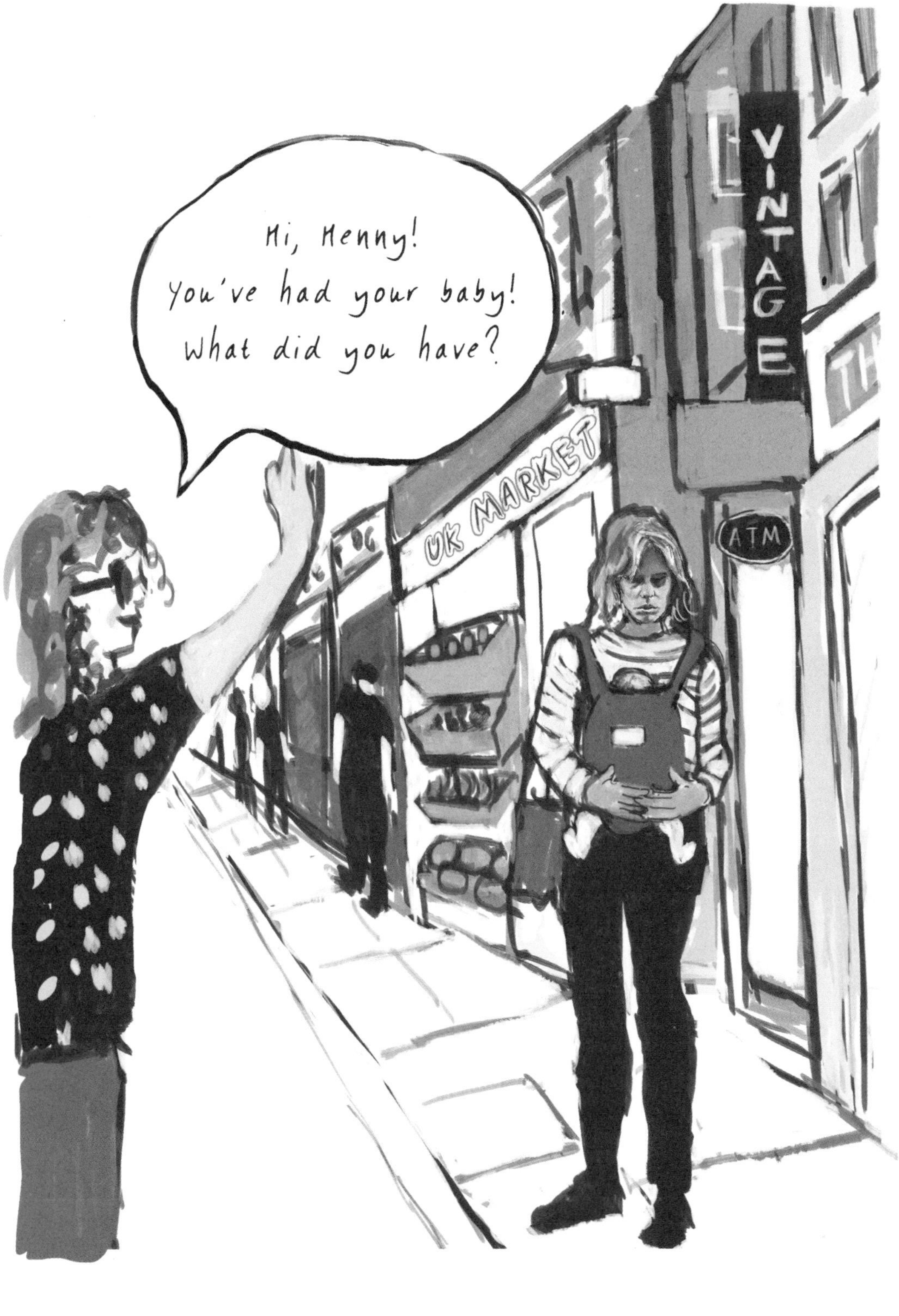
Hi, Henny!
You've had your baby!
What did you have?
VINTAGE
TH
UK MARKET
ATM

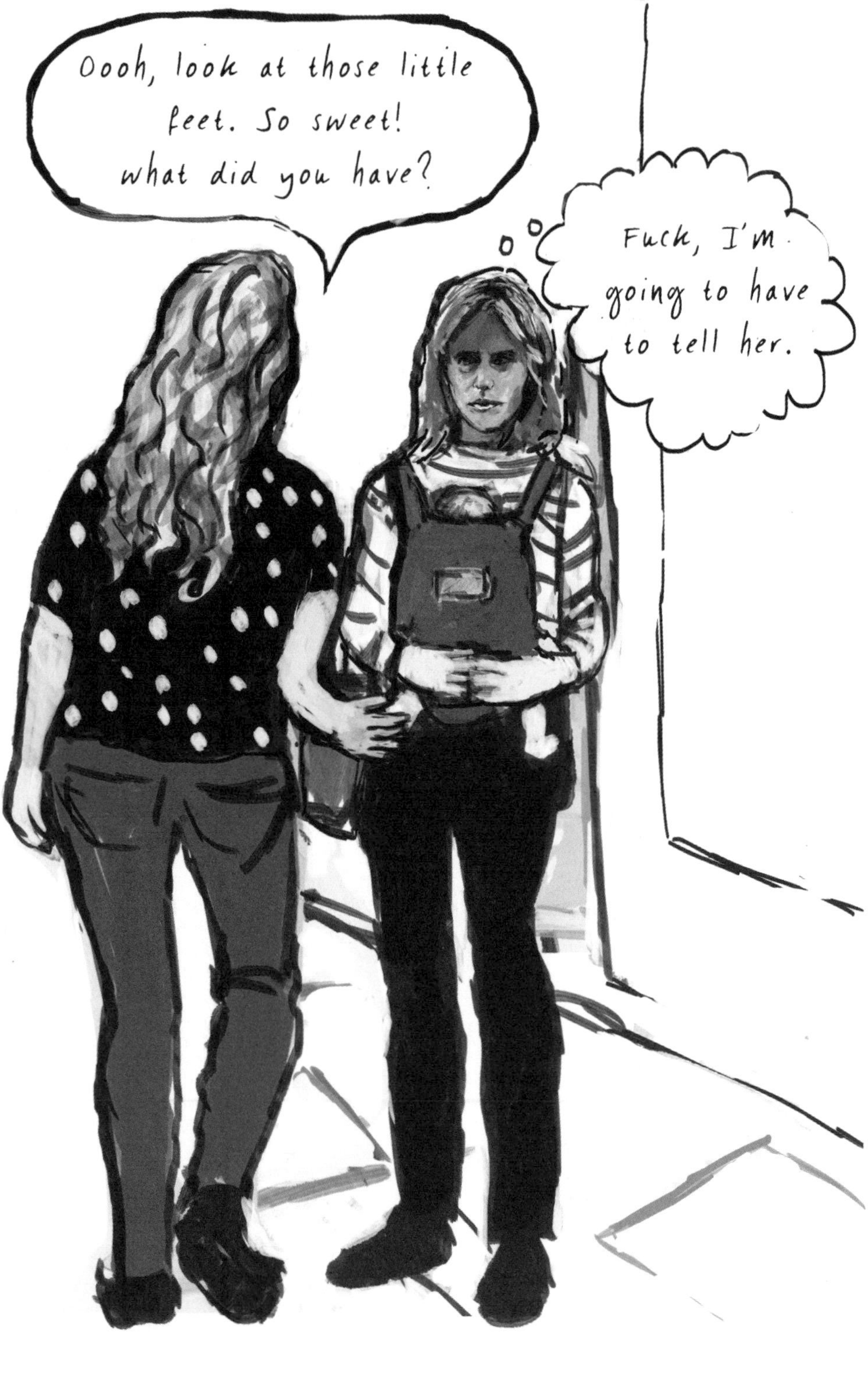
Oooh, look at those little feet. So sweet! what did you have?
Fuck, I'm going to have to tell her.

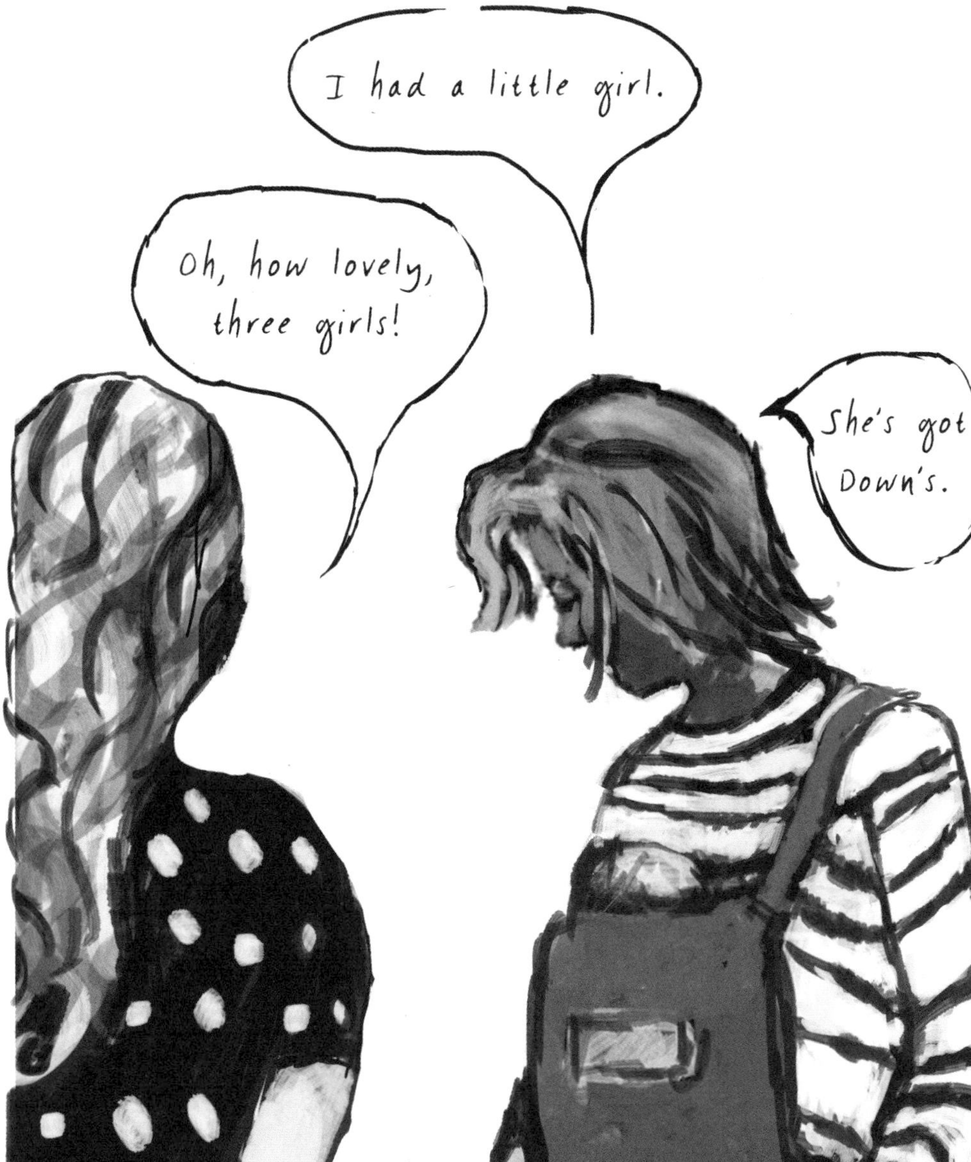
I had a little girl.
Oh, how lovely, three girls!
She's got Down's.

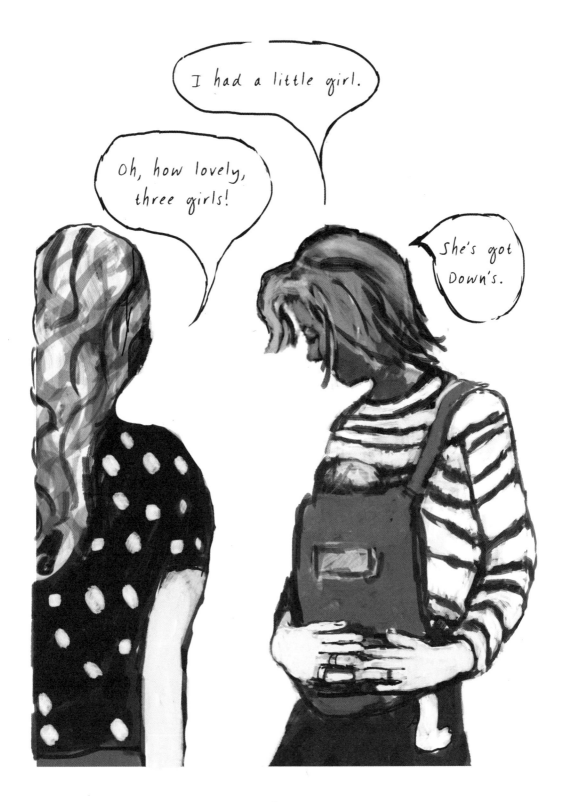

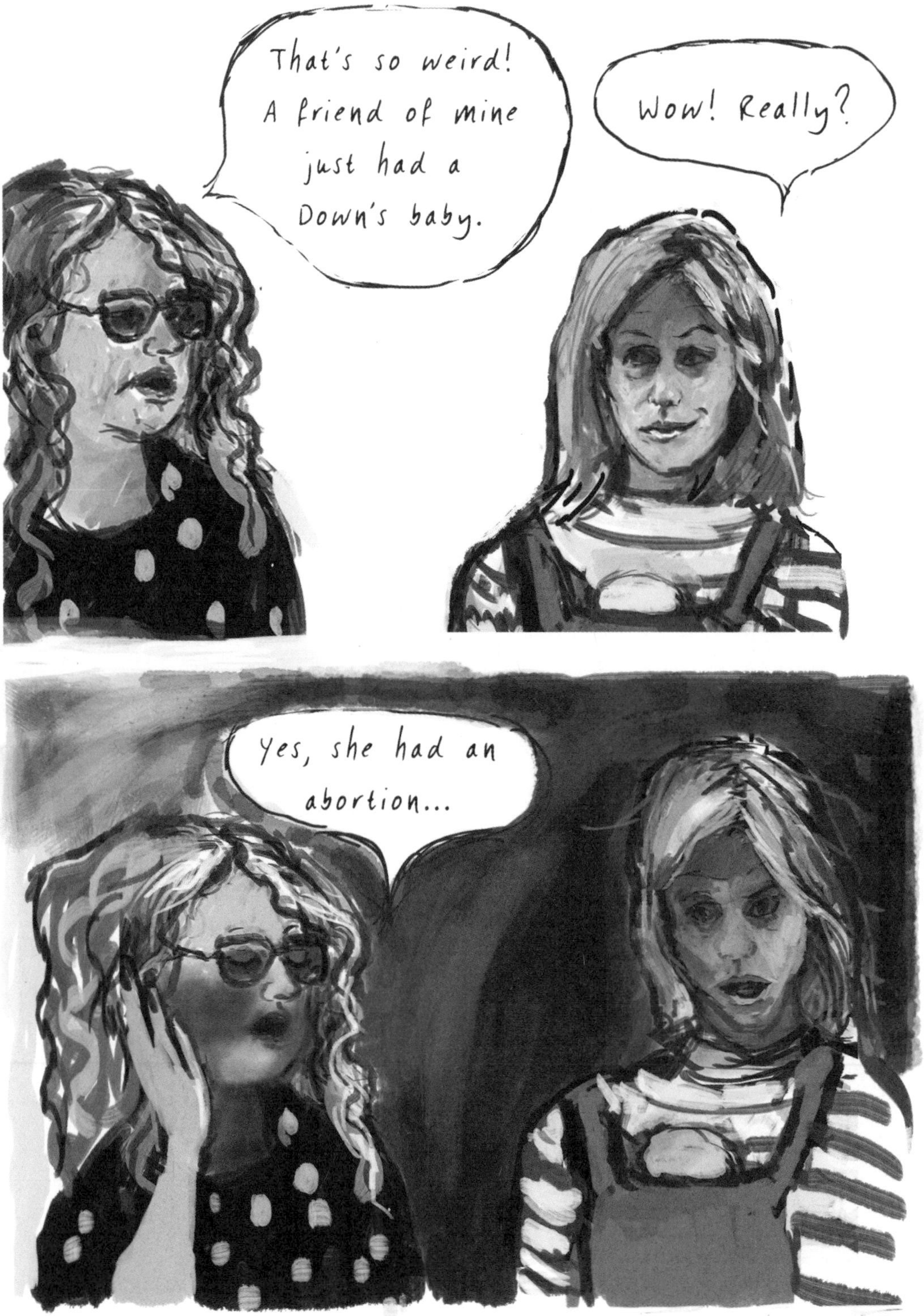
That's so weird! A friend of mine just had a Down's baby.
Wow! Really?
Yes, she had an abortion...

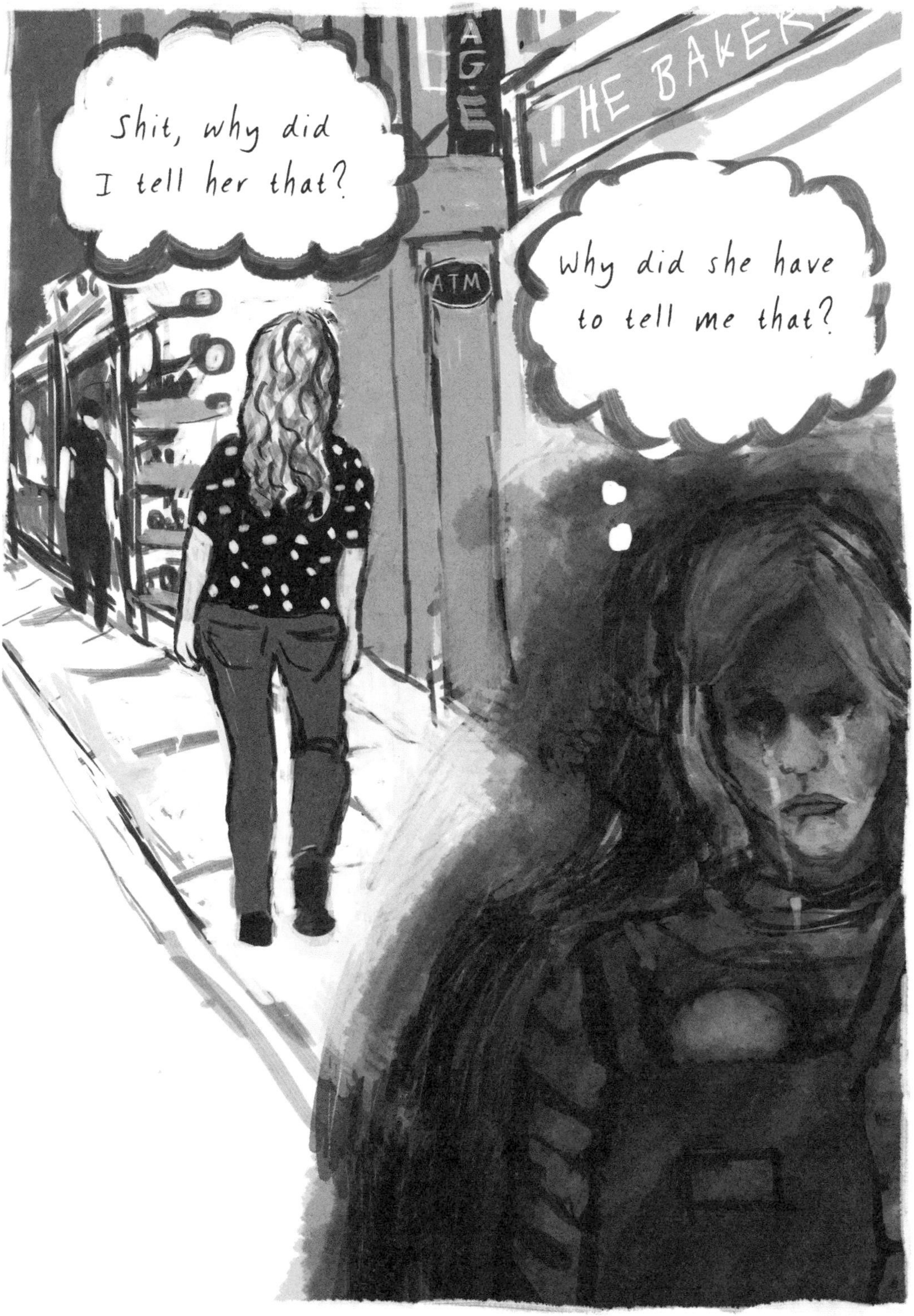
AGE
THE BAKER
ATM
Shit, why did I tell her that?
Why did she have to tell me that?

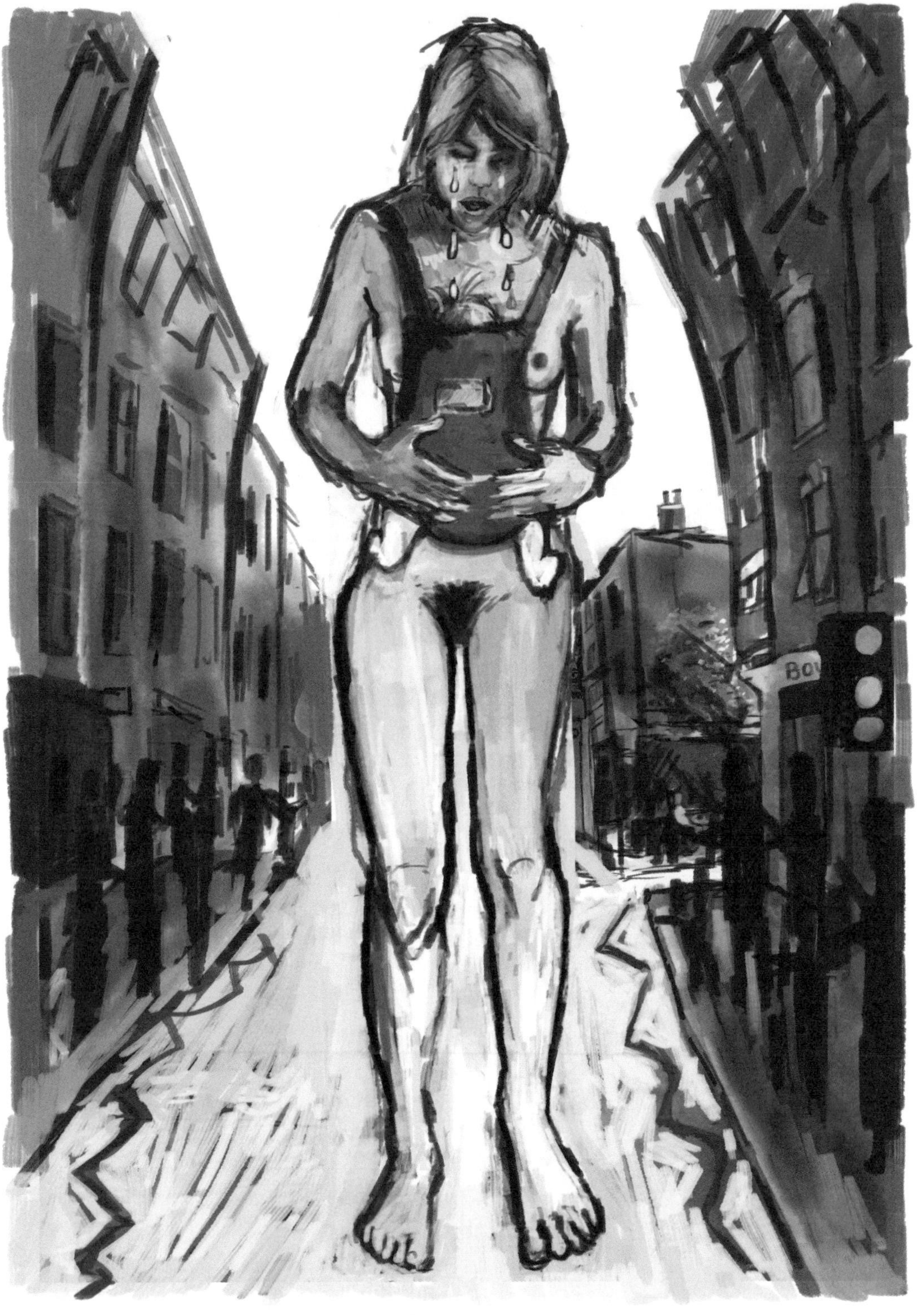

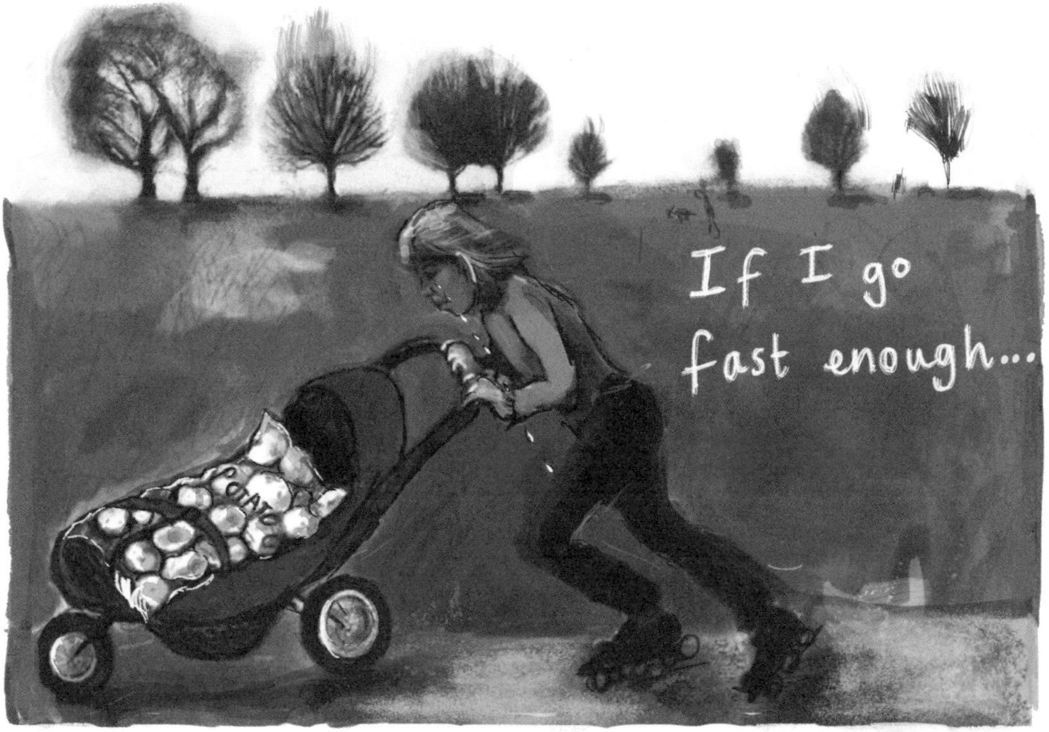
If I go
fast enough...

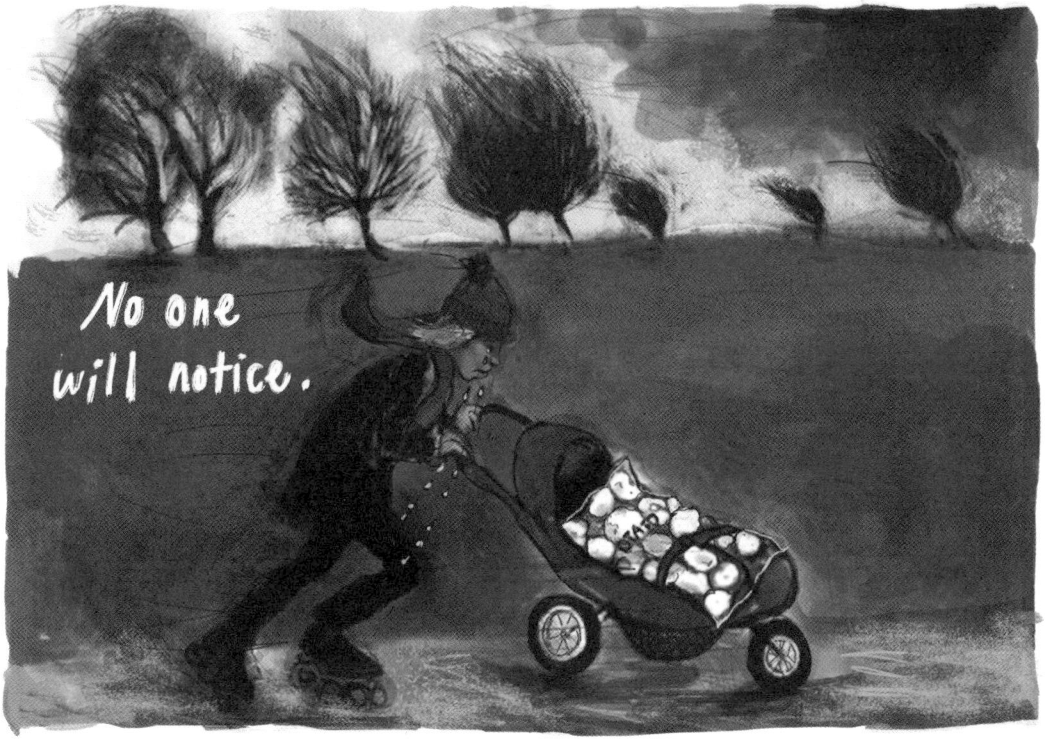
No one
will notice.

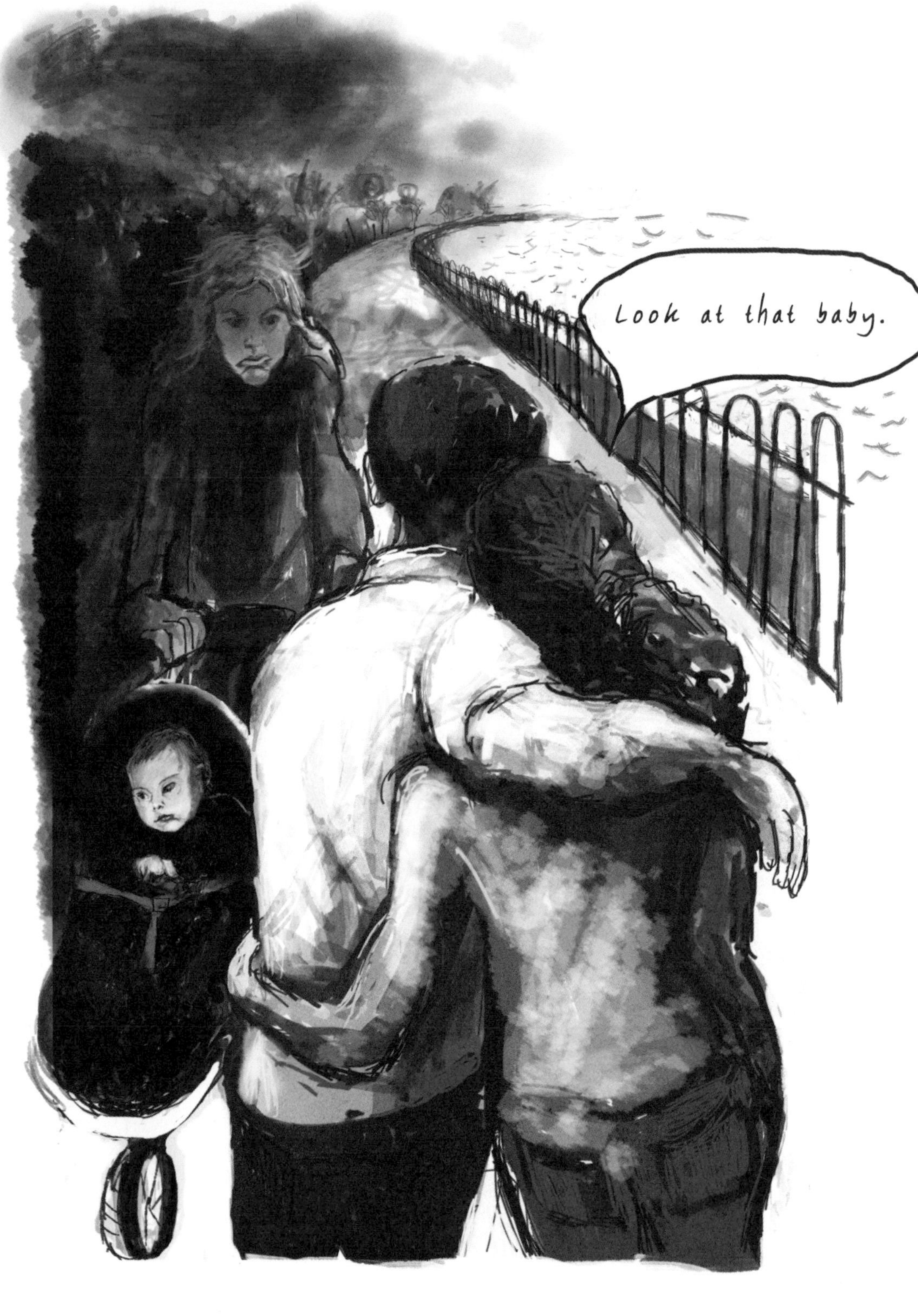
Look at that baby.

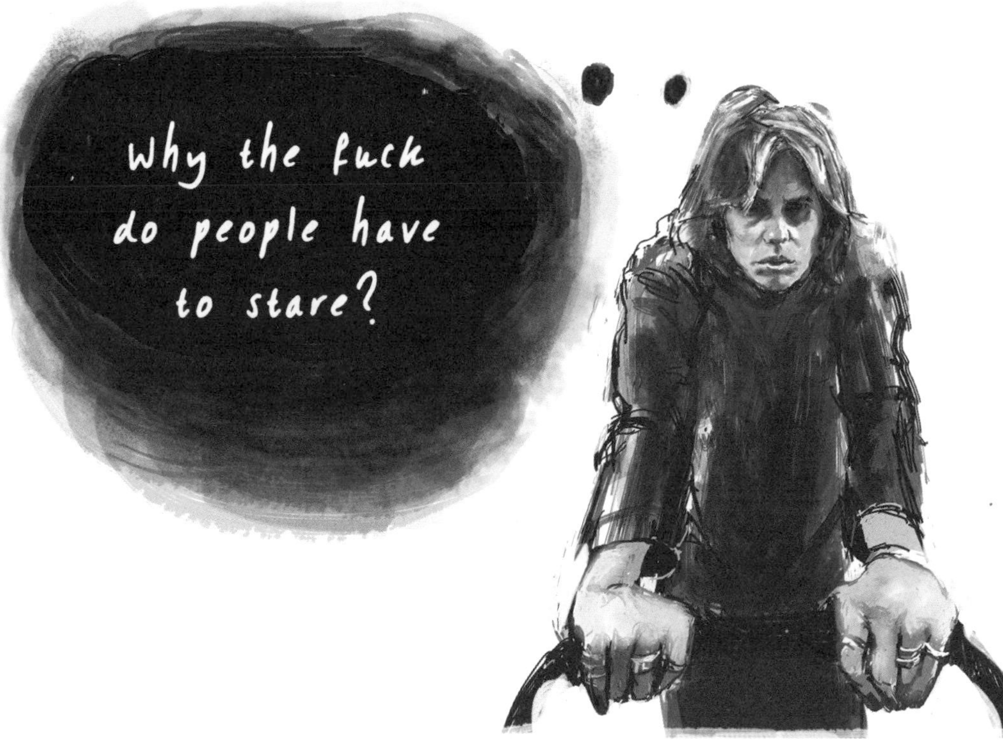
Why the fuck do people have to stare?

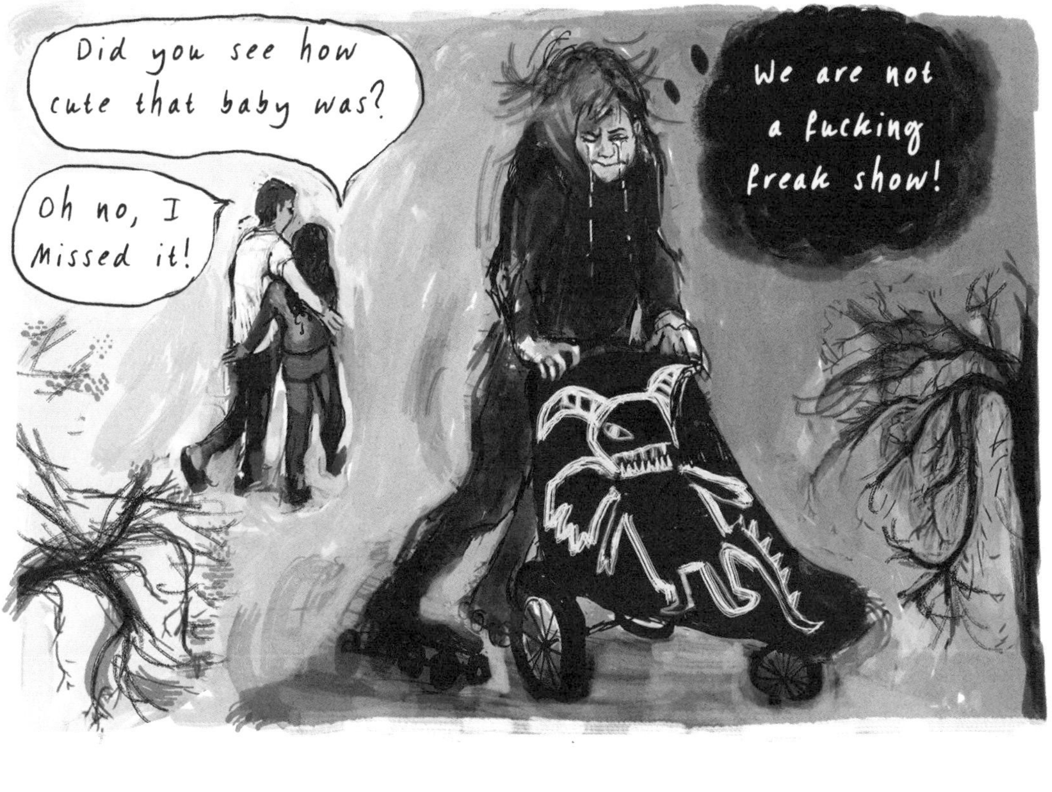
Did you see how cute that baby was?
Oh no, I missed it!
We are not a fucking freak show!

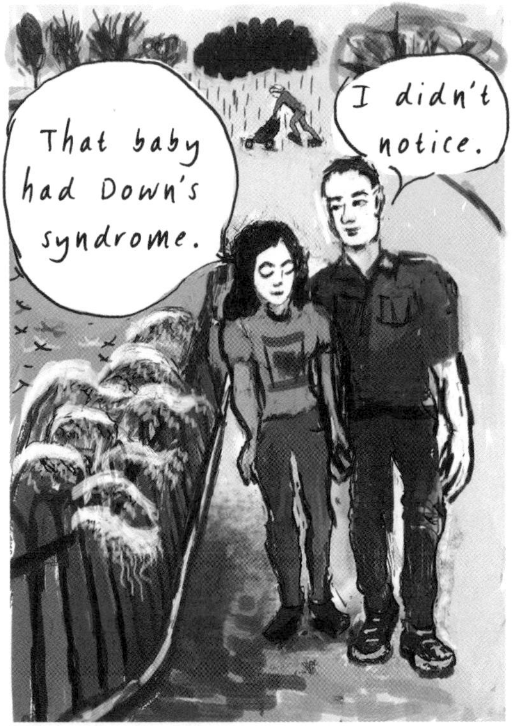
That baby had Down's syndrome.
I didn't notice.

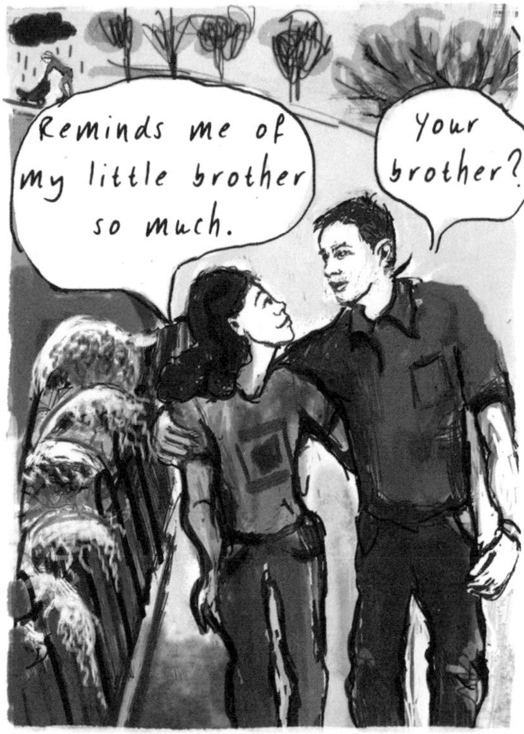
Reminds me of my little brother so much.
Your brother?

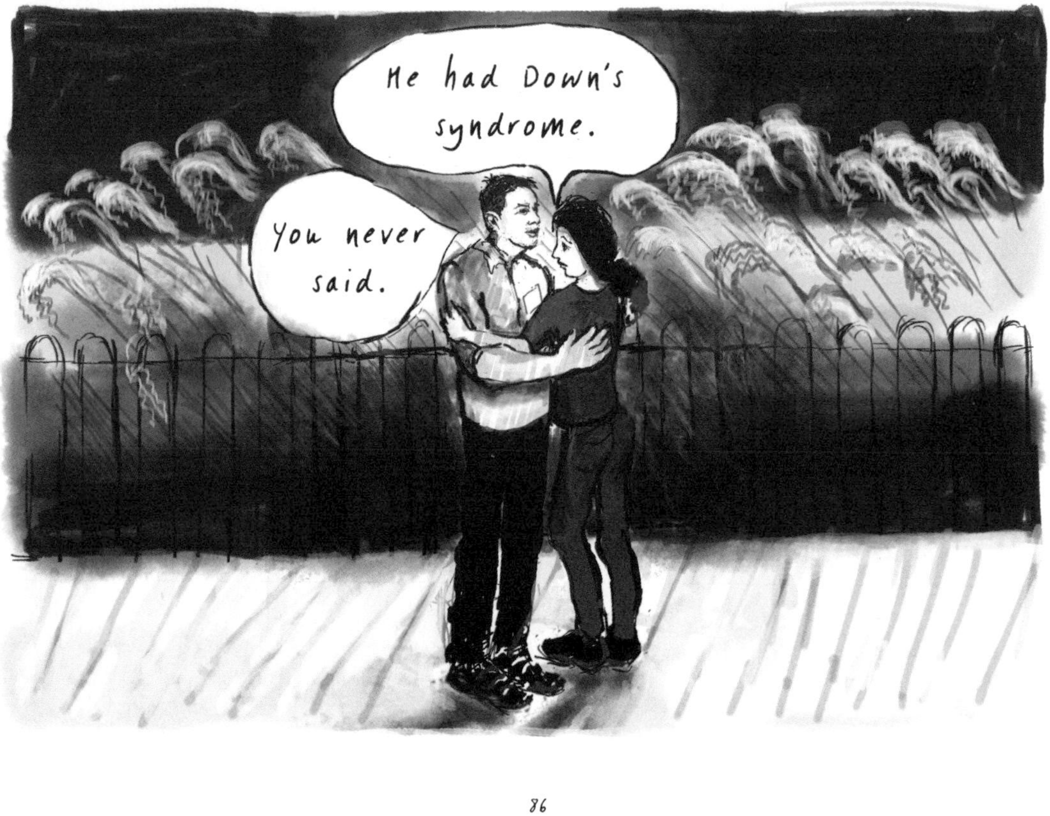
He had Down's syndrome.
You never said.

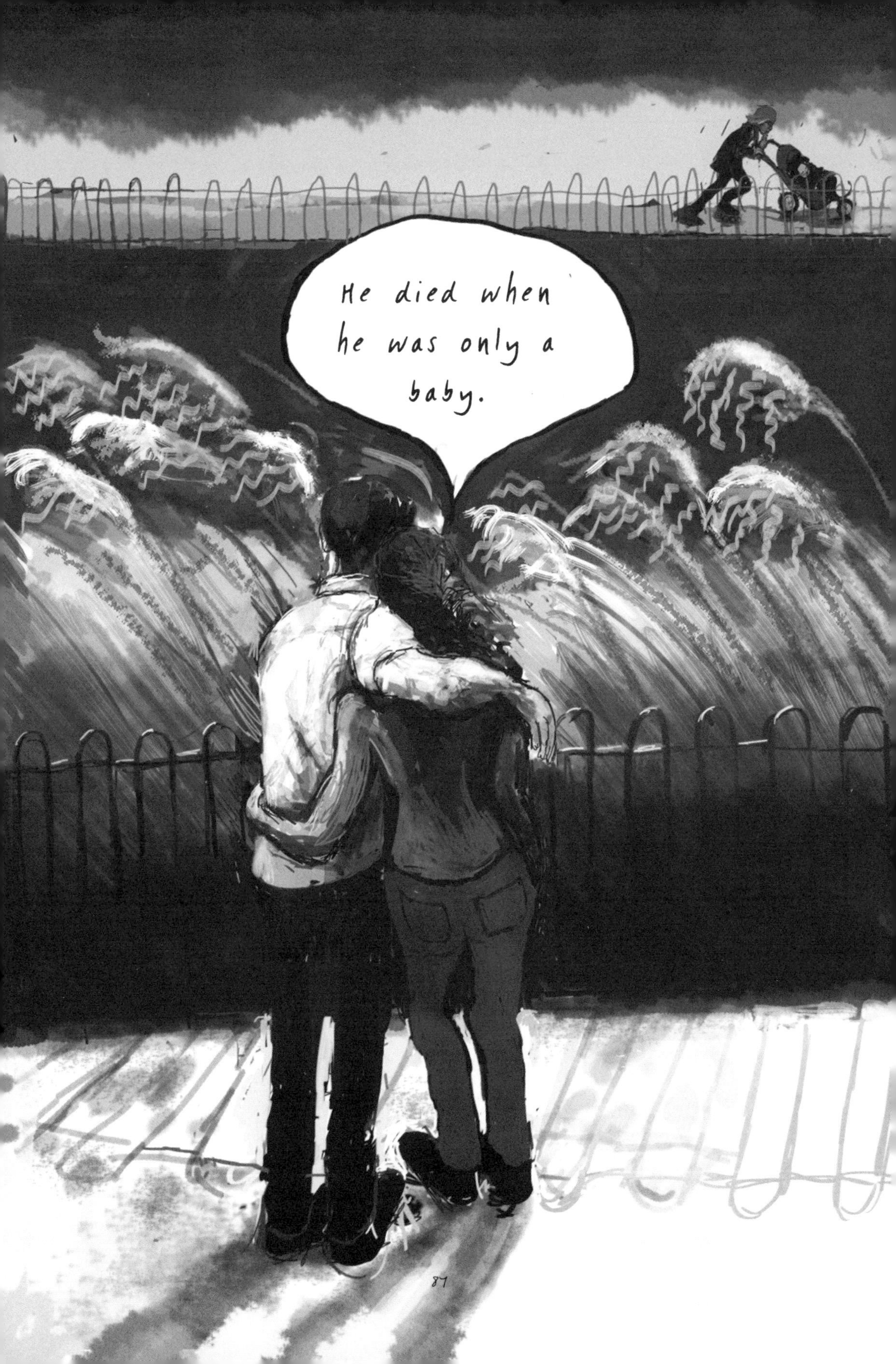
He died when he was only a baby.

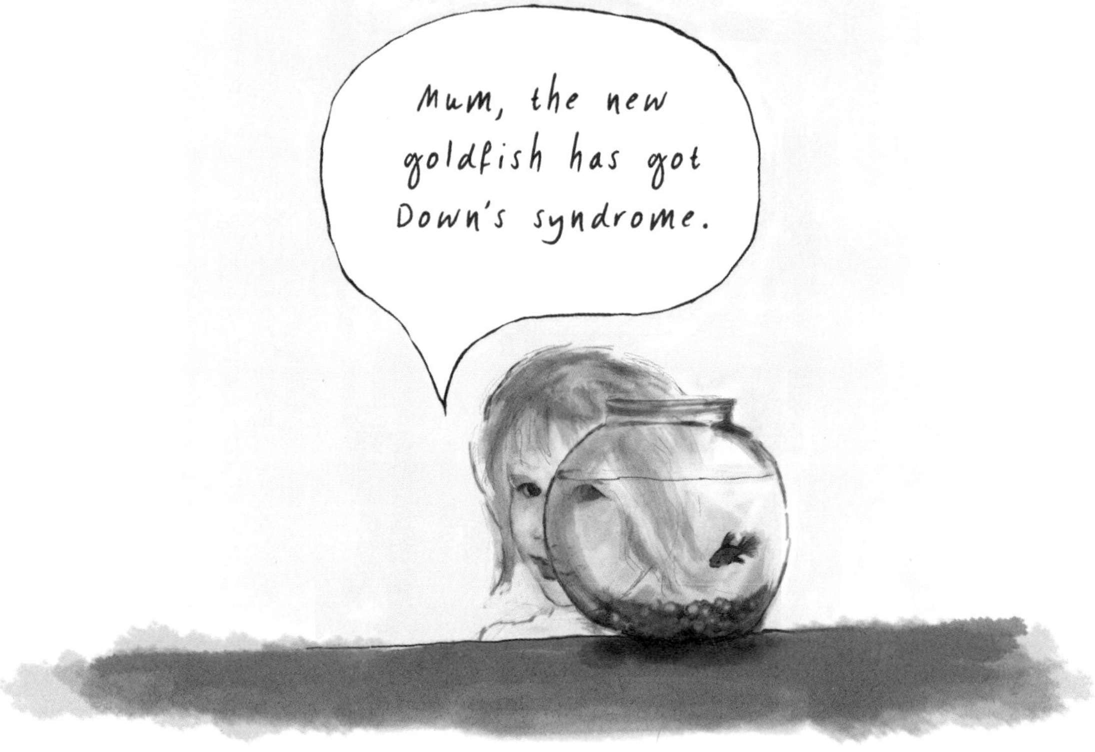
Mum, the new goldfish has got Down's syndrome.

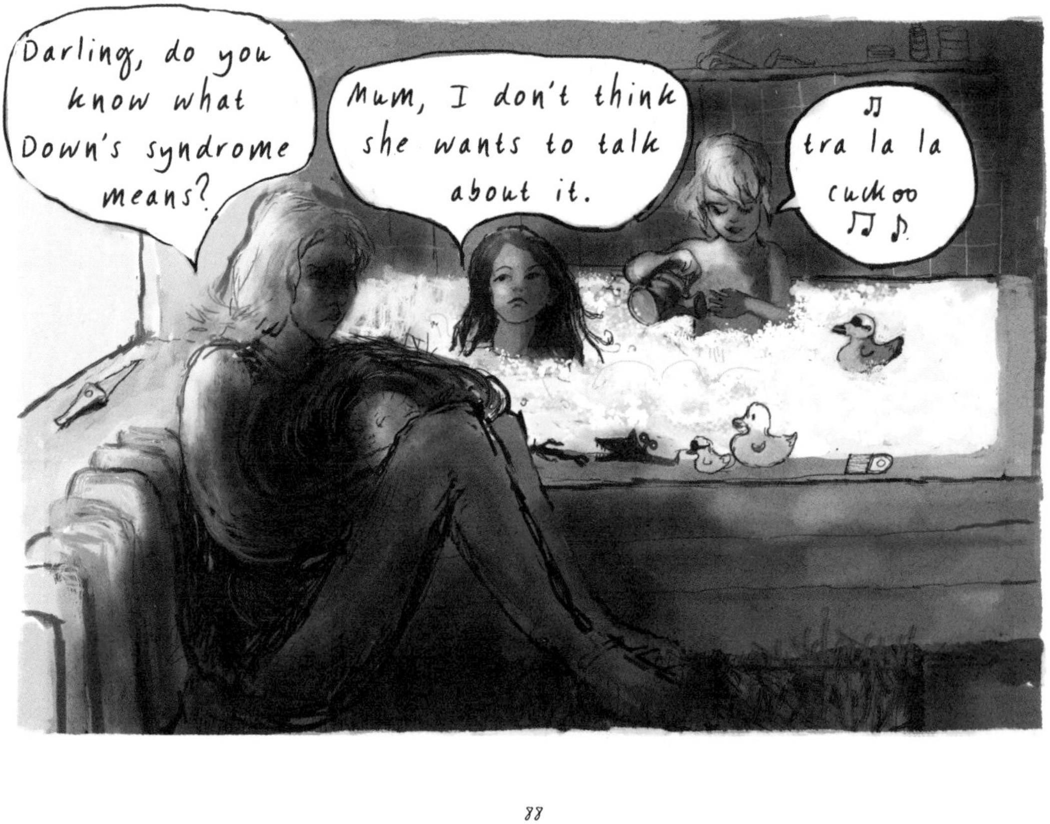
Darling, do you know what Down's syndrome means?
Mum, I don't think she wants to talk about it.
♫ tra la la cuckoo ♫ ♪

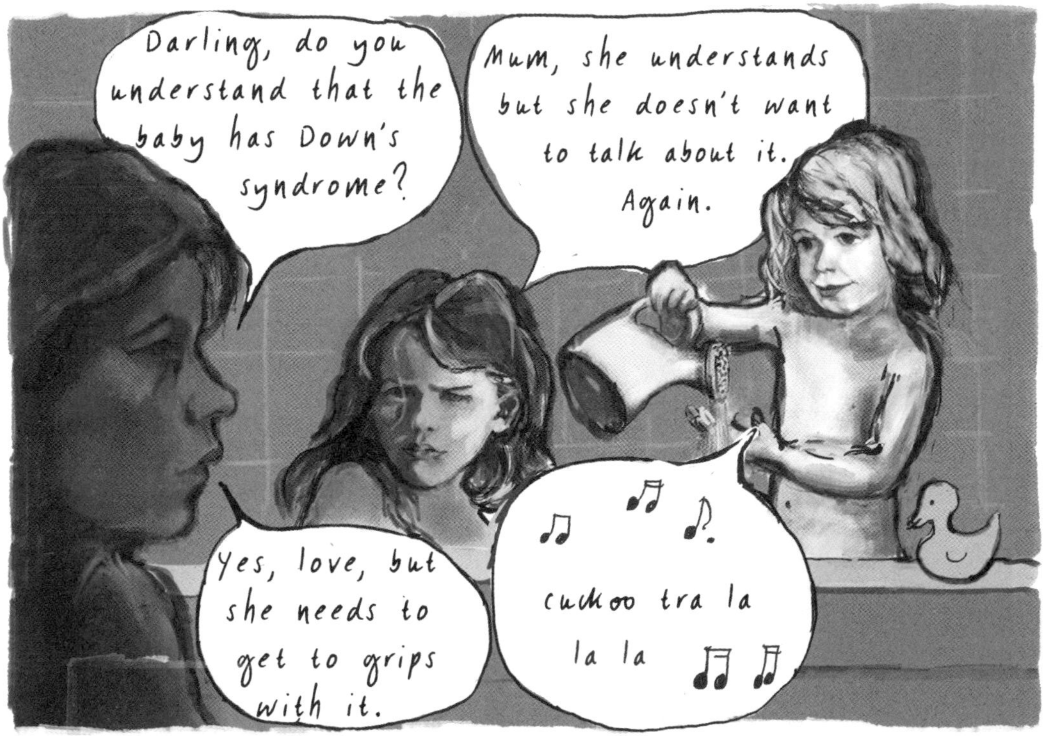
Darling, do you understand that the baby has Down's syndrome?
Mum, she understands but she doesn't want to talk about it. Again.
Yes, love, but she needs to get to grips with it.
cuckoo tra la la la

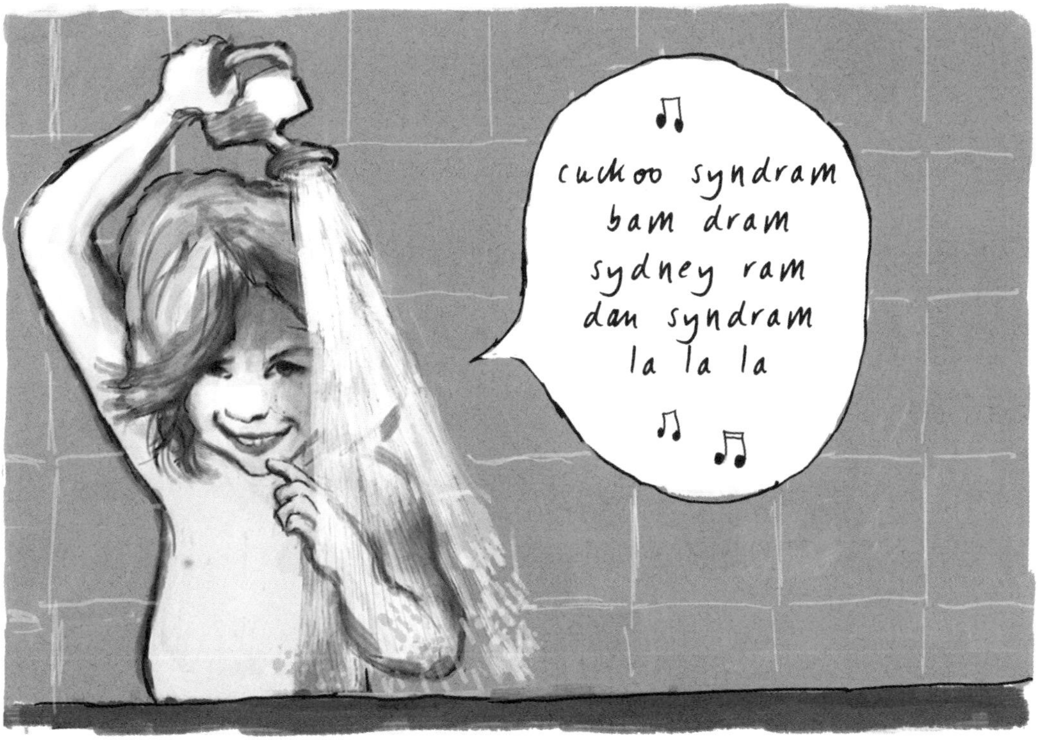
cuckoo syndram bam dram sydney ram dan syndram la la la

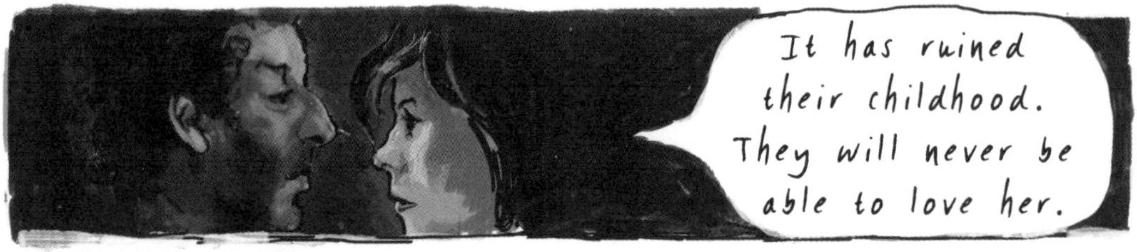
It has ruined their childhood. They will never be able to love her.

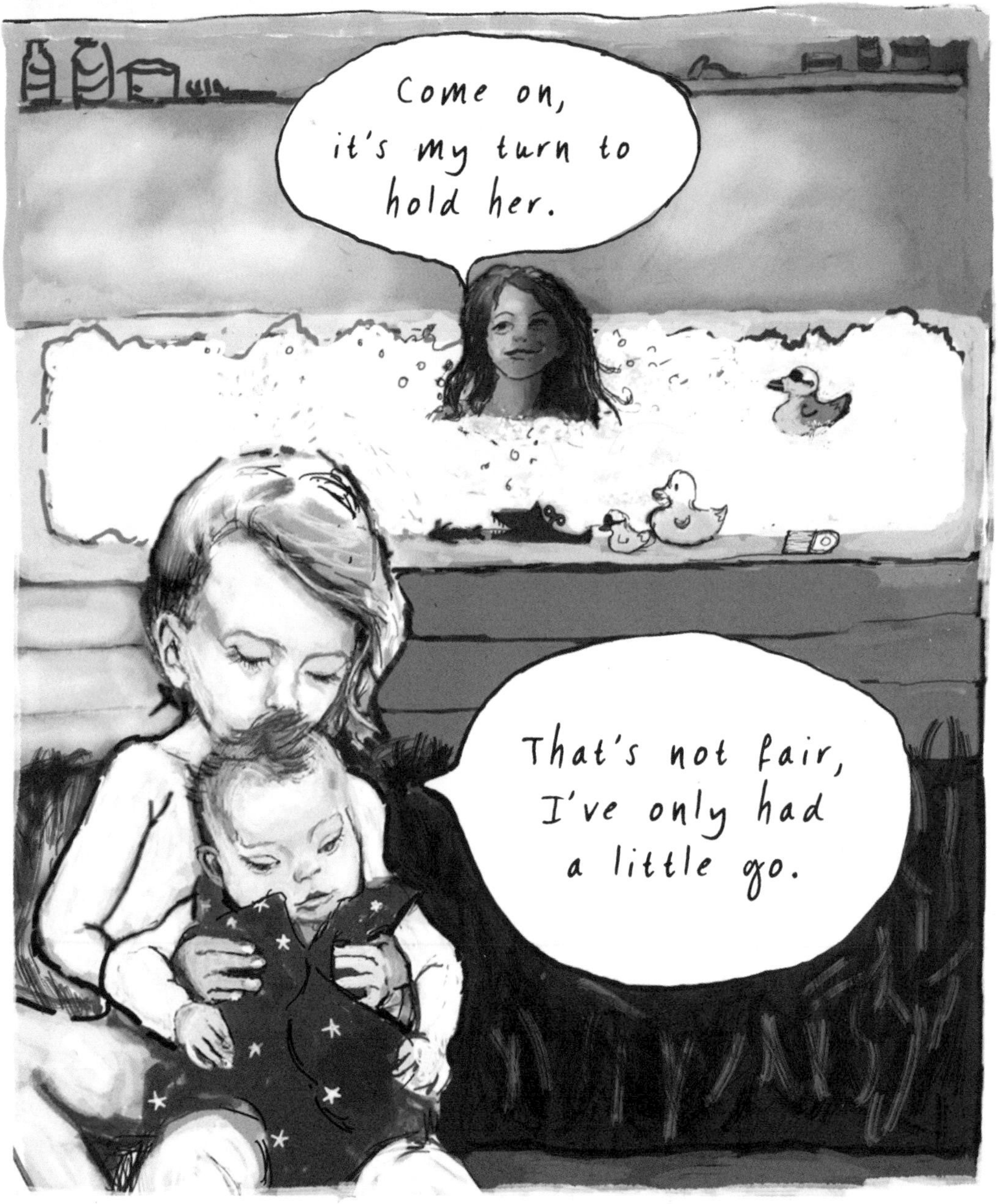
Come on, it's my turn to hold her.
That's not fair, I've only had a little go.

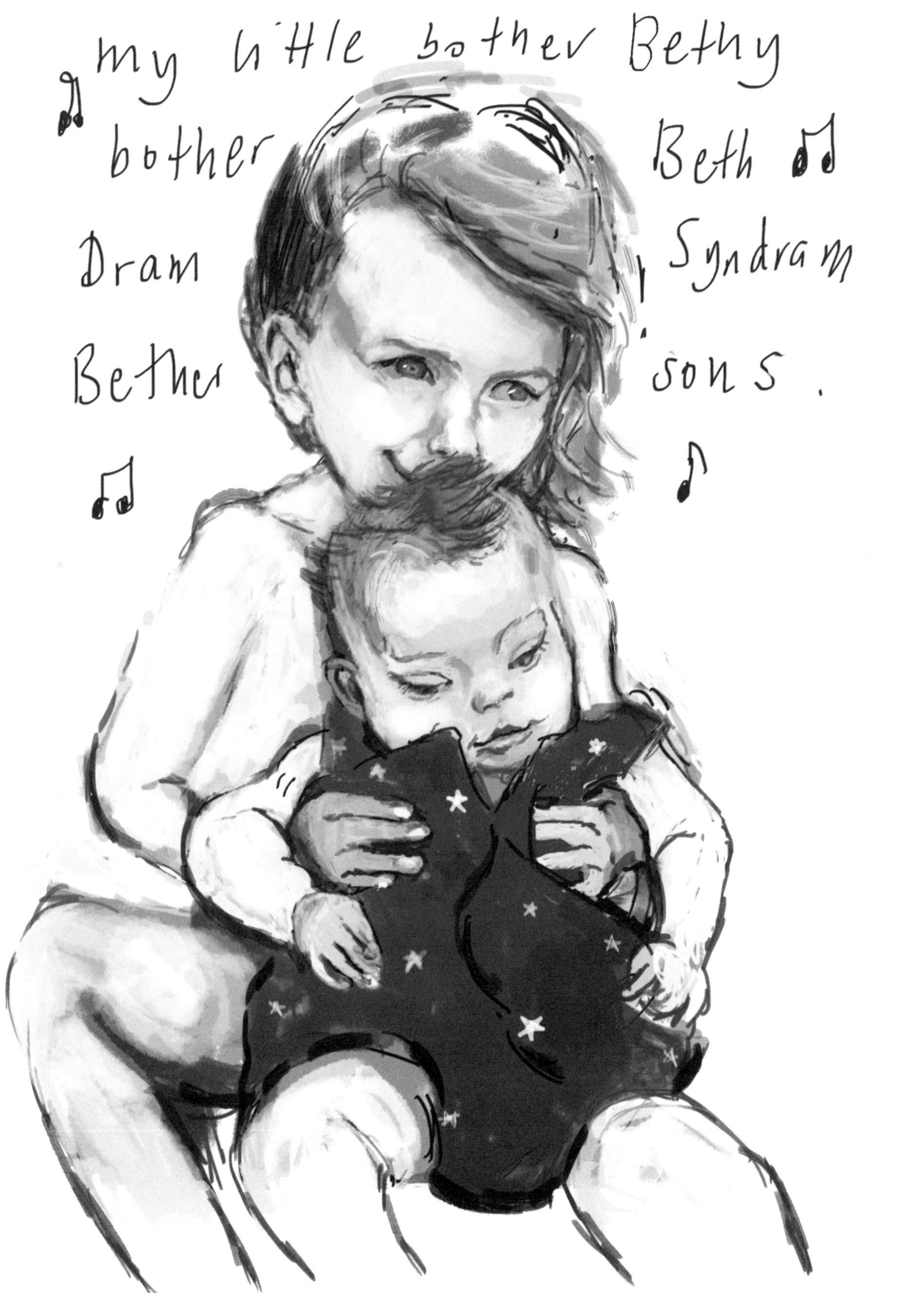
My little bother Bethy
bother Beth
Dram Syndram
Bether sons.

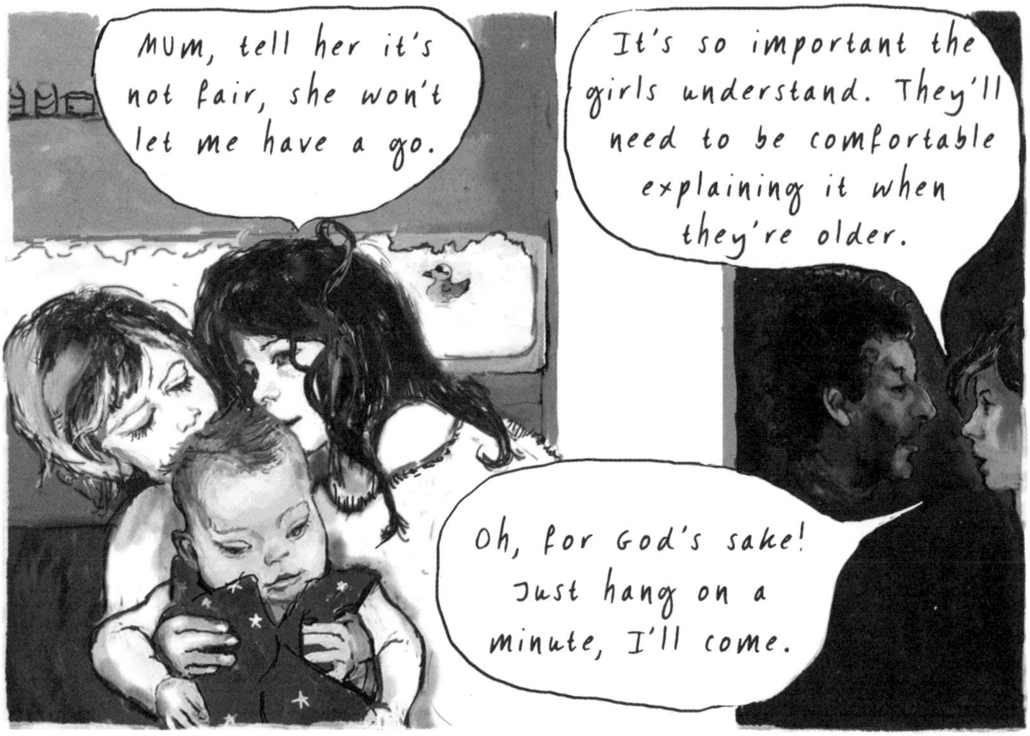
MUM, tell her it's not fair, she won't let me have a go.
It's so important the girls understand. They'll need to be comfortable explaining it when they're older.
Oh, for God's sake! Just hang on a minute, I'll come.

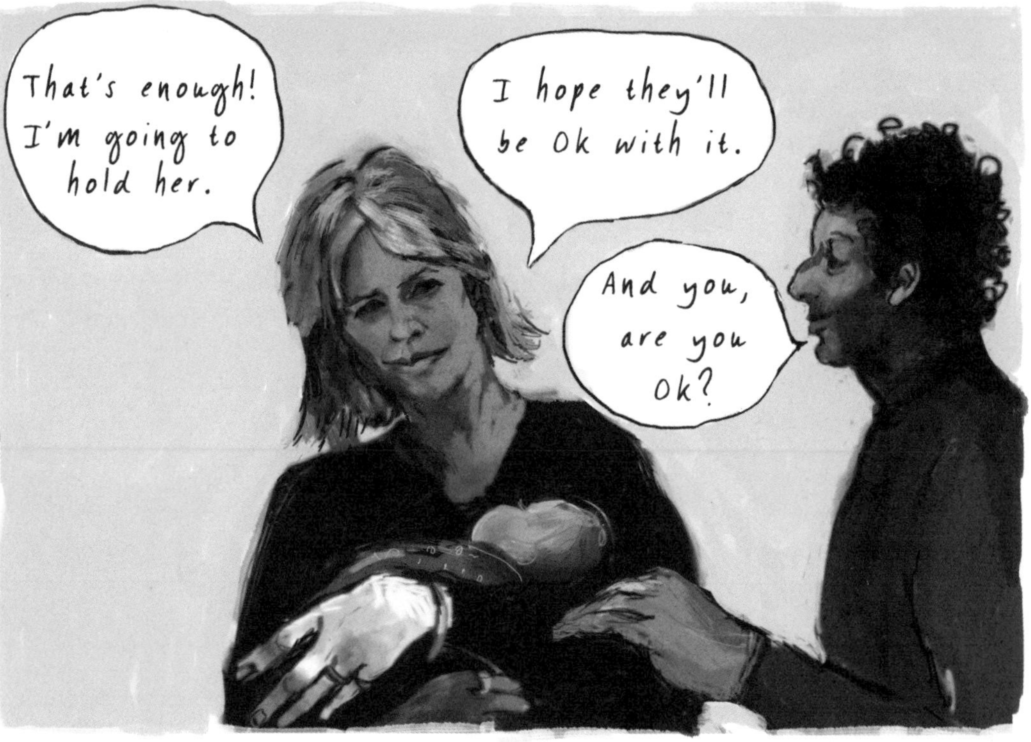
That's enough! I'm going to hold her.
I hope they'll be Ok with it.
And you, are you Ok?

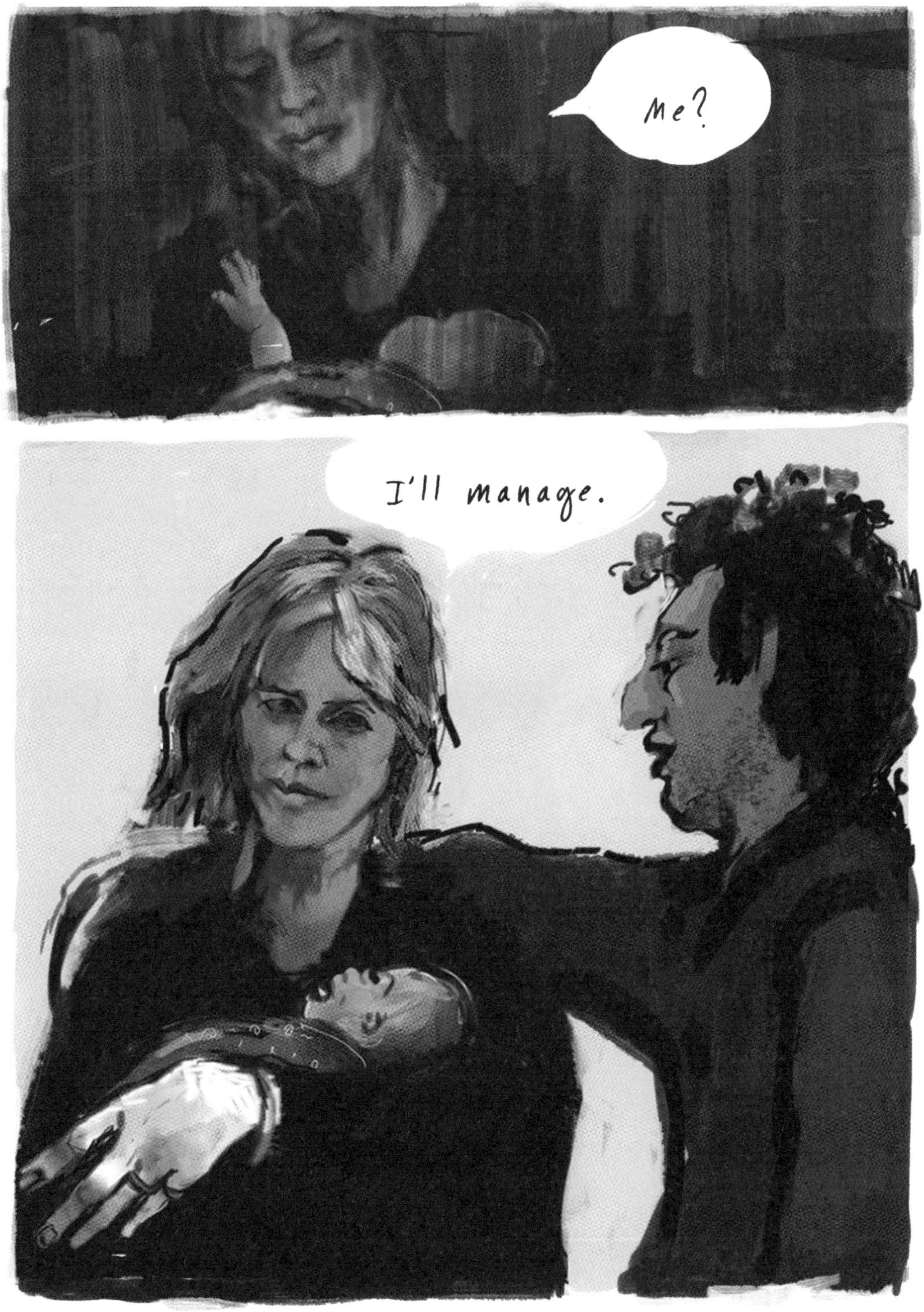
Me?
I'll manage.

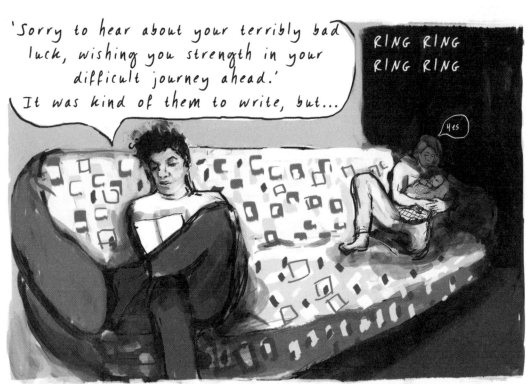

'Sorry to hear about your terribly bad luck, wishing you strength in your difficult journey ahead.'
It was kind of them to write, but...

RING RING
RING RING

yes

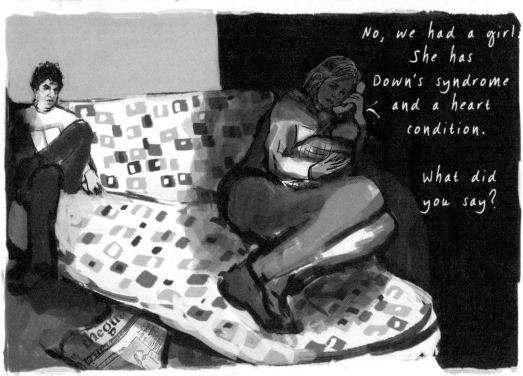

No, we had a girl. She has Down's syndrome and a heart condition.

What did you say?

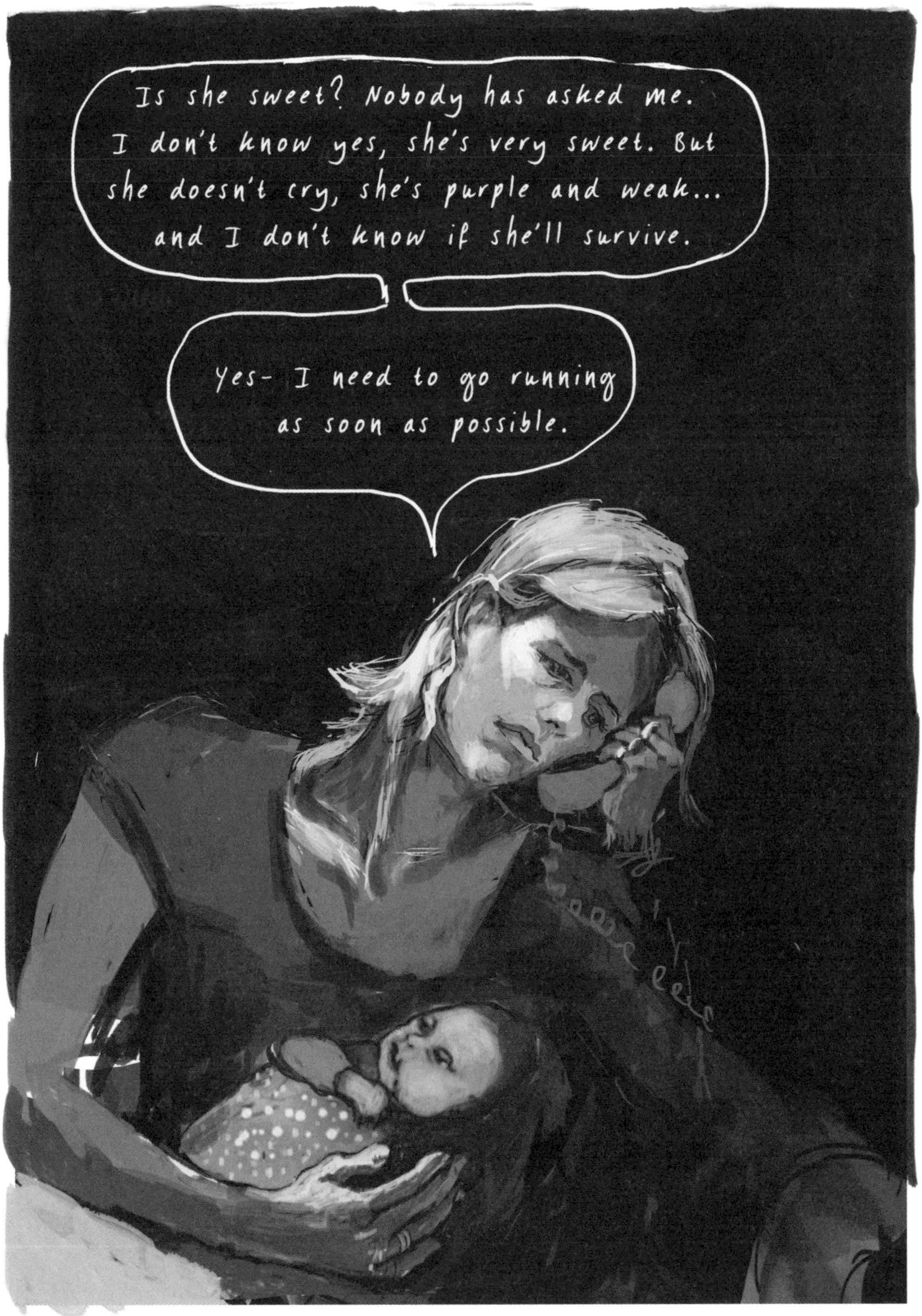
Is she sweet? Nobody has asked me. I don't know yes, she's very sweet. But she doesn't cry, she's purple and weak... and I don't know if she'll survive.
Yes- I need to go running as soon as possible.

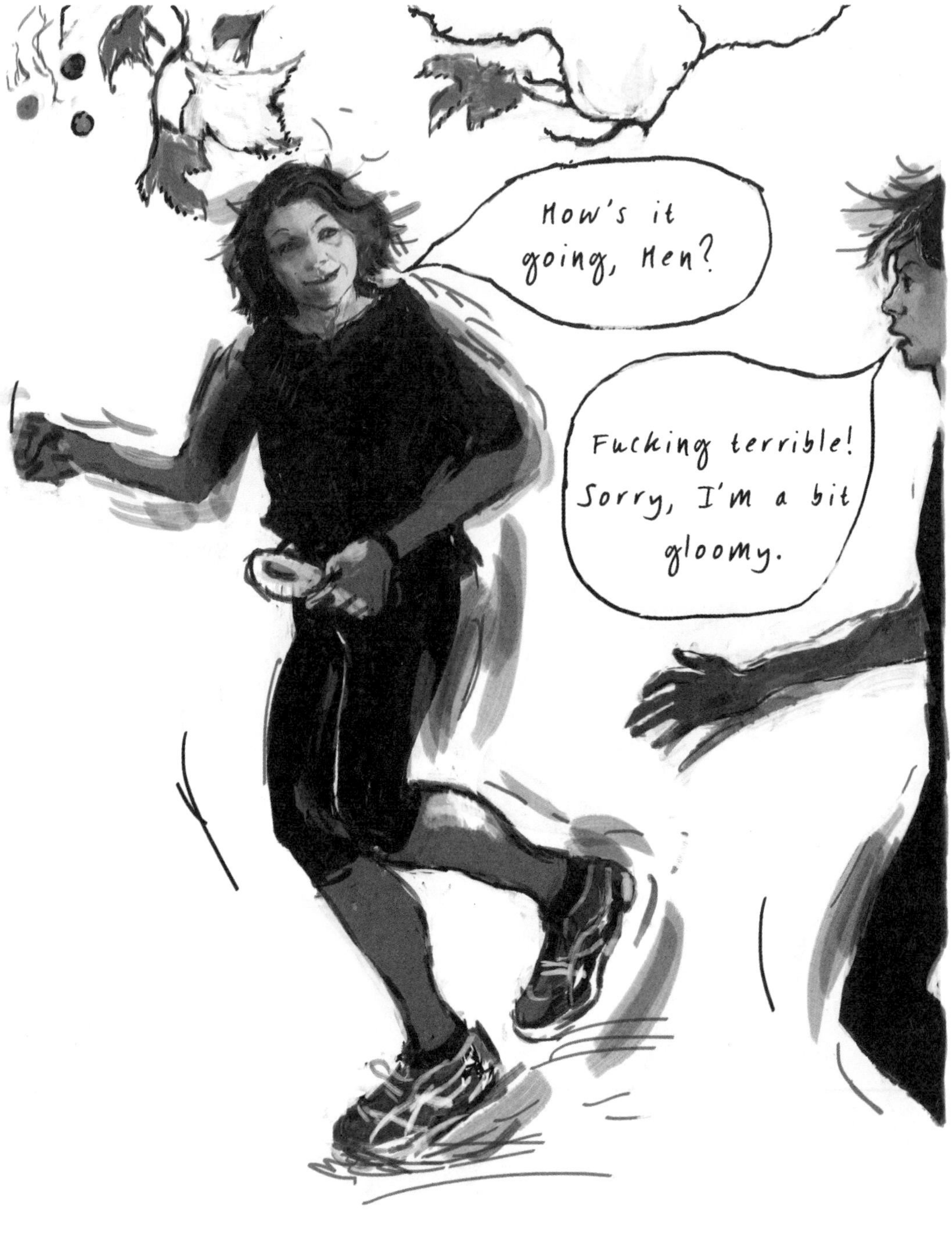
How's it going, Hen?
Fucking terrible! Sorry, I'm a bit gloomy.

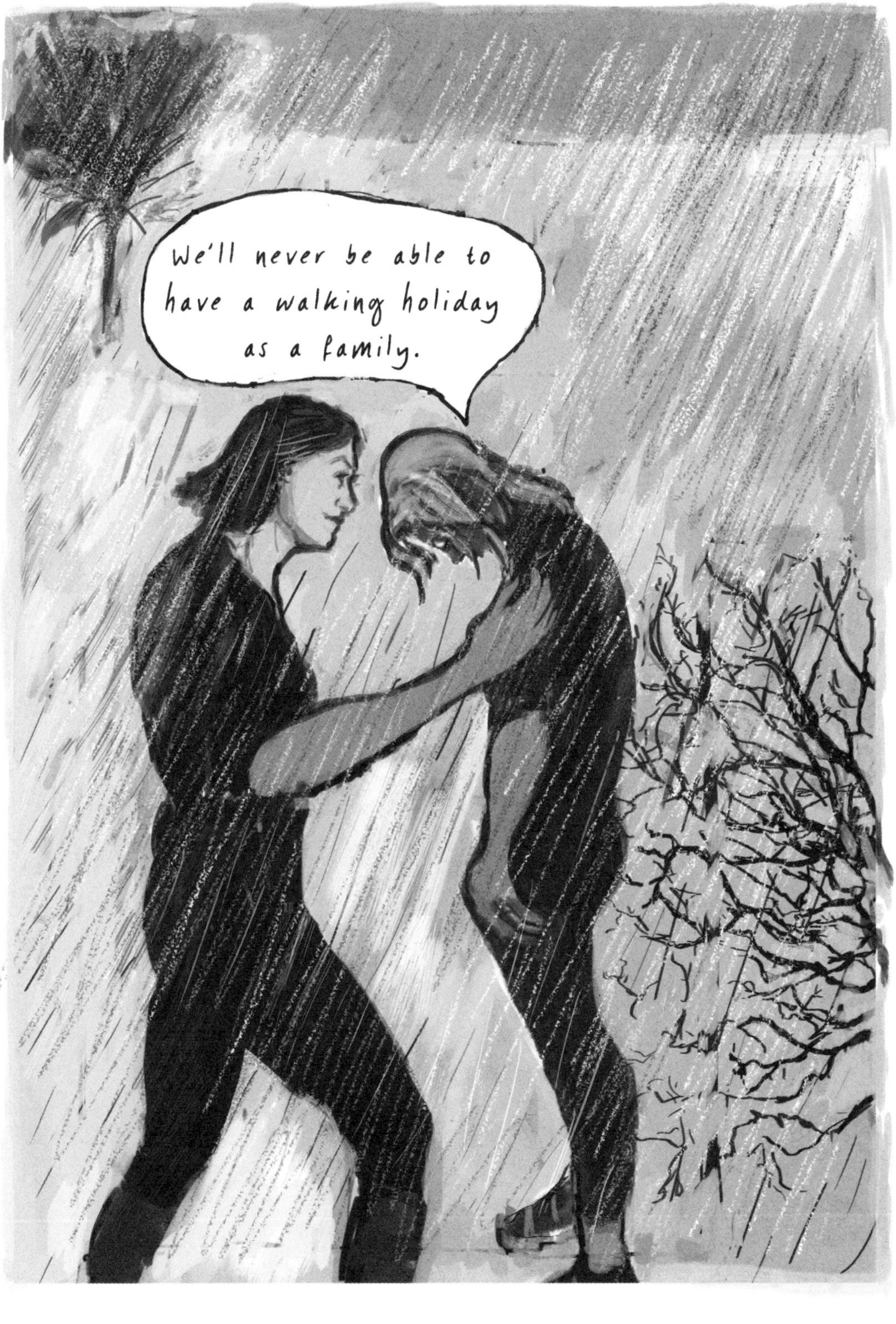
We'll never be able to have a walking holiday as a family.

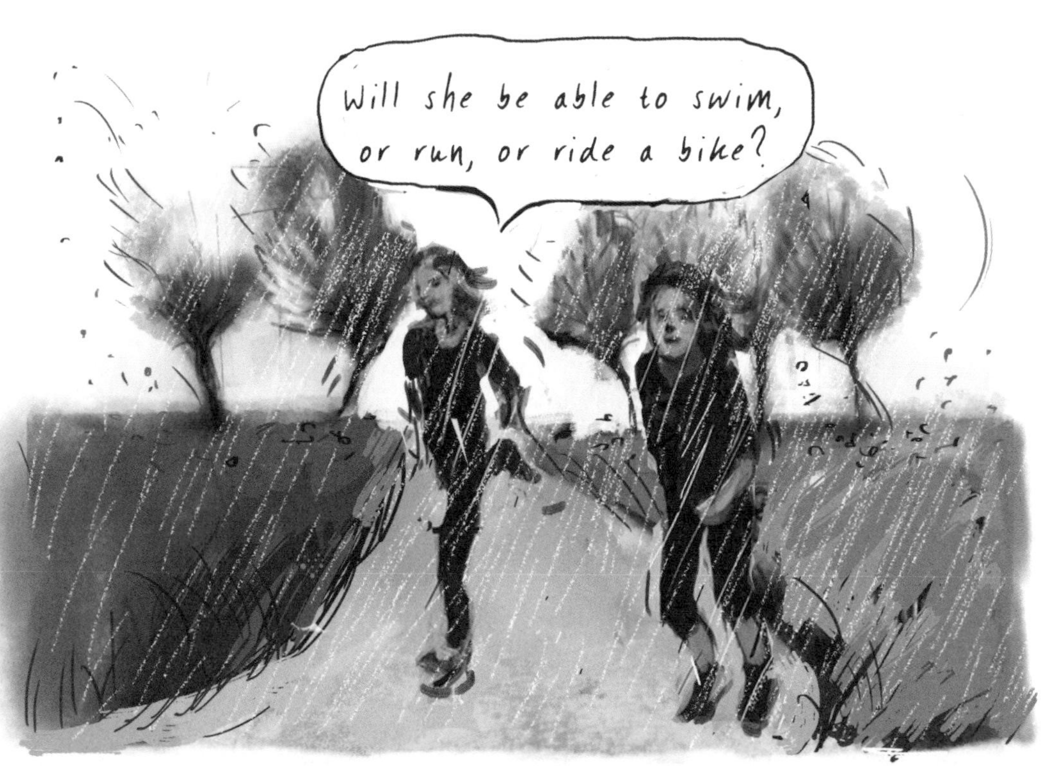
Will she be able to swim,
or run, or ride a bike?

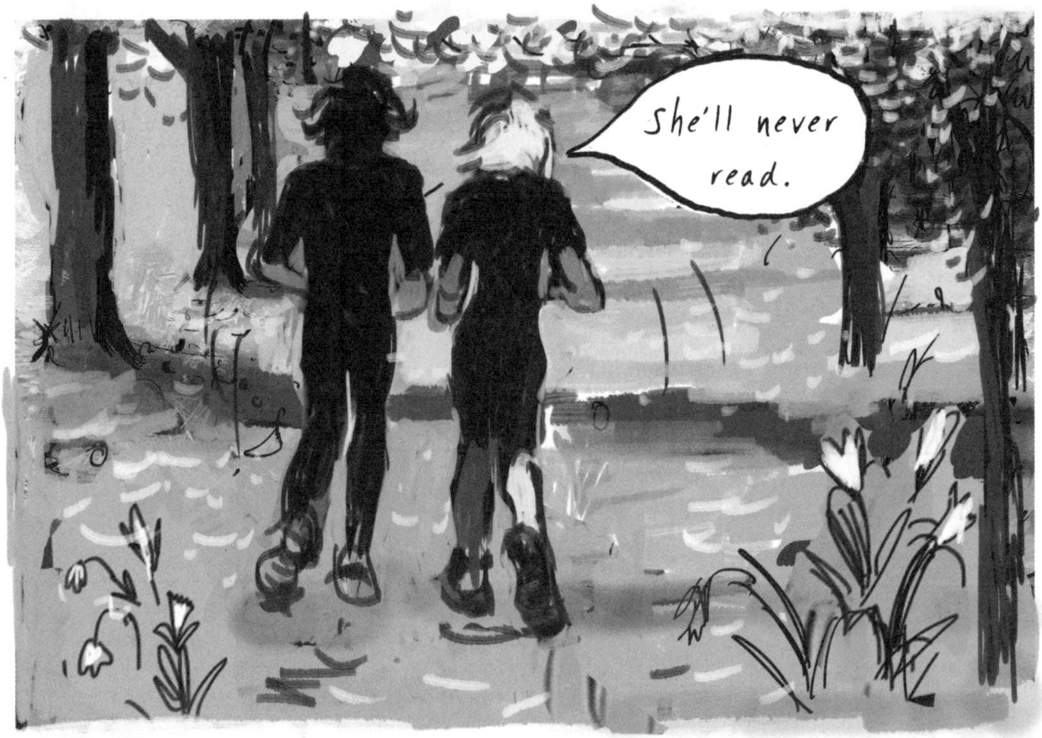
She'll never
read.

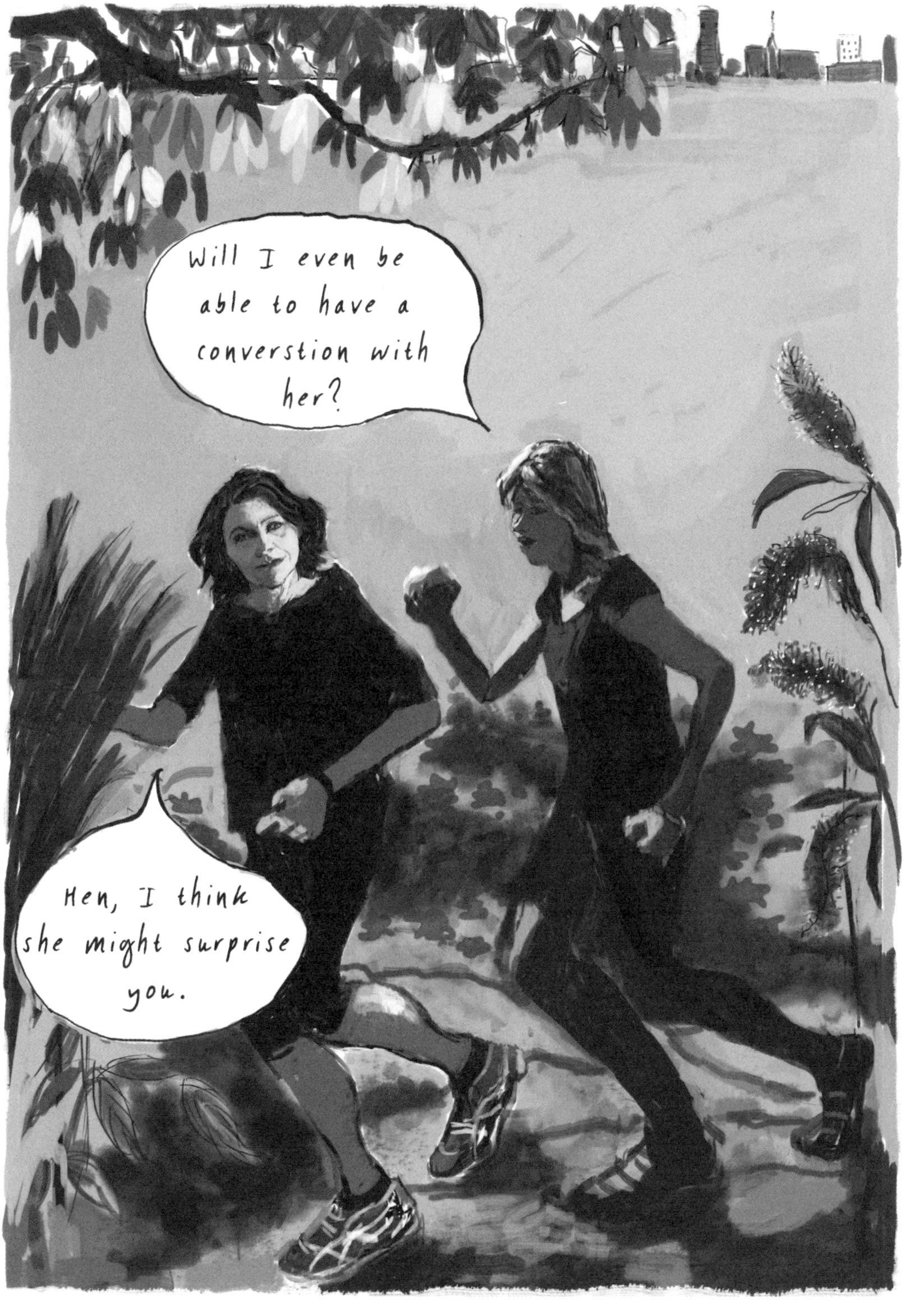
Will I even be able to have a converstion with her?
Hen, I think she might surprise you.

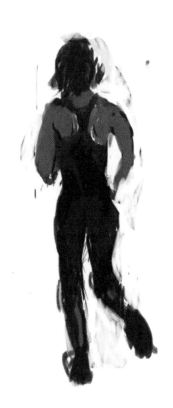

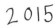

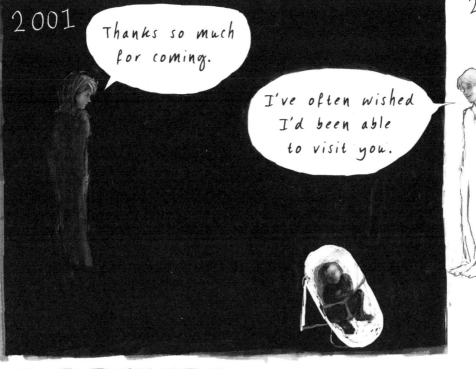

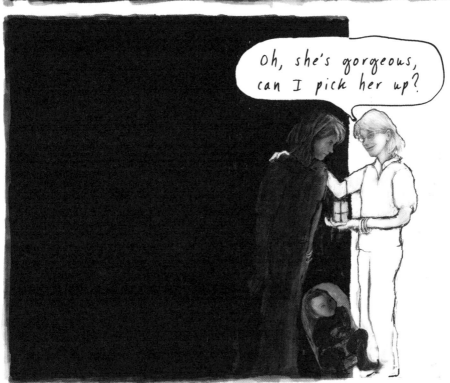

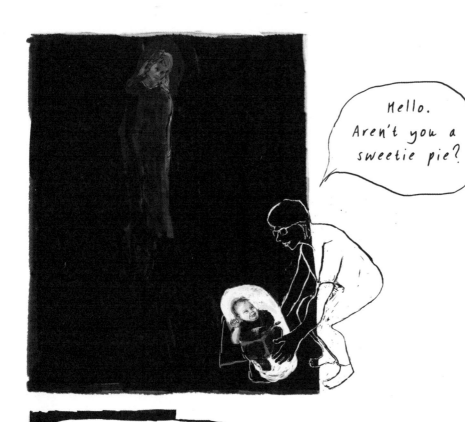

Hello.
Aren't you a
sweetie pie?

If I could love
her it would be Ok.

I HATED my daughter
when she was born.

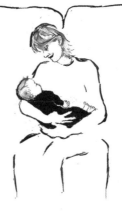

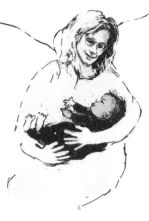

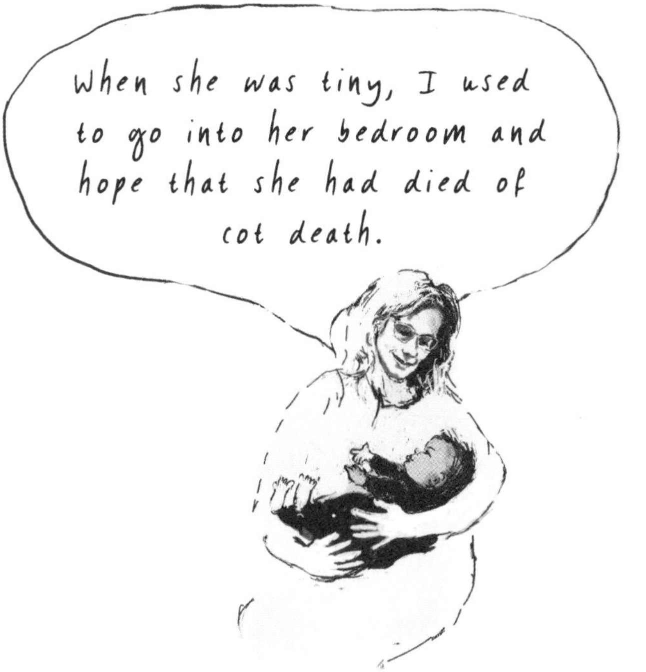

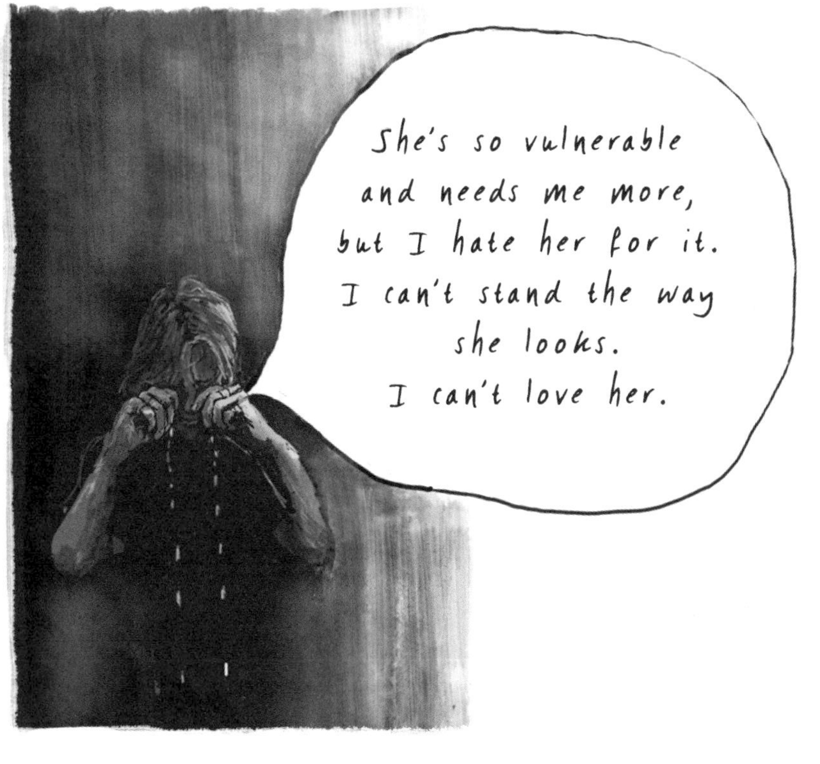

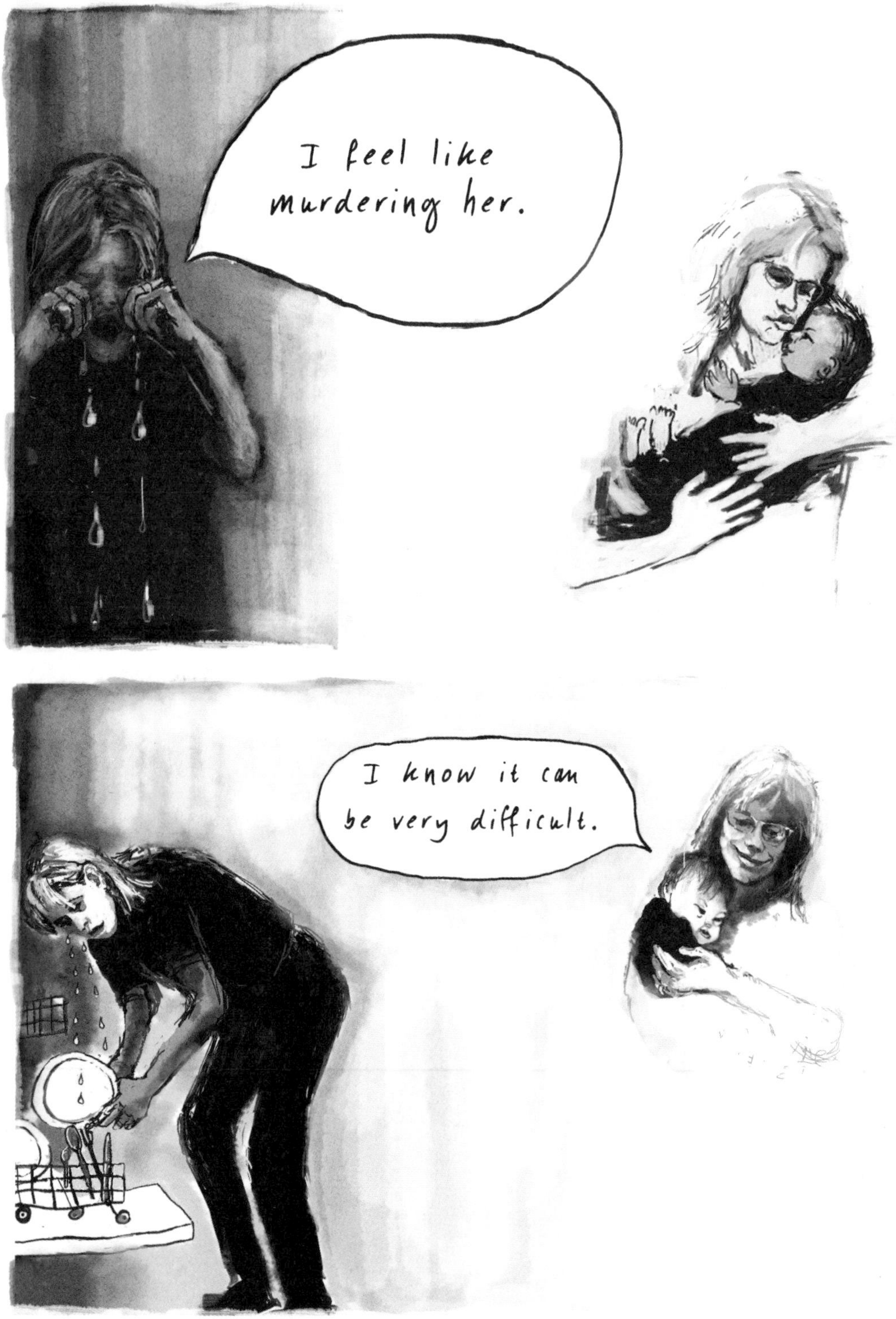
I feel like murdering her.
I know it can be very difficult.

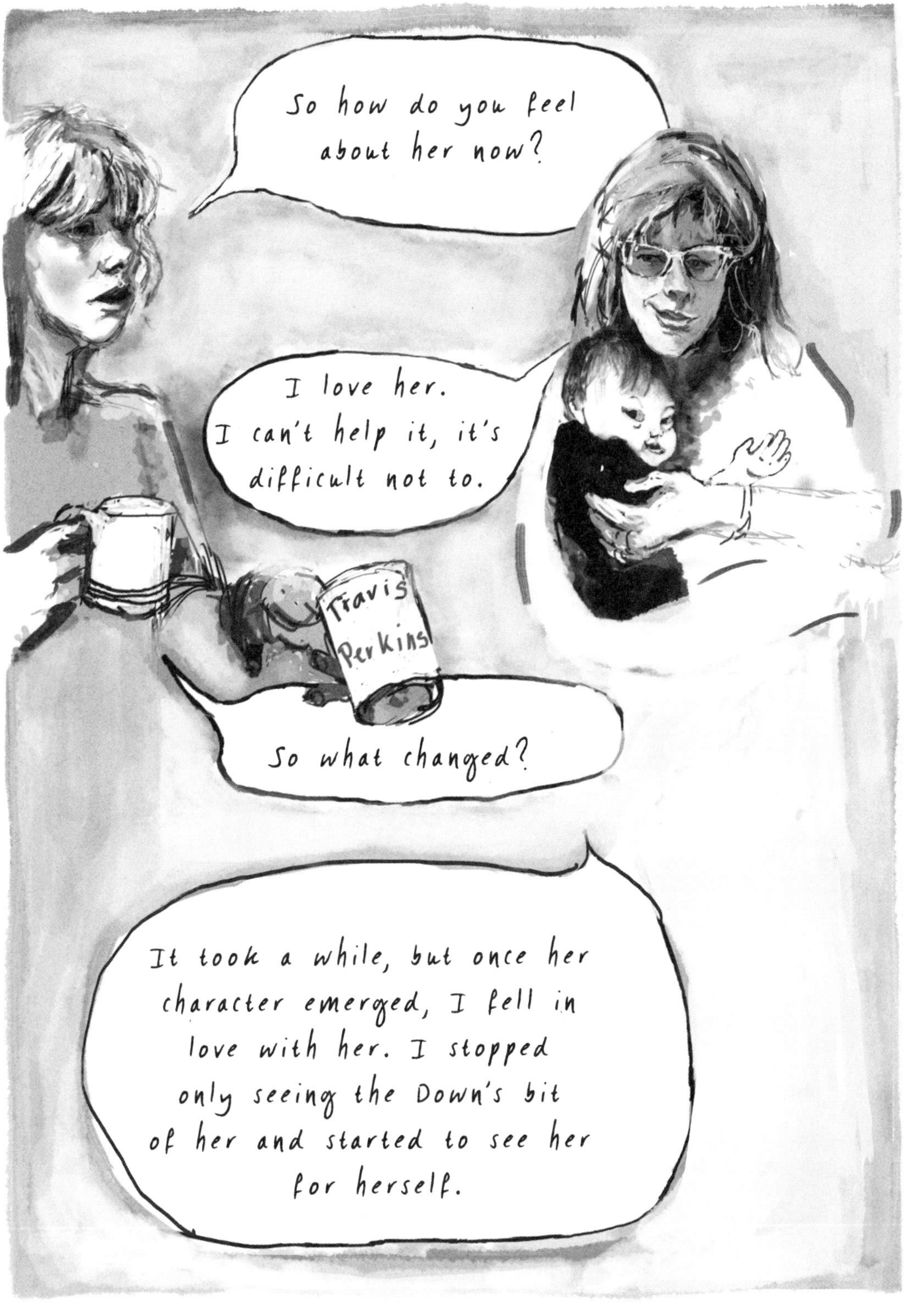
So how do you feel about her now?
I love her. I can't help it, it's difficult not to.
Travis Perkins
So what changed?
It took a while, but once her character emerged, I fell in love with her. I stopped only seeing the Down's bit of her and started to see her for herself.

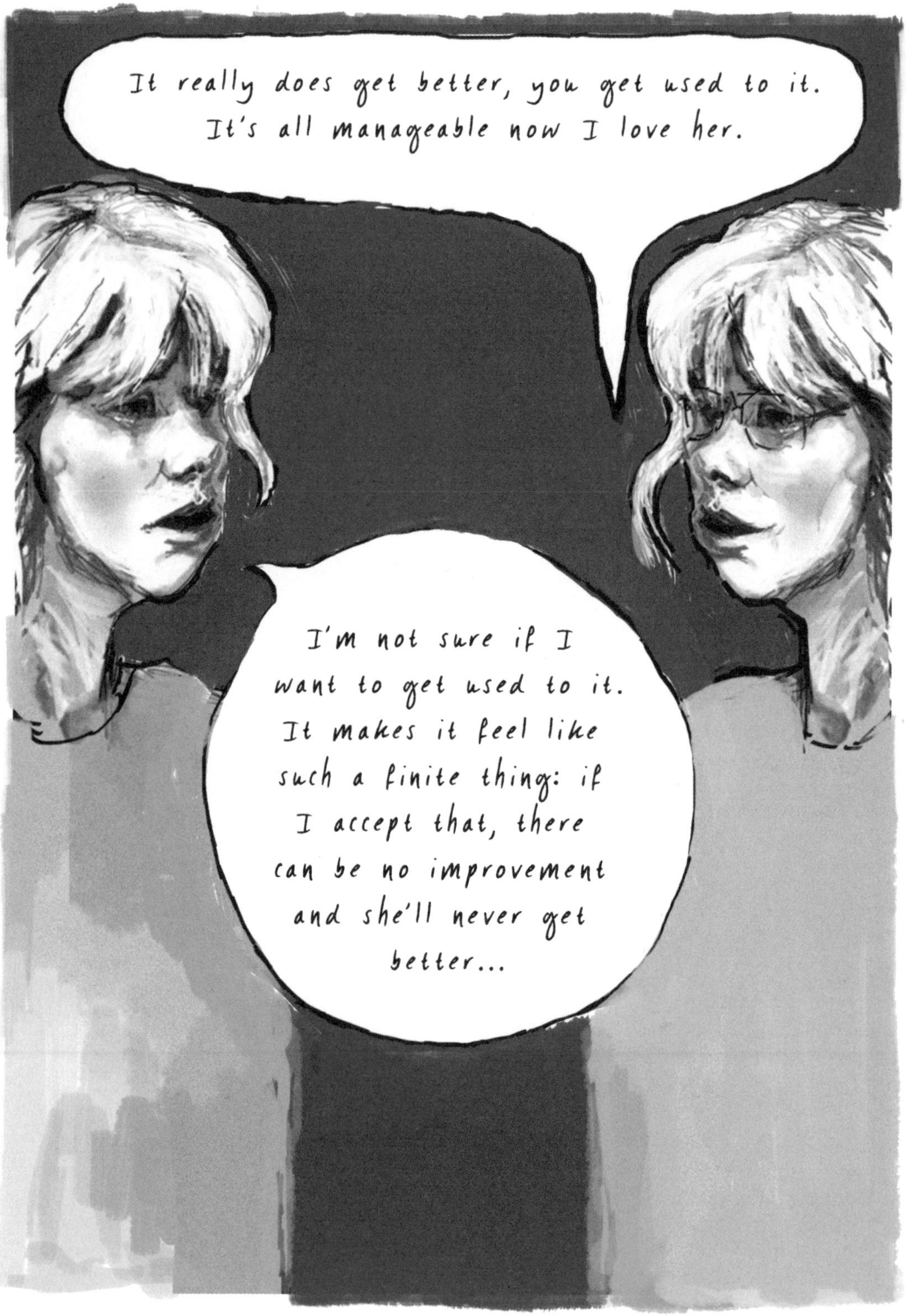
It really does get better, you get used to it. It's all manageable now I love her.
I'm not sure if I want to get used to it. It makes it feel like such a finite thing: if I accept that, there can be no improvement and she'll never get better...

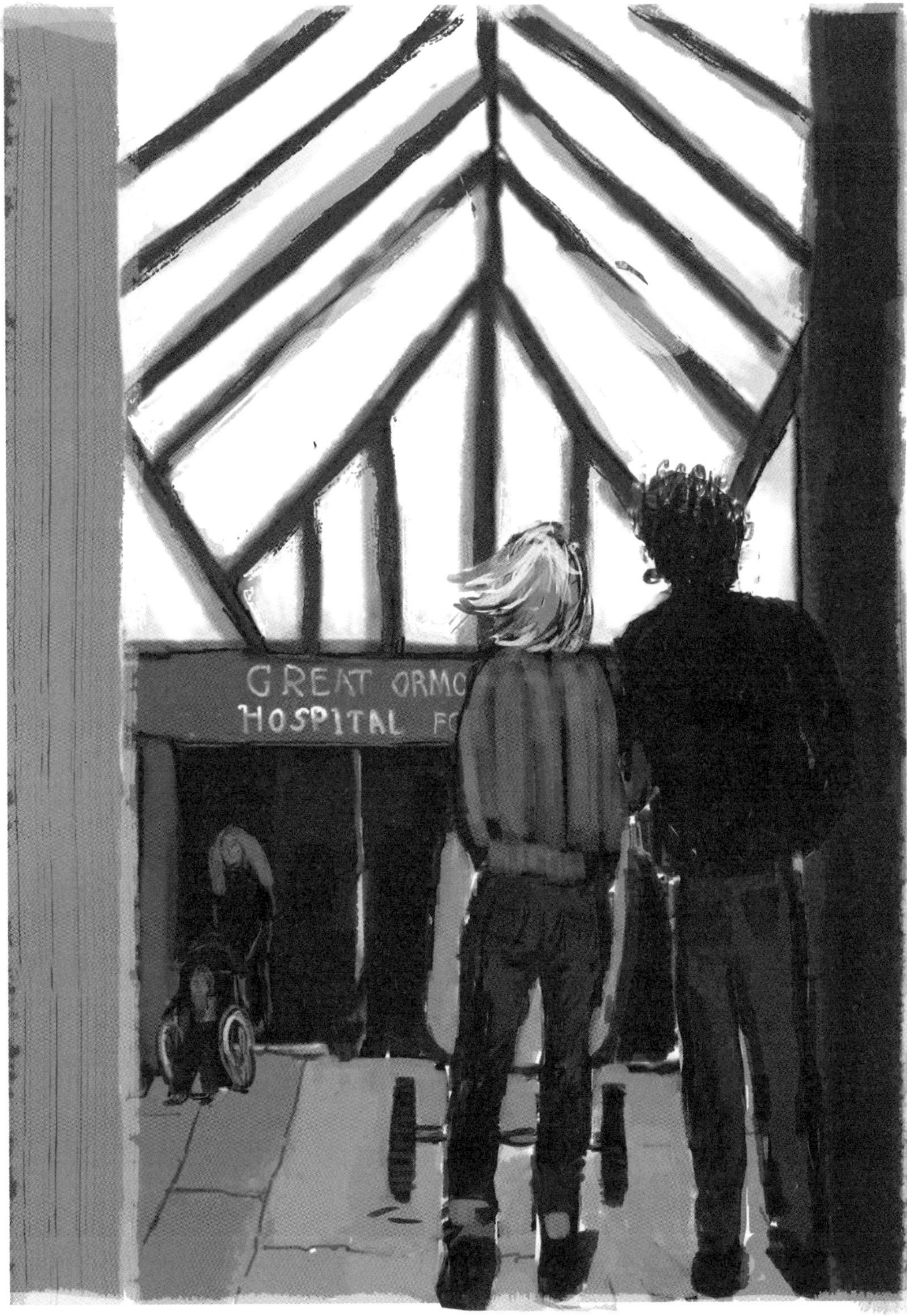
GREAT ORMO
HOSPITAL FO

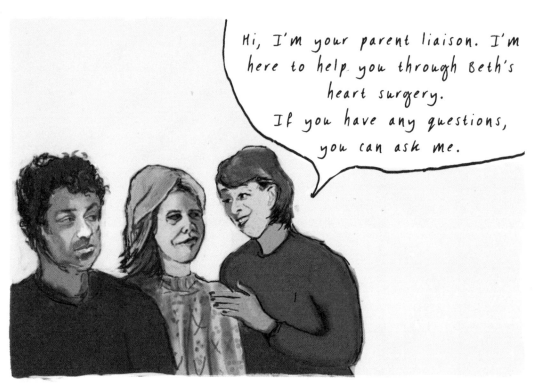

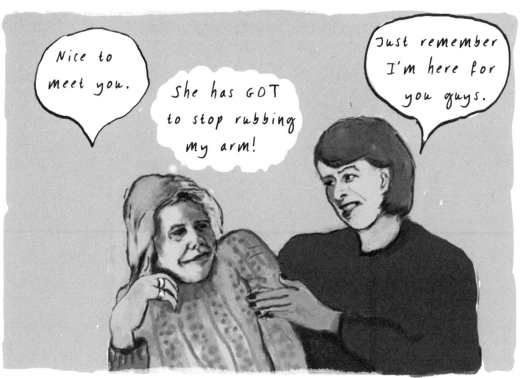

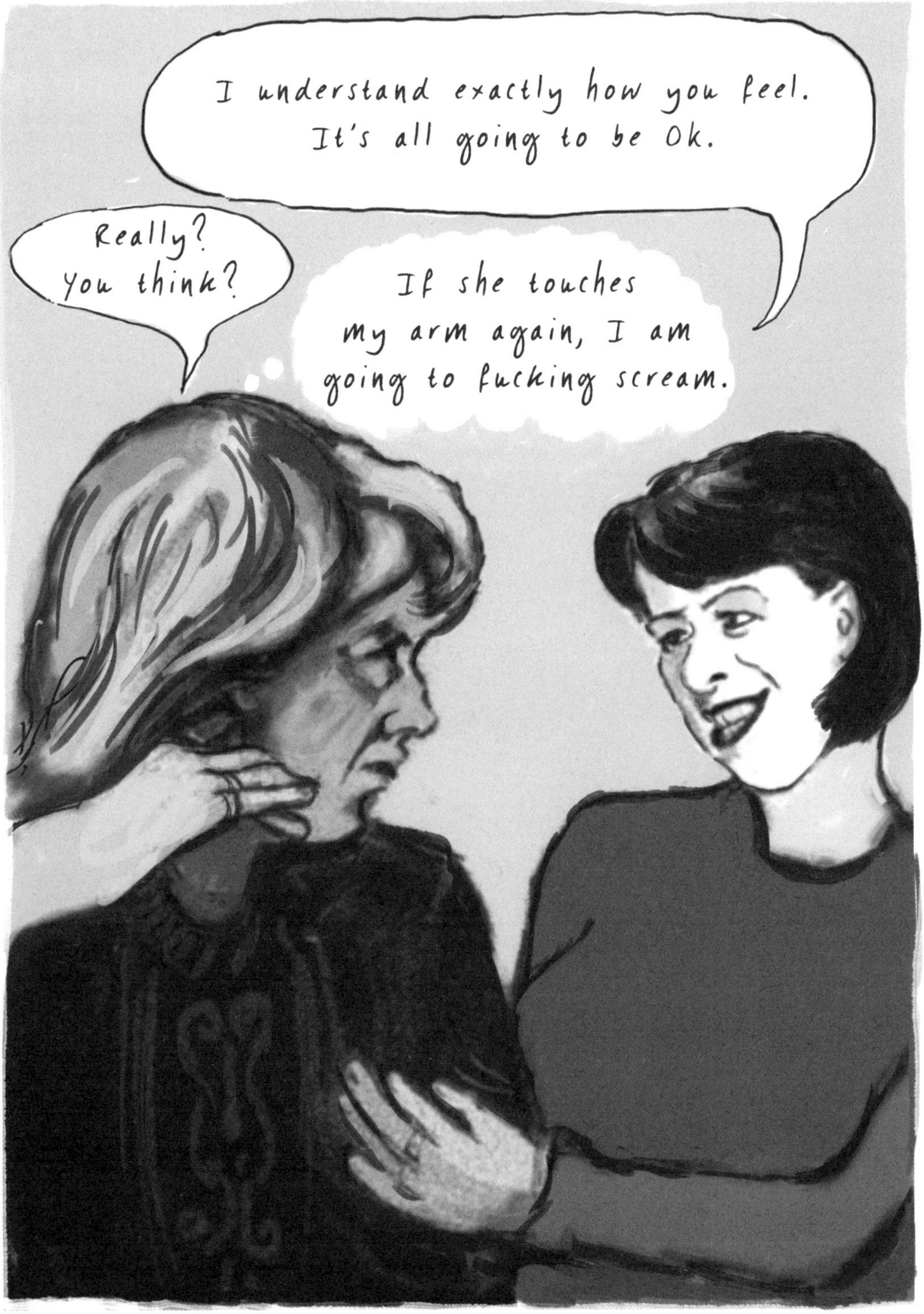
I understand exactly how you feel. It's all going to be Ok.
Really? you think?
If she touches my arm again, I am going to fucking scream.

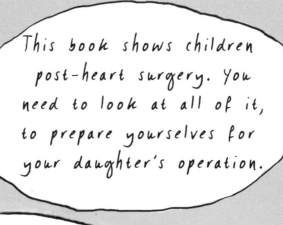

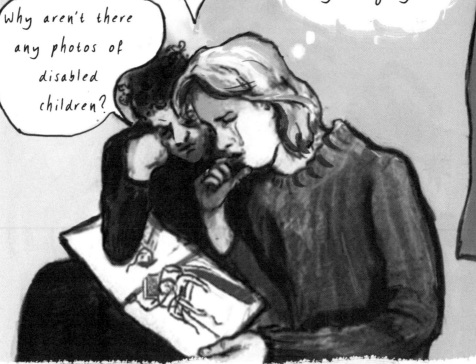

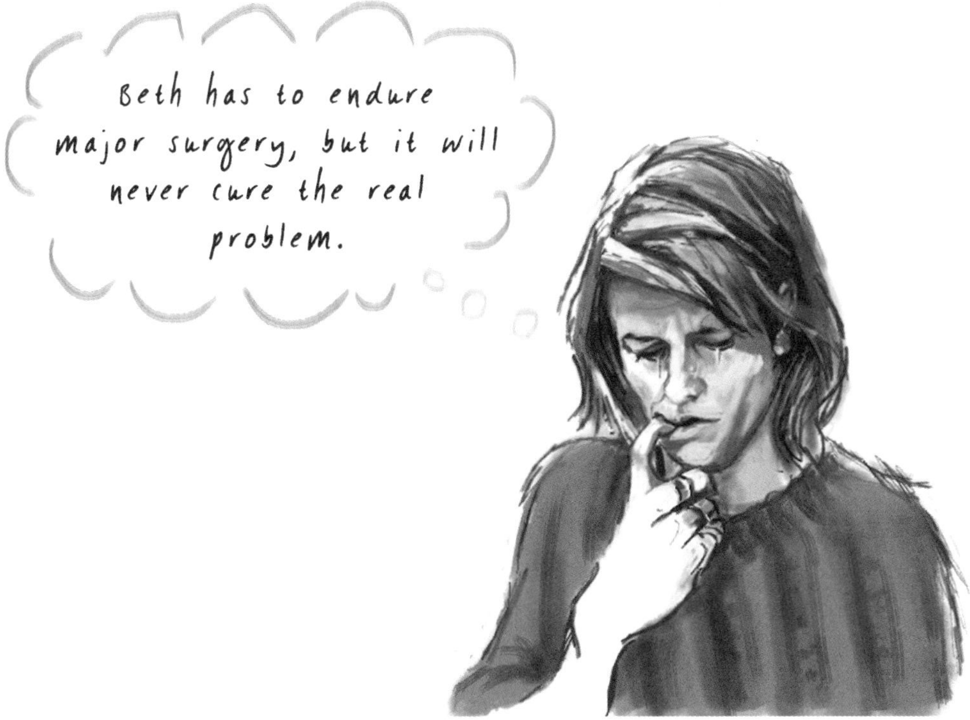
Beth has to endure major surgery, but it will never cure the real problem.

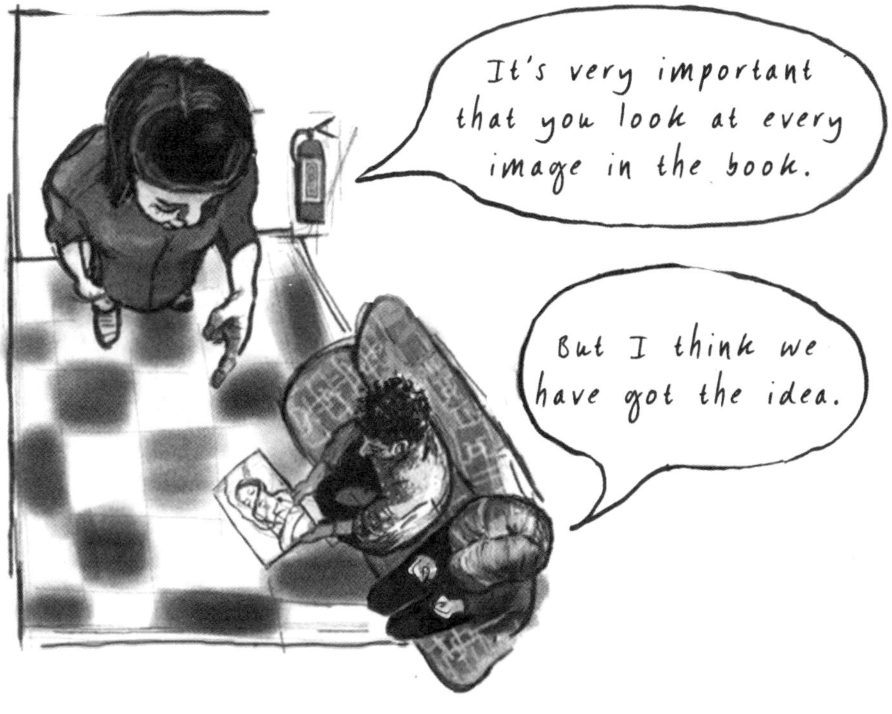
It's very important that you look at every image in the book.
But I think we have got the idea.

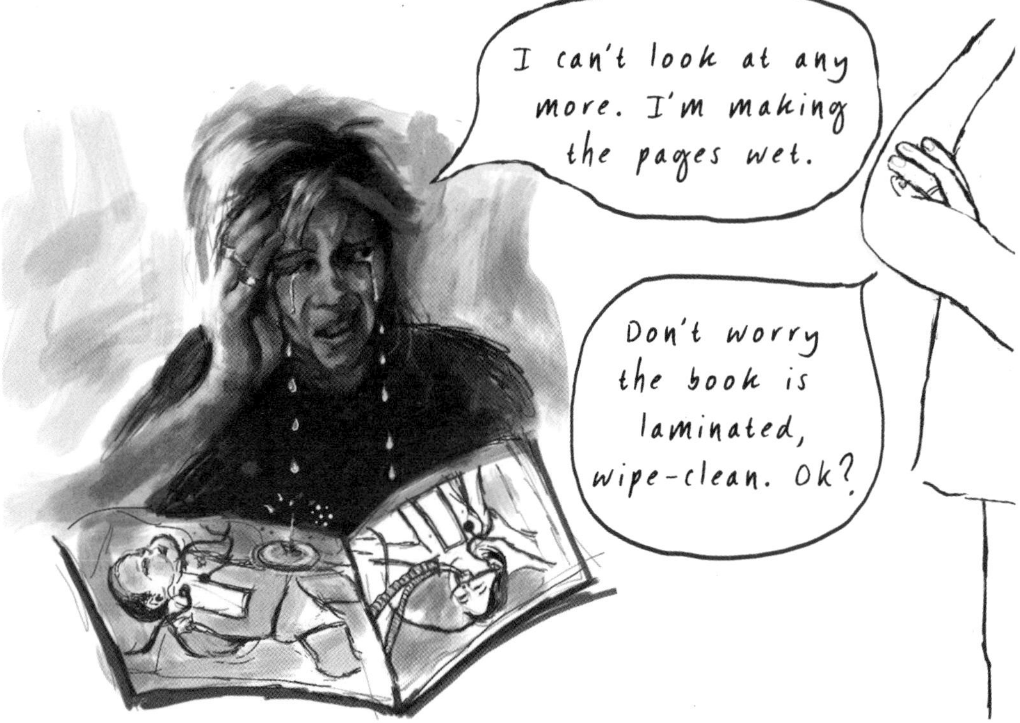
I can't look at any more. I'm making the pages wet.
Don't worry the book is laminated, wipe-clean. Ok?

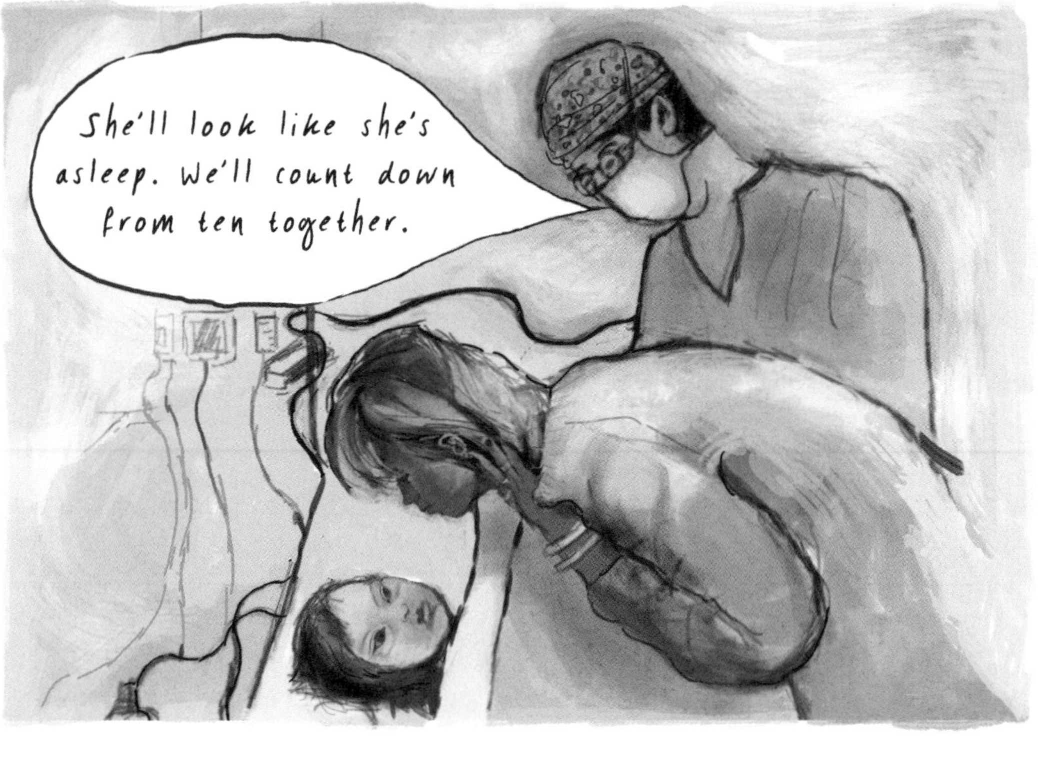
She'll look like she's asleep. We'll count down from ten together.

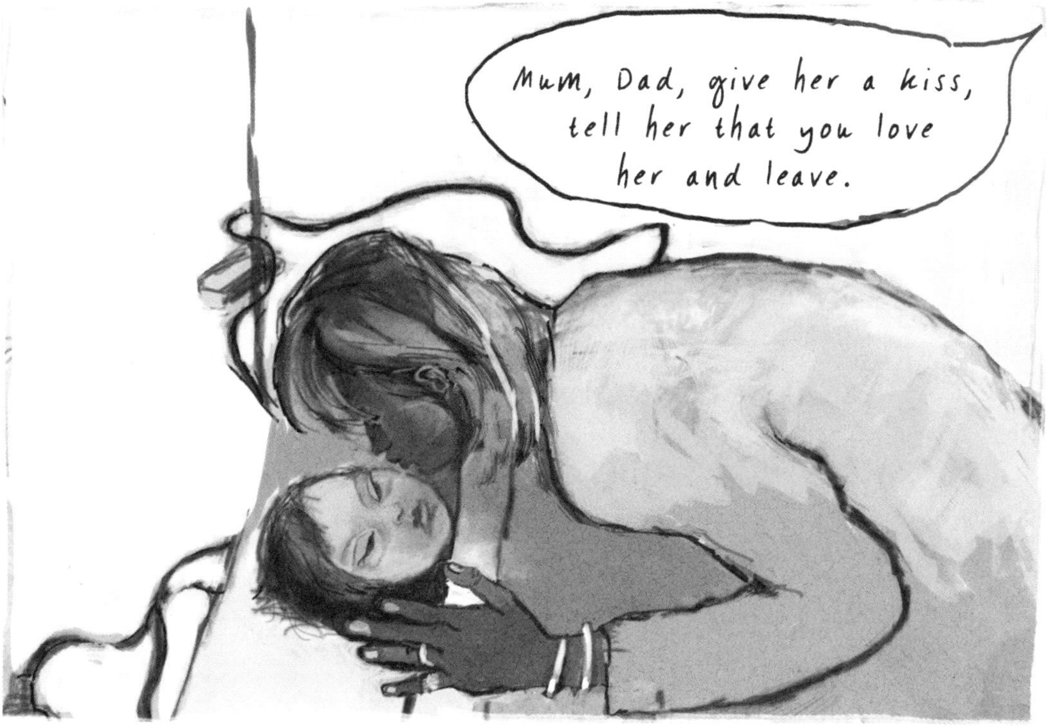
Mum, Dad, give her a kiss, tell her that you love her and leave.

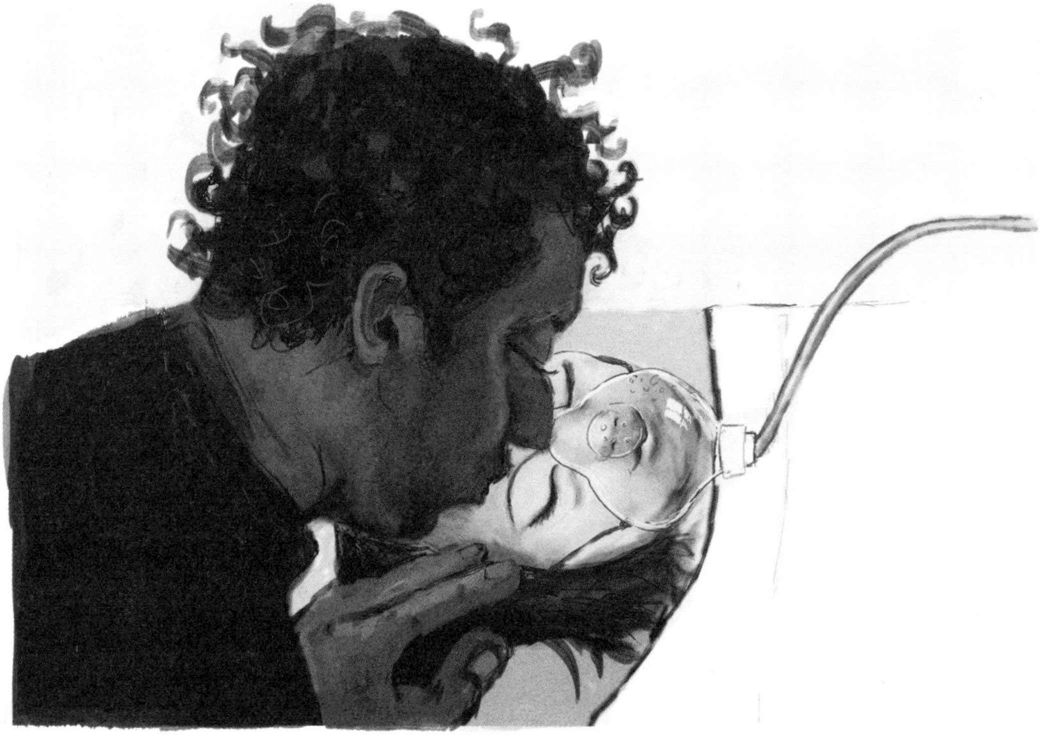

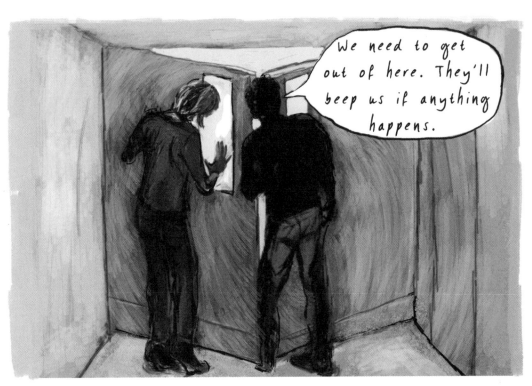

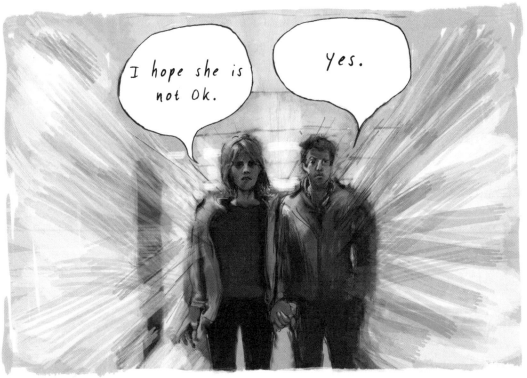

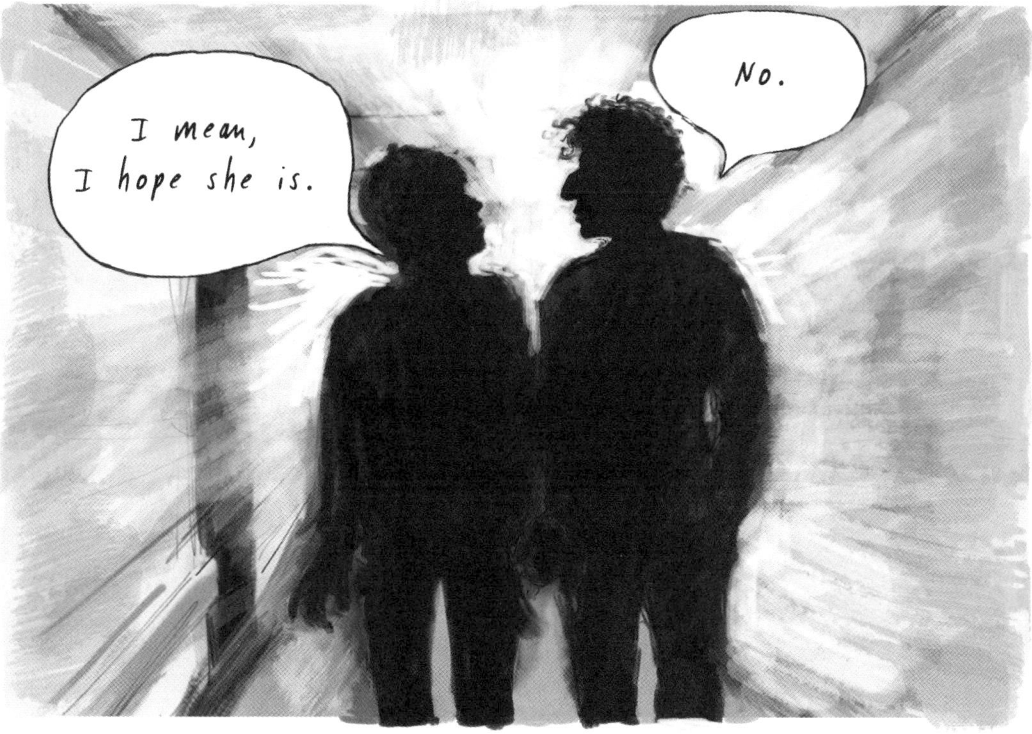
I mean, I hope she is.
No.

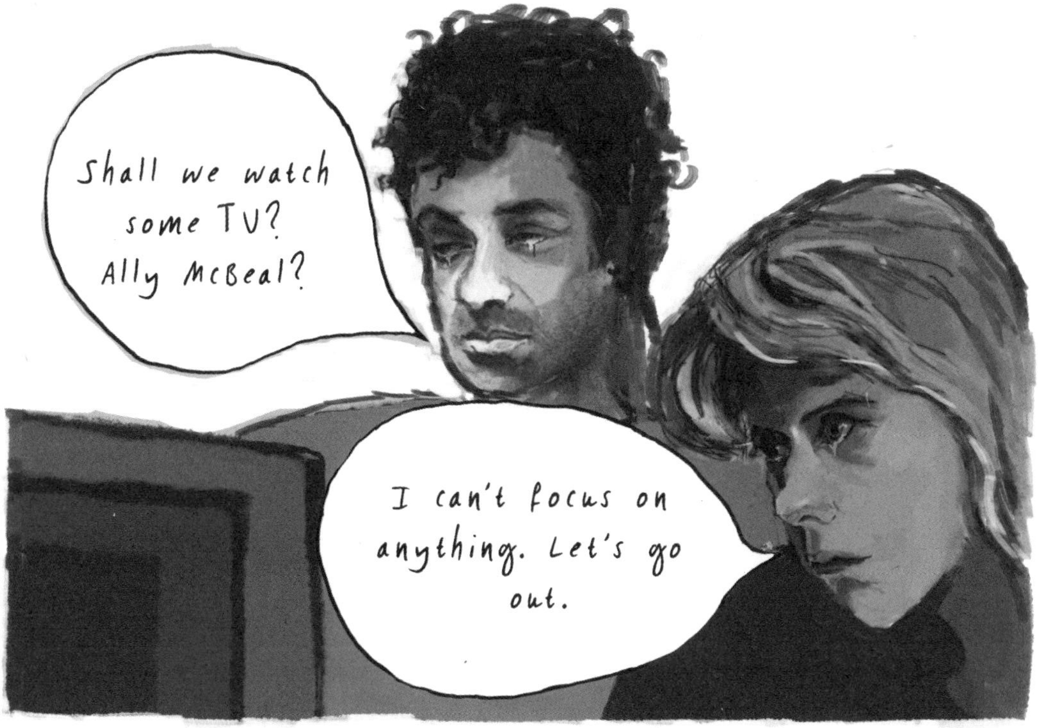
Shall we watch some TV? Ally McBeal?
I can't focus on anything. Let's go out.

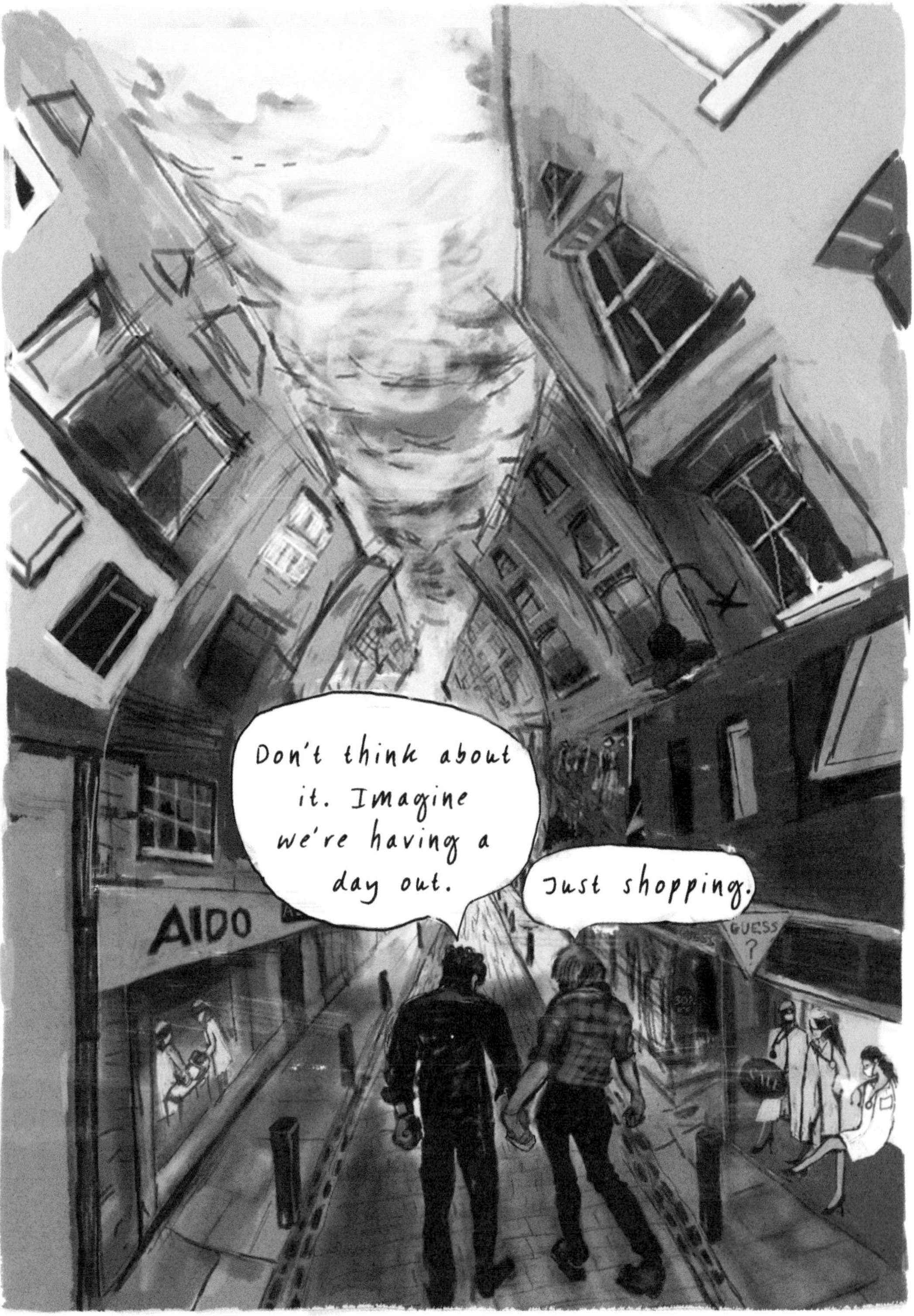
Don't think about it. Imagine we're having a day out.
Just shopping.
AIDO
GUESS
?

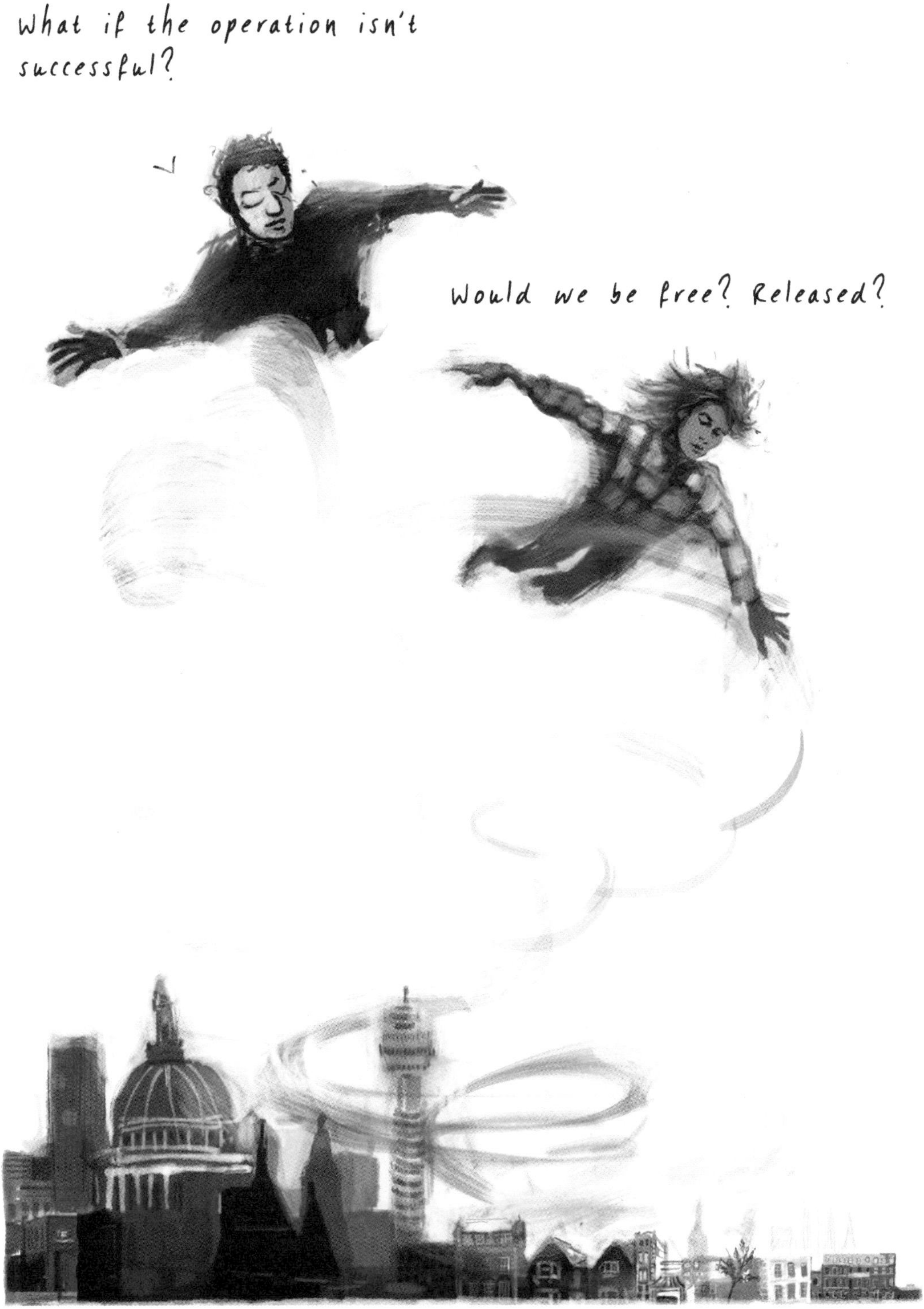
What if the operation isn't successful?
Would we be free? Released?

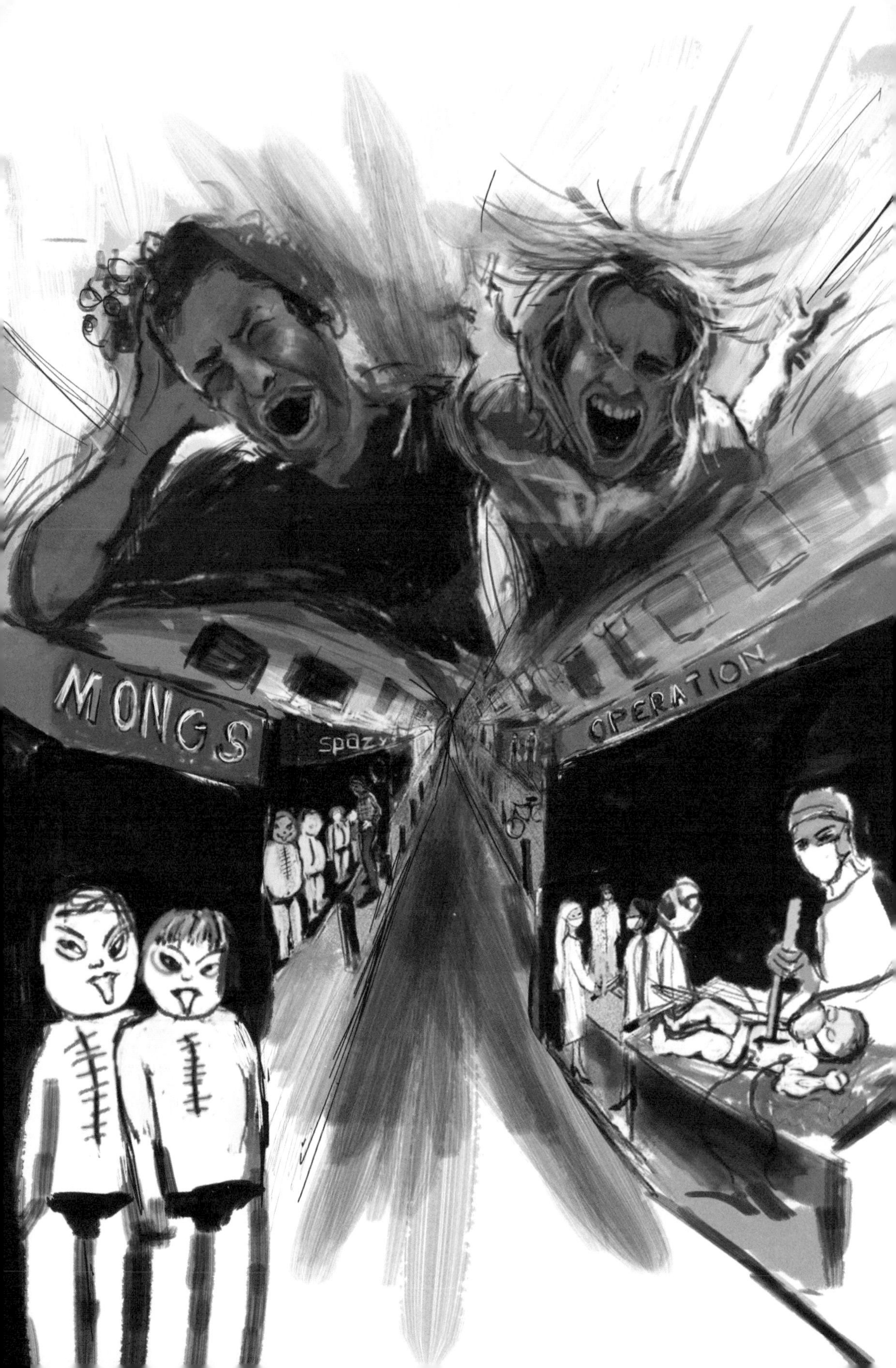
MONGS
spazy
OPERATION

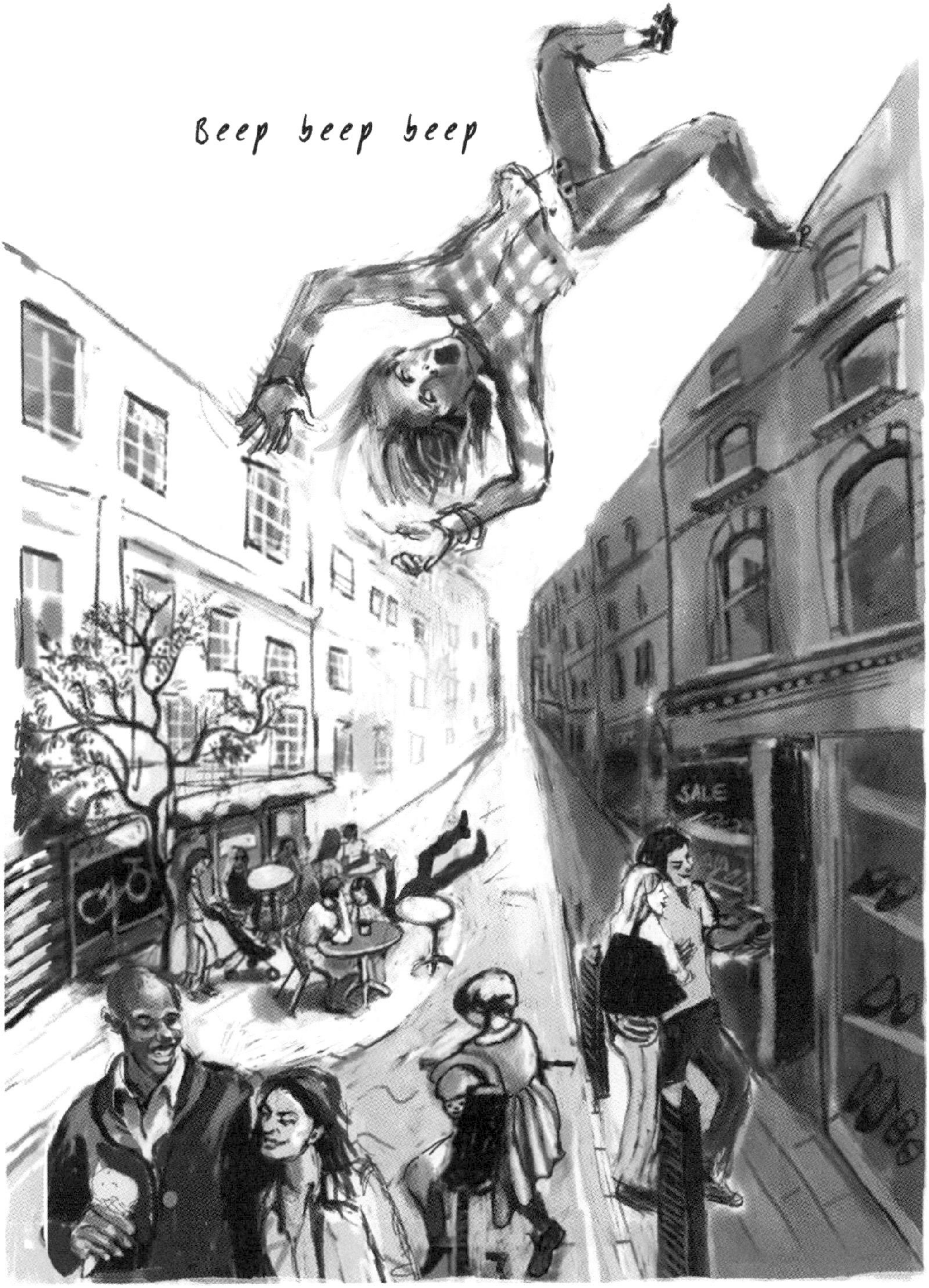
Beep beep beep
SALE

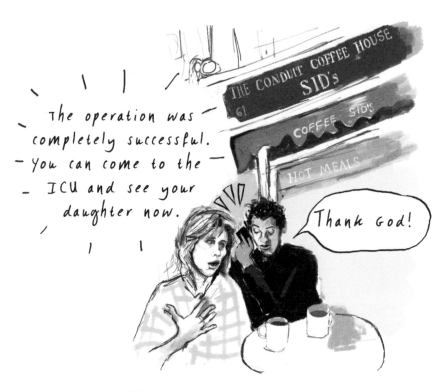

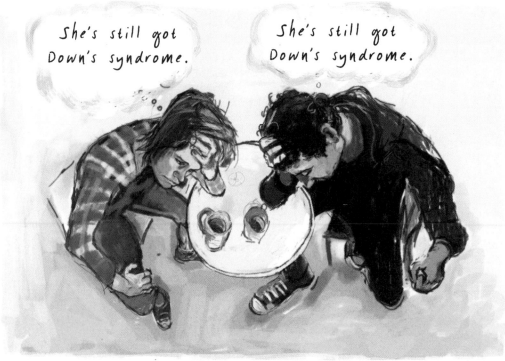

Part Three

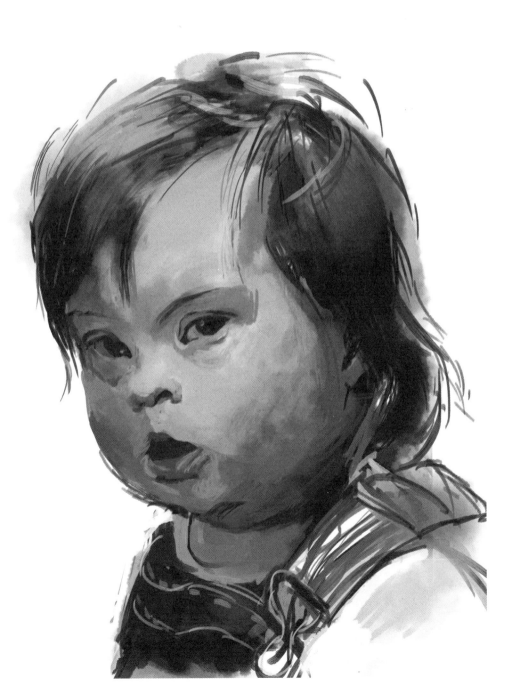

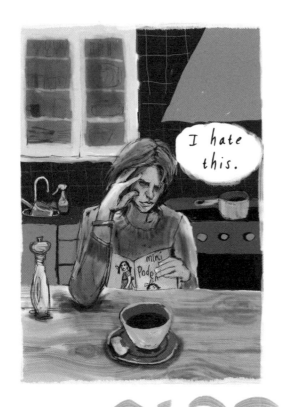

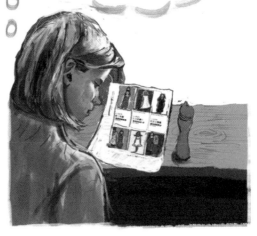

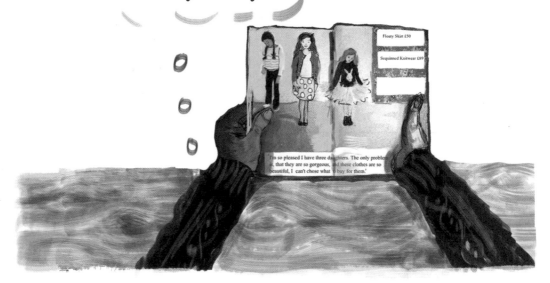

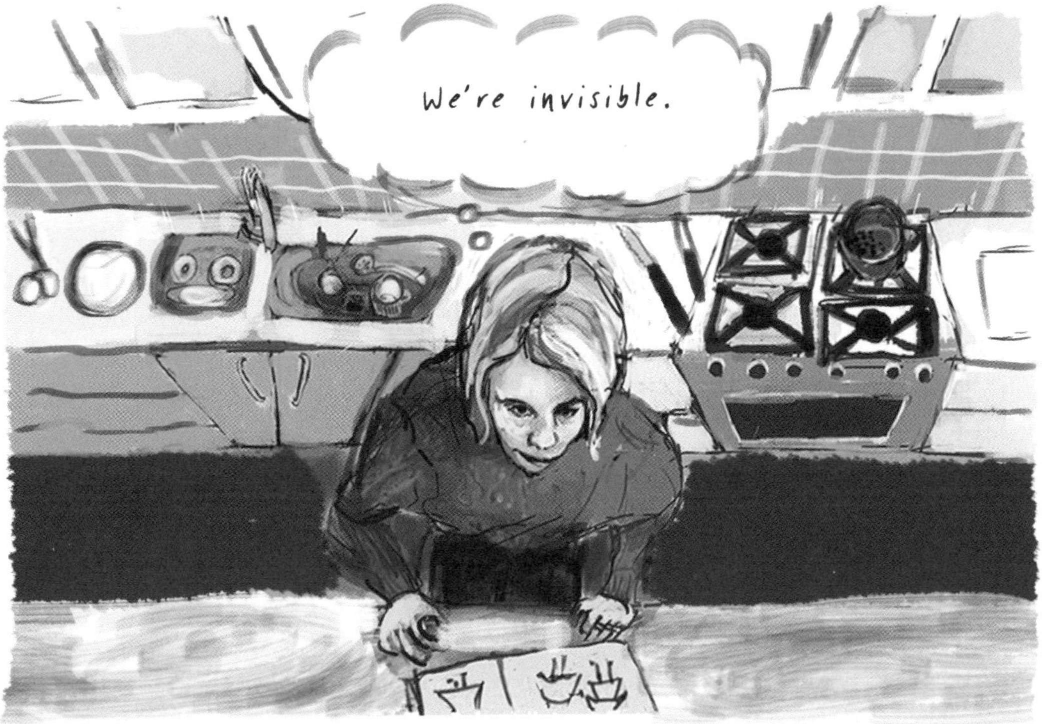
We're invisible.

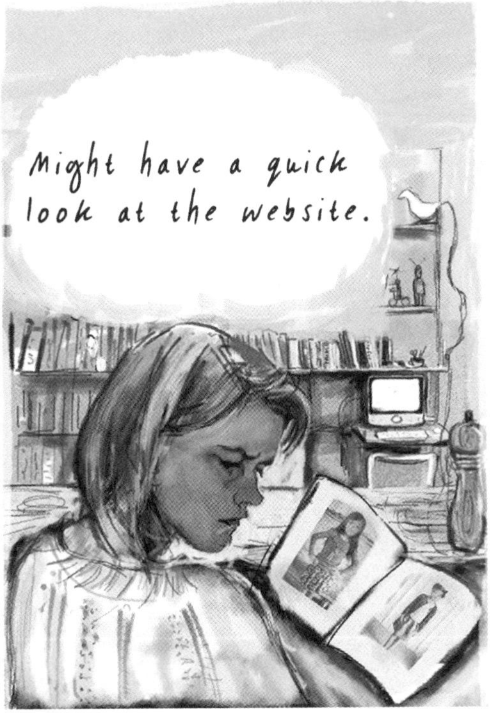
Might have a quick look at the website.

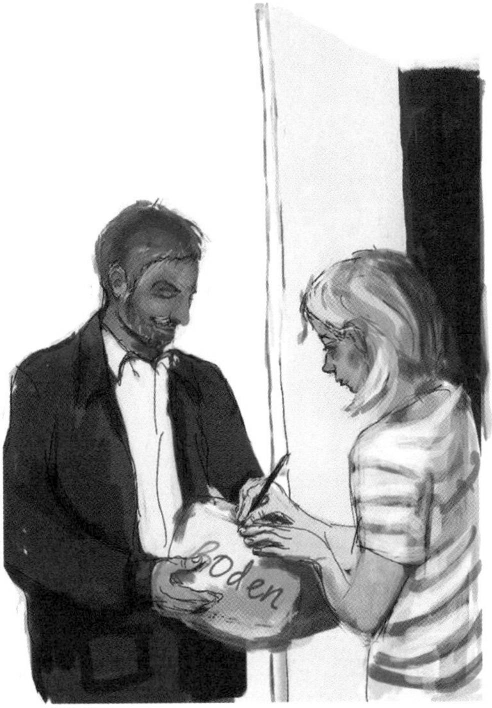
boden

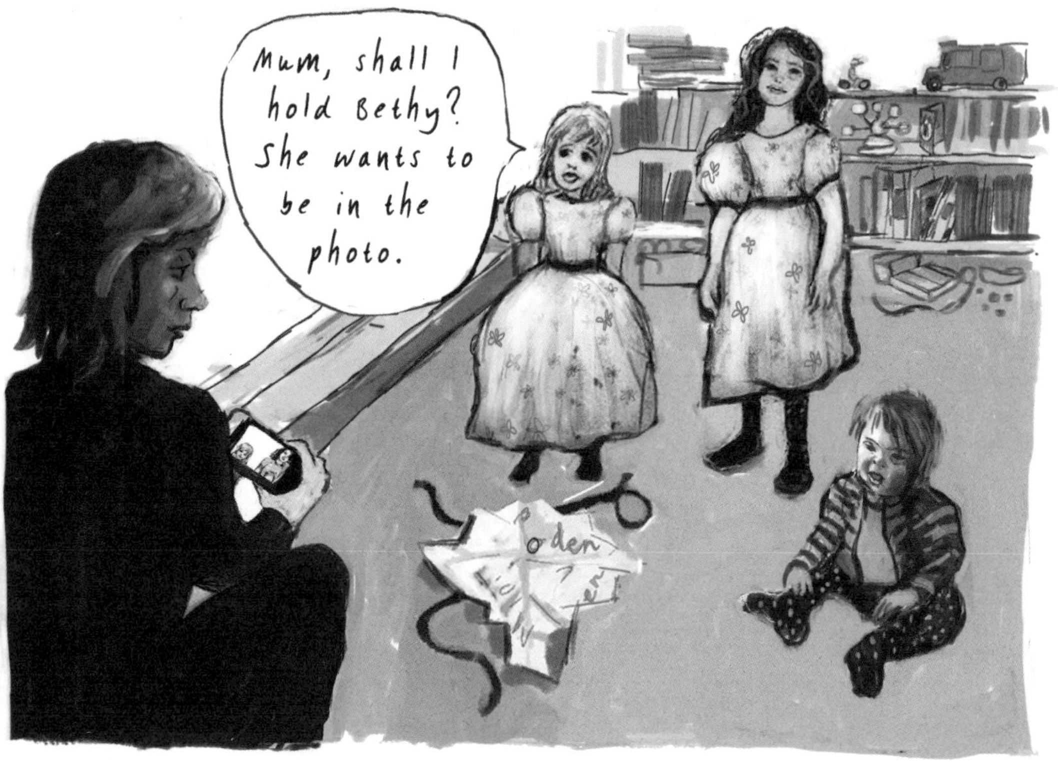
Mum, shall I hold Bethy? She wants to be in the photo.

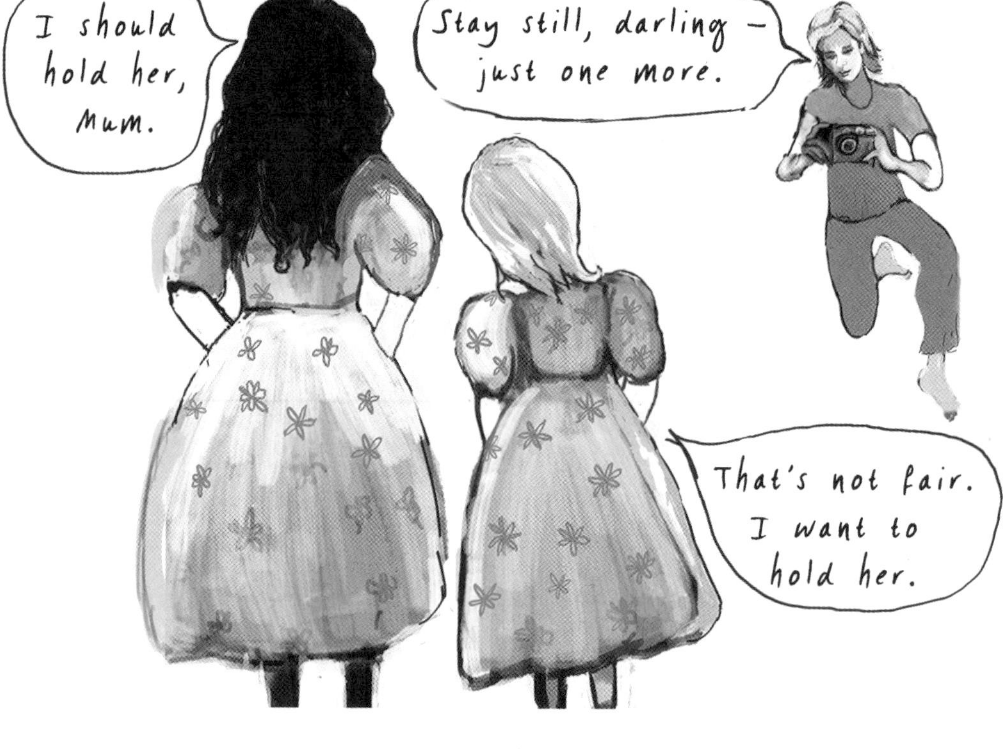
I should hold her, Mum.
Stay still, darling – just one more.
That's not fair. I want to hold her.

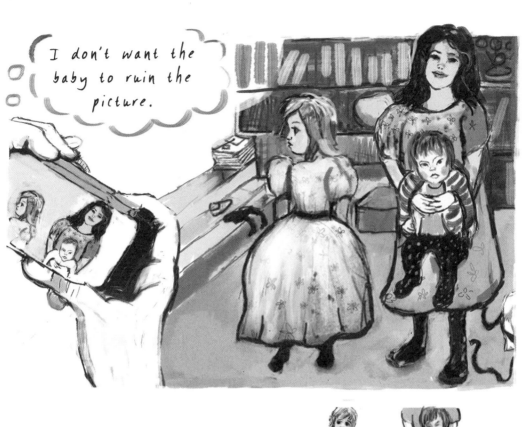

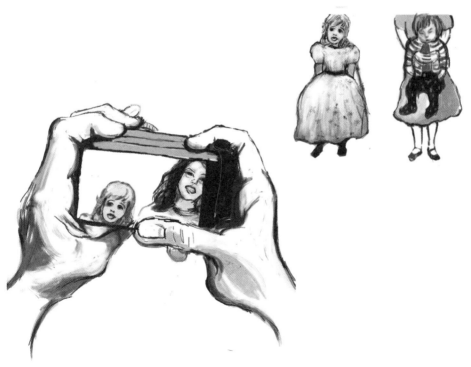

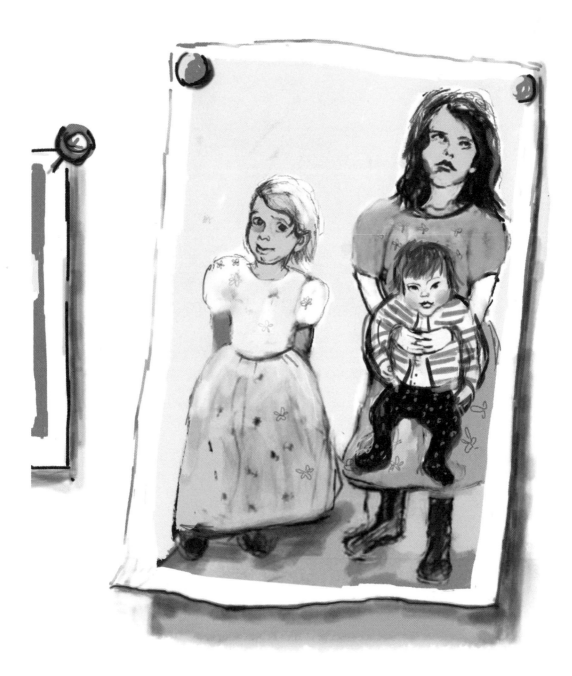

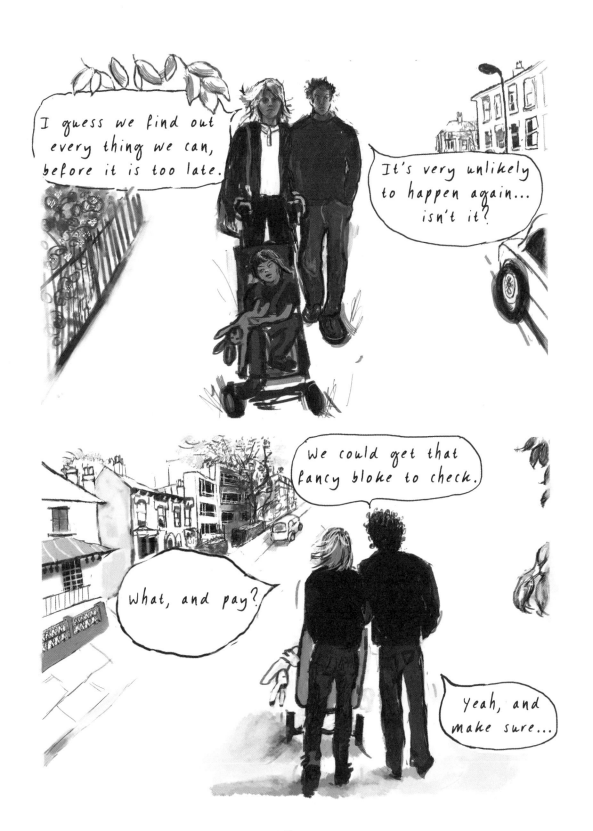

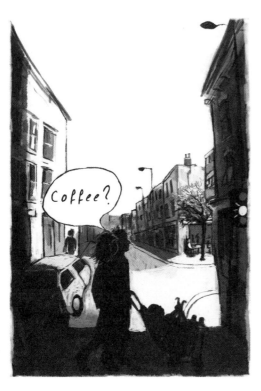

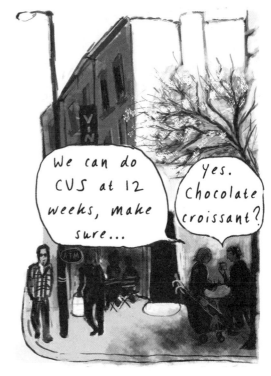

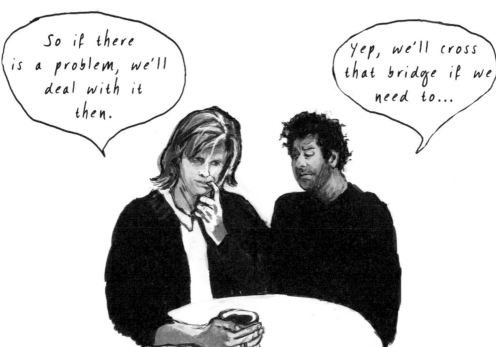

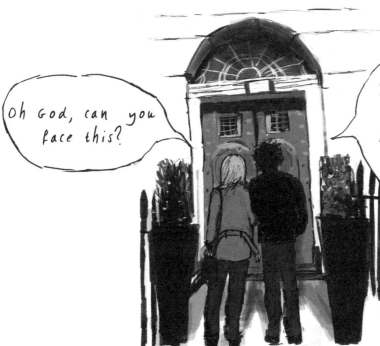

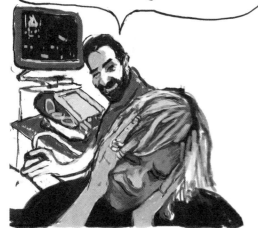

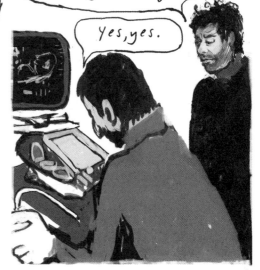

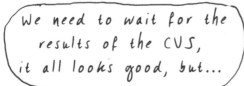

We need to wait for the results of the CVS, it all looks good, but...

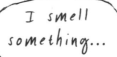

I smell something...

But?

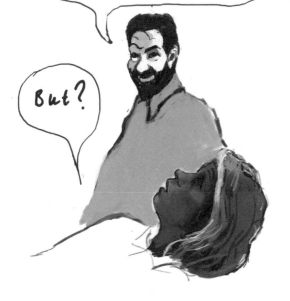

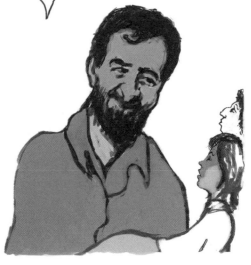

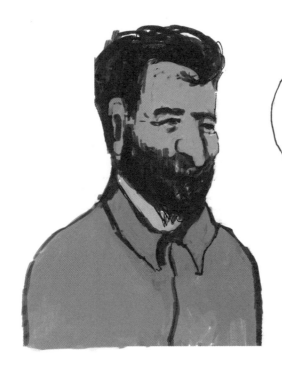

What can you smell?

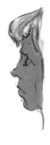

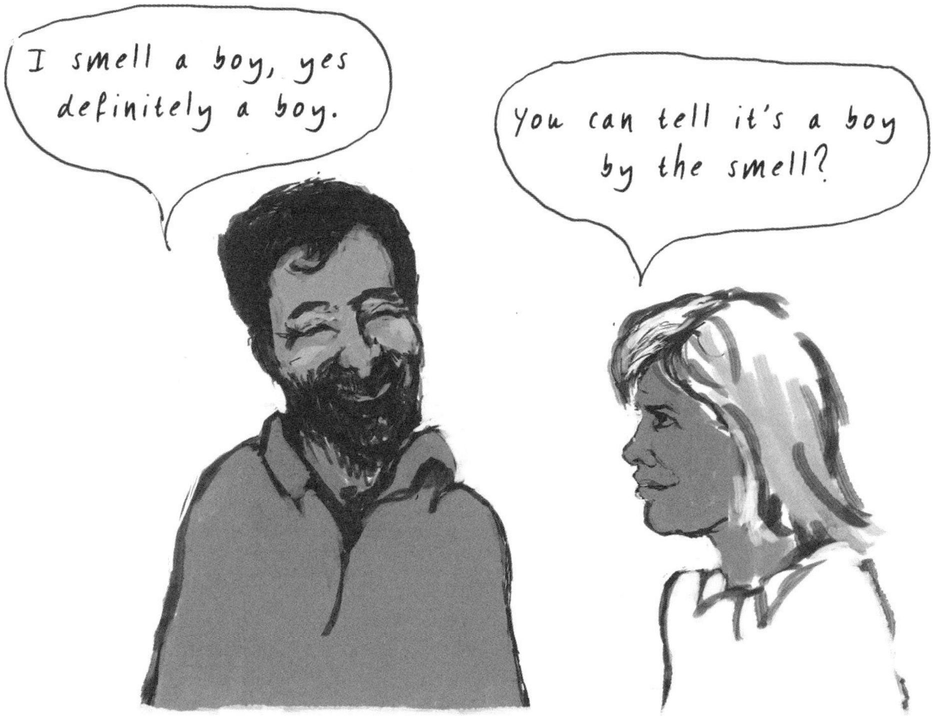
I smell a boy, yes definitely a boy.
You can tell it's a boy by the smell?

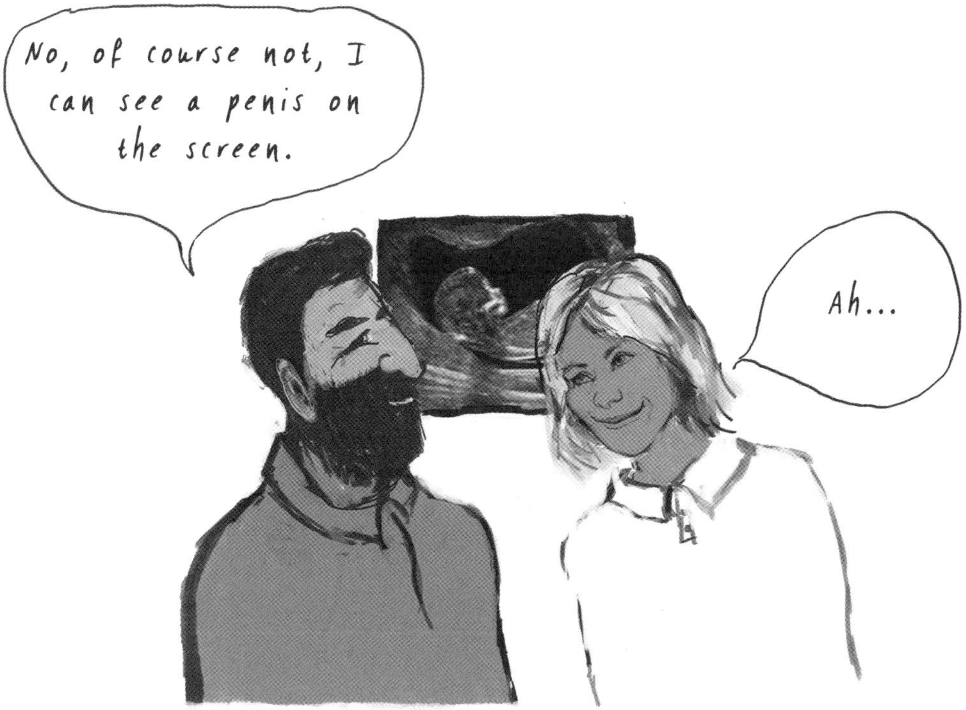
No, of course not, I can see a penis on the screen.
Ah...

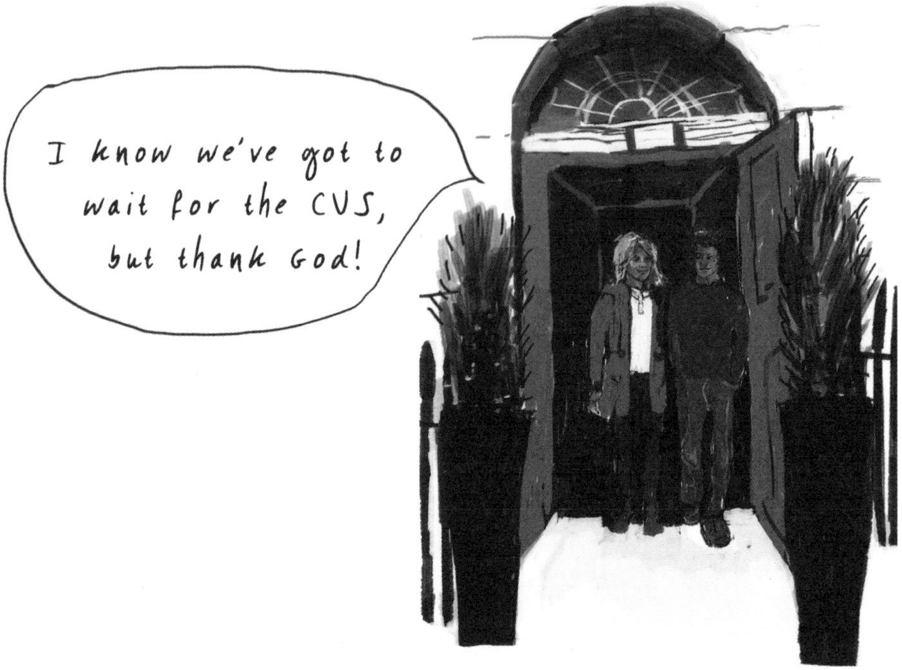
I know we've got to wait for the CVS, but thank God!

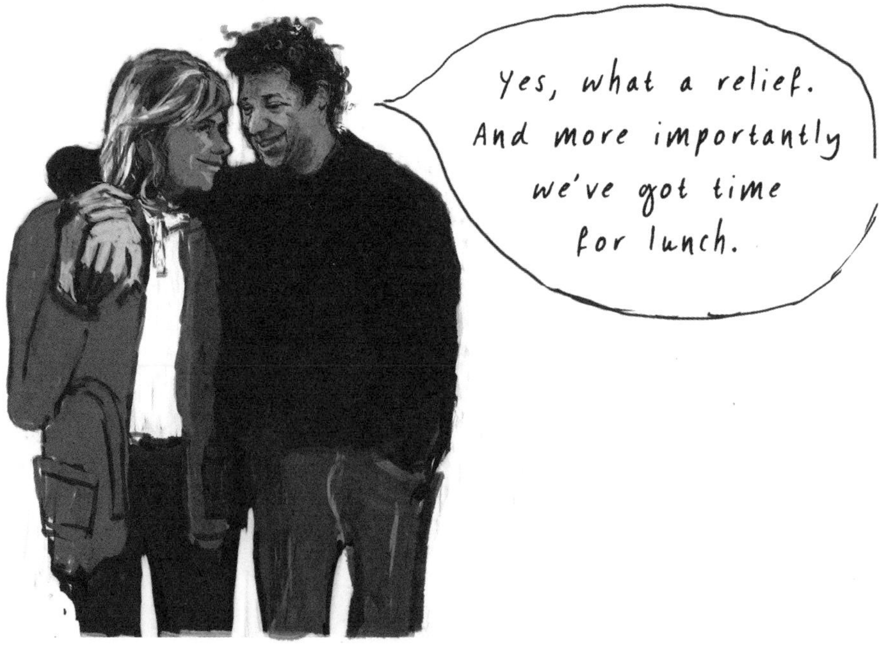
Yes, what a relief. And more importantly we've got time for lunch.

September 2003

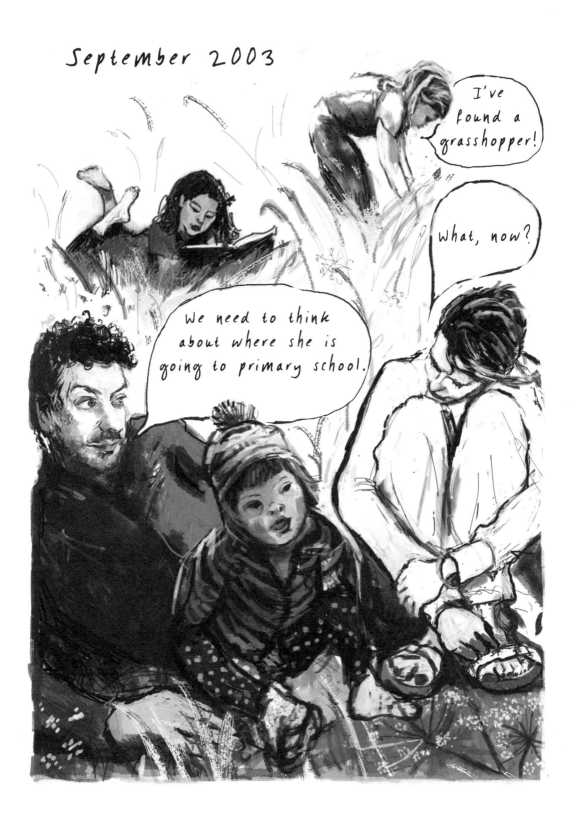

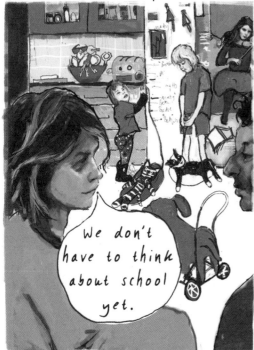

We don't have to think about school yet.

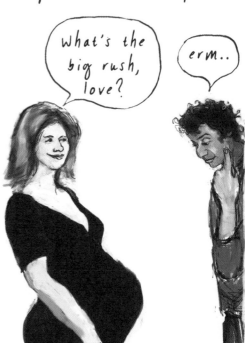

What's the big rush, love?

erm..

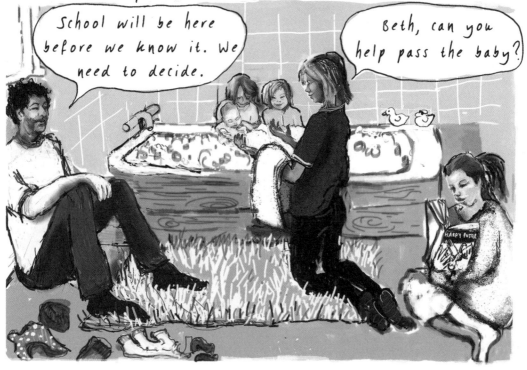

School will be here before we know it. We need to decide.

Beth, can you help pass the baby?

July 2005

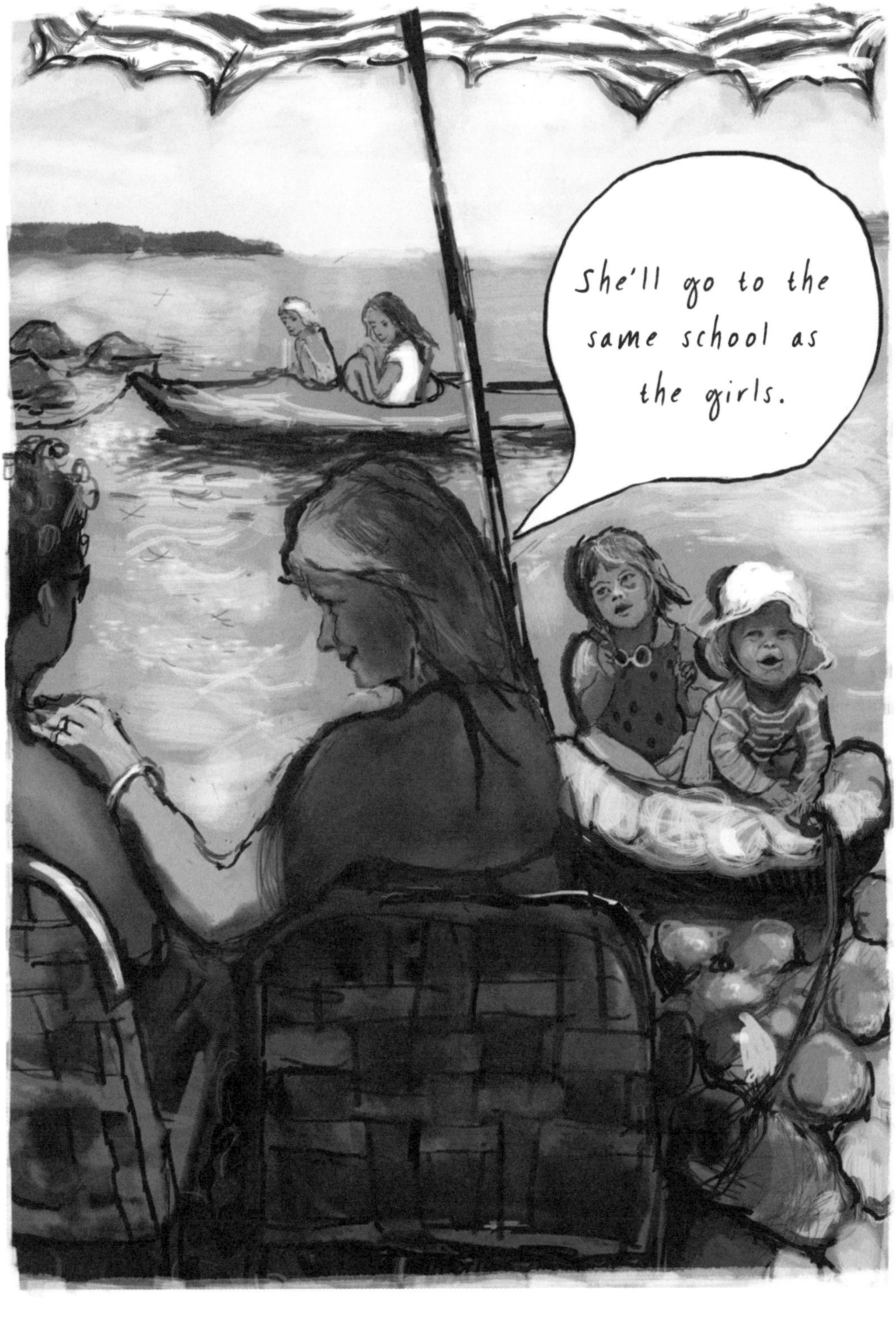
She'll go to the same school as the girls.

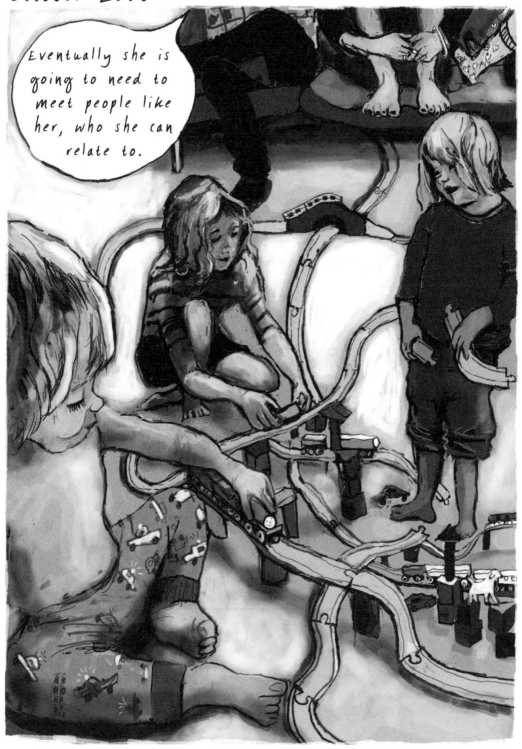

December 2006

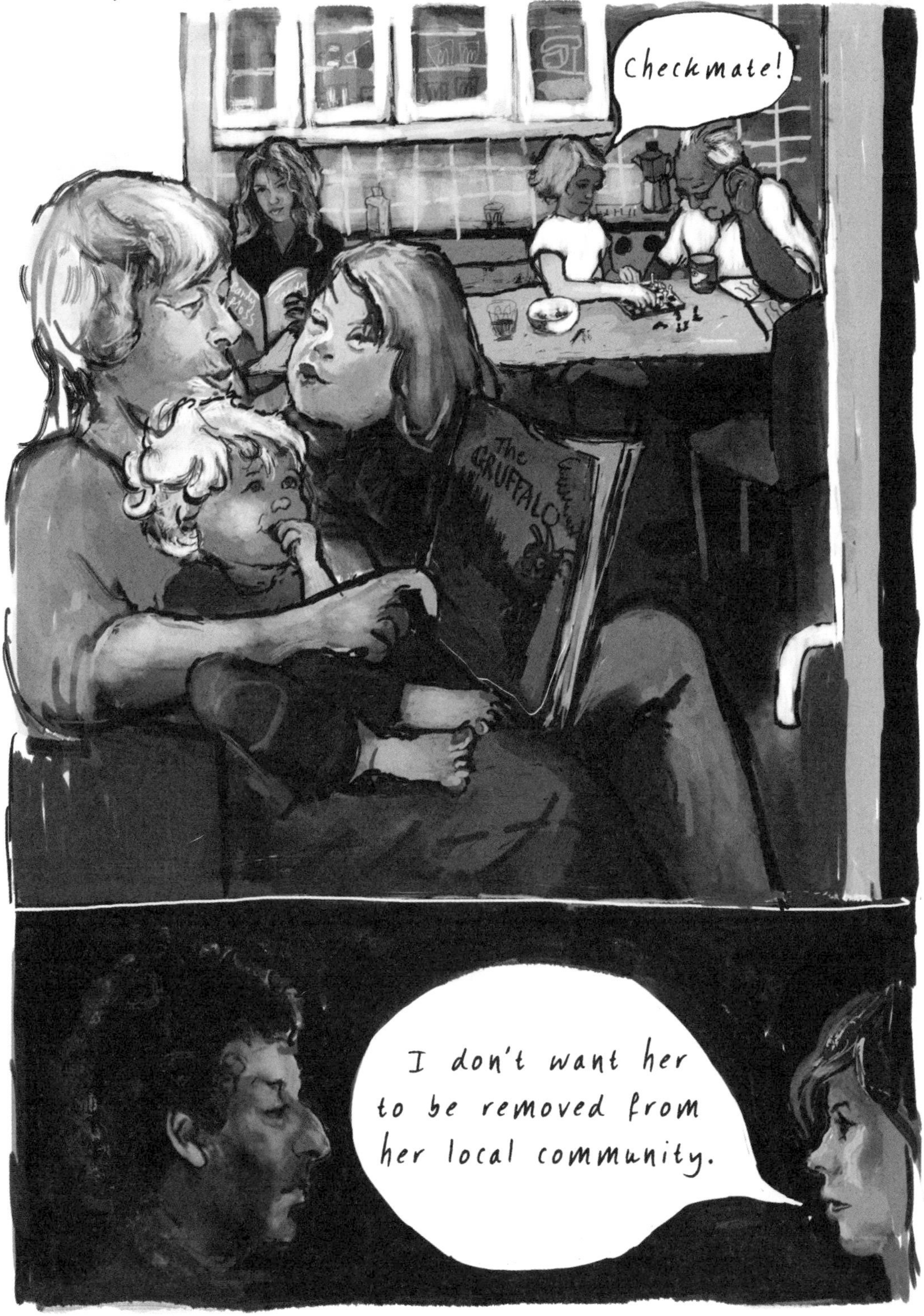
Checkmate!
The GRUFFALO
I don't want her to be removed from her local community.

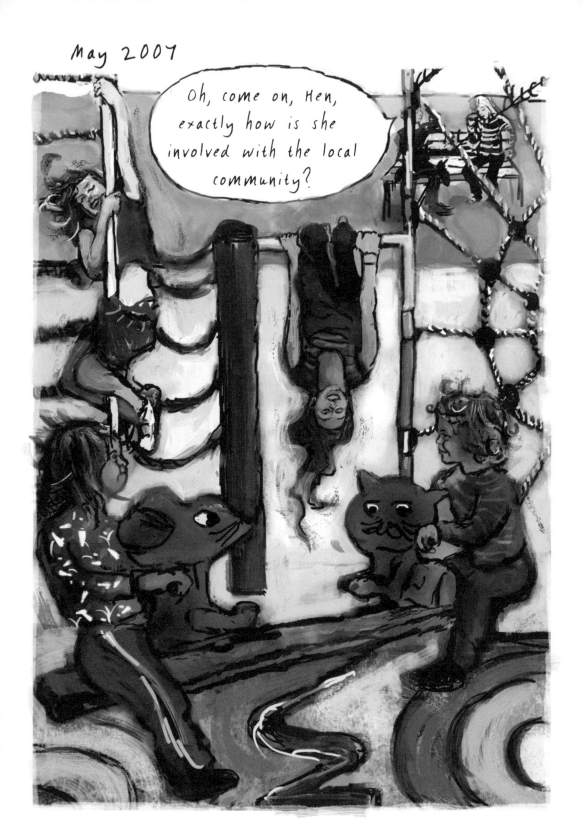

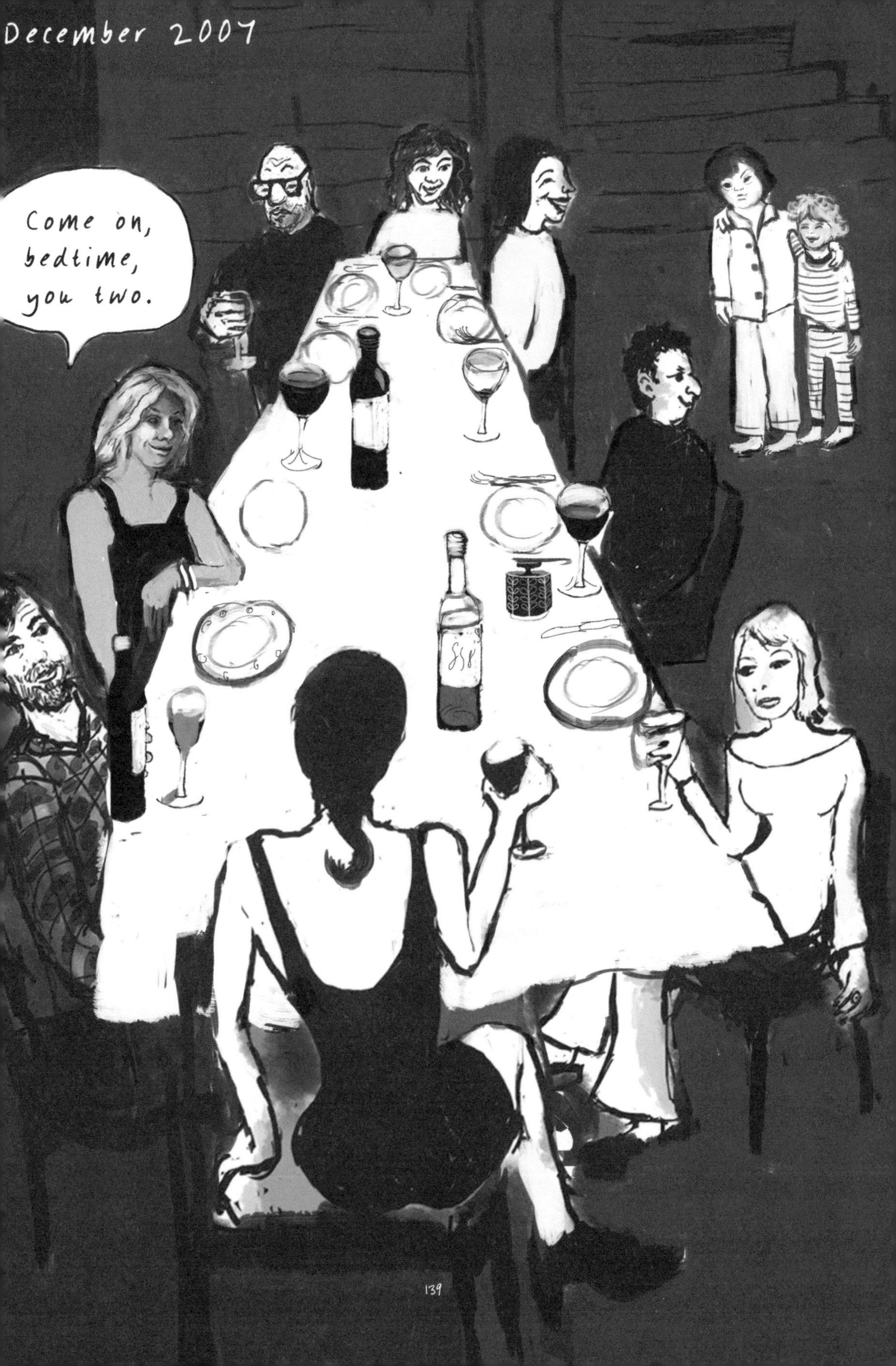
December 2007
Come on, bedtime, you two.

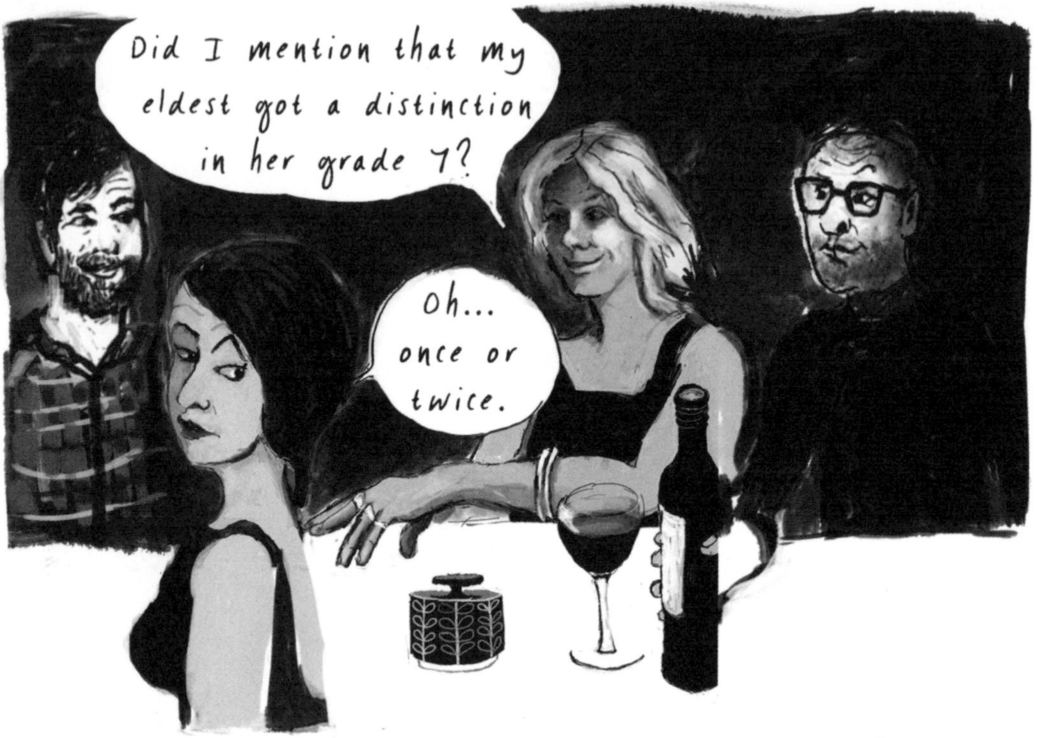
Did I mention that my eldest got a distinction in her grade 7?
Oh... once or twice.

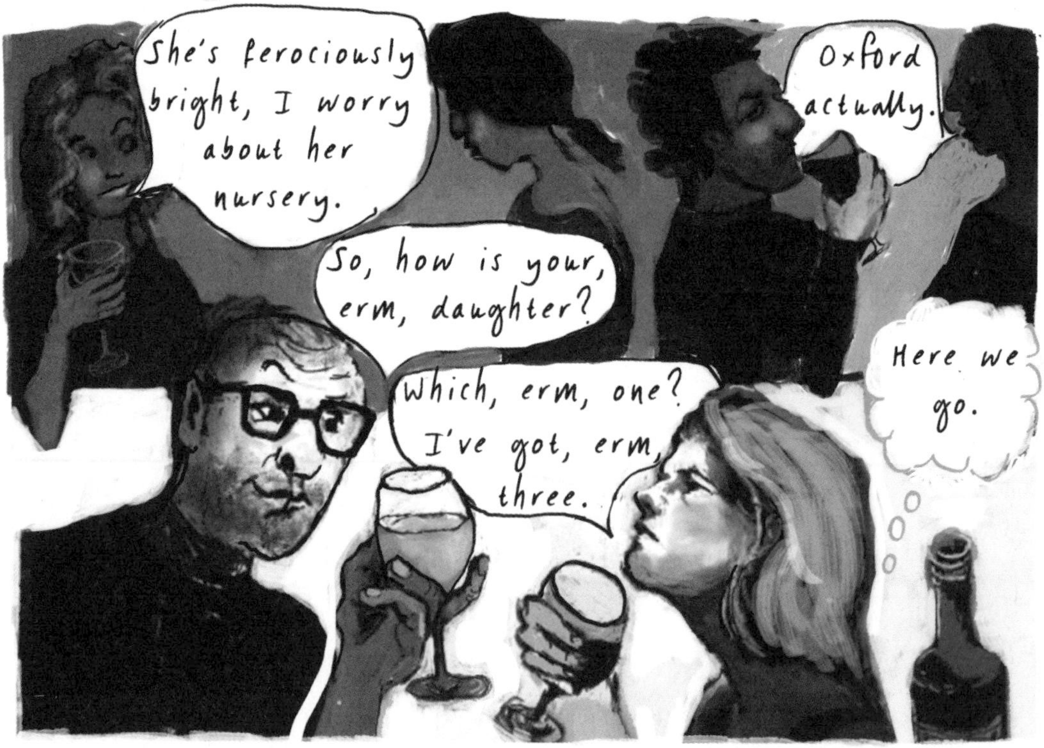
She's ferociously bright, I worry about her nursery.
Oxford actually.
So, how is your, erm, daughter?
Which, erm, one? I've got, erm, three.
Here we go.

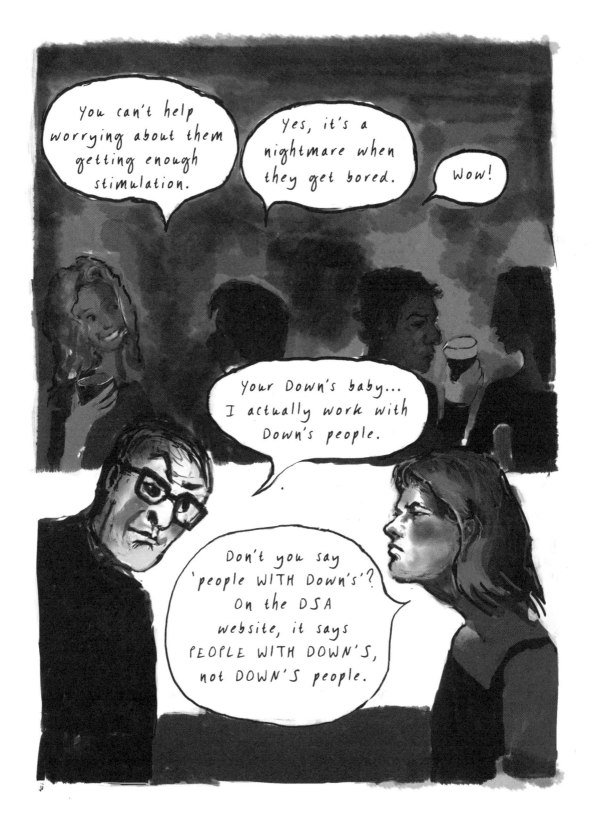

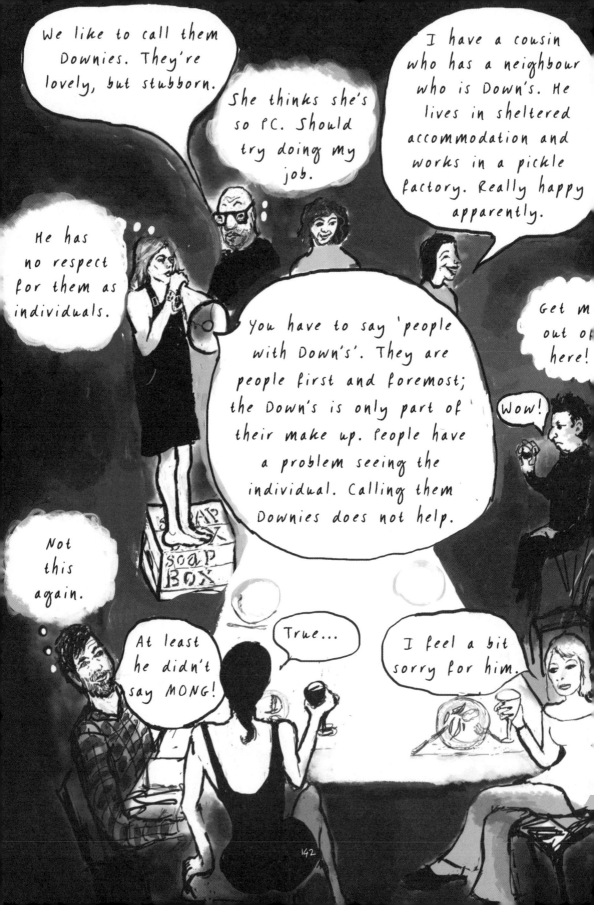

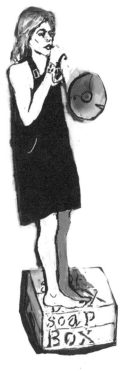

What we call people makes a huge difference to how we see them. It makes a big difference to me, as a mother of a child WITH Down's and my ability to love her.

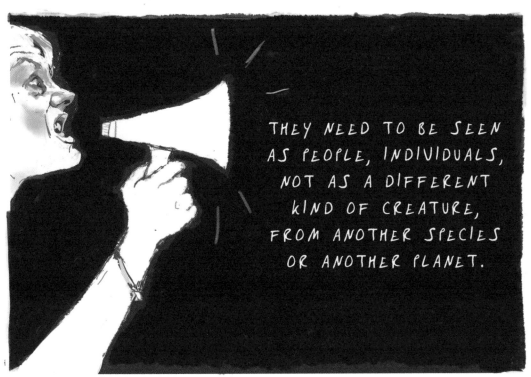

THEY NEED TO BE SEEN AS PEOPLE, INDIVIDUALS, NOT AS A DIFFERENT KIND OF CREATURE, FROM ANOTHER SPECIES OR ANOTHER PLANET.

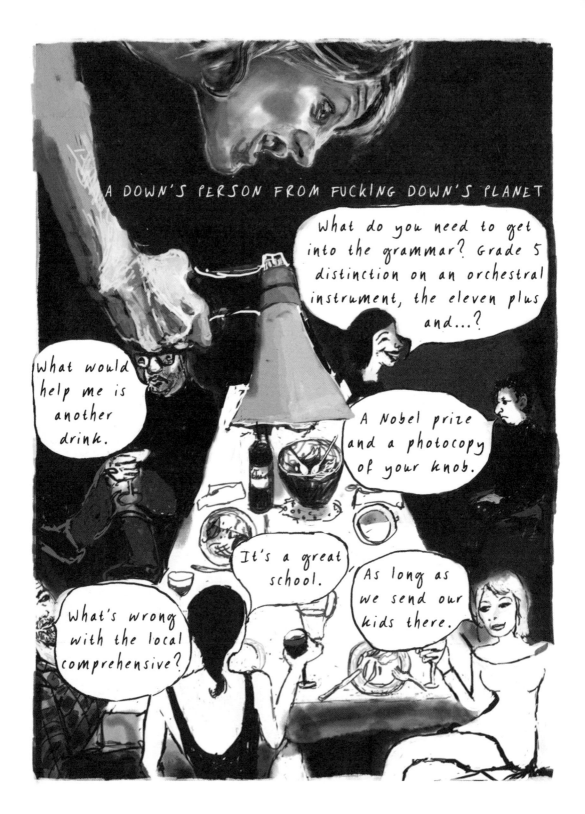

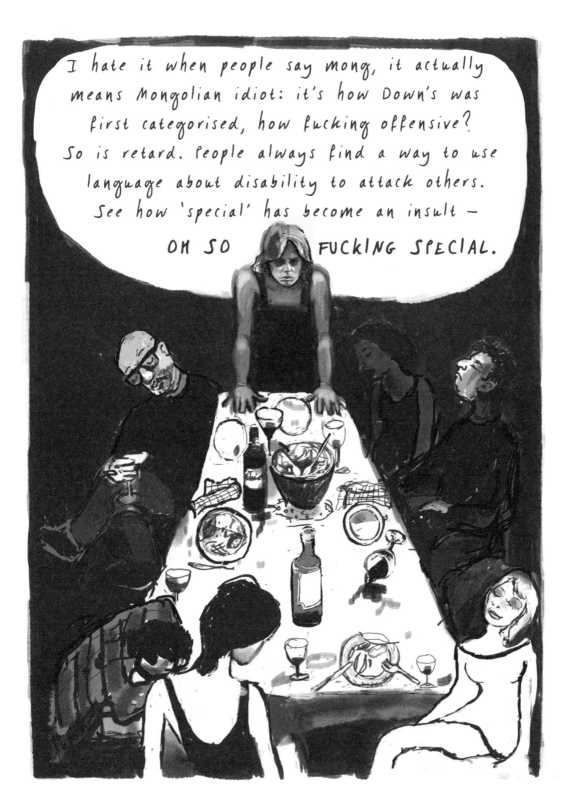

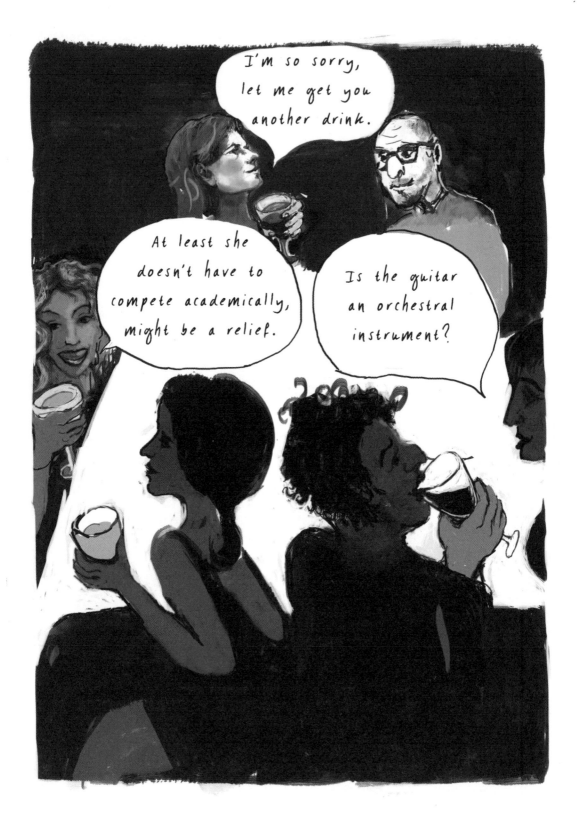

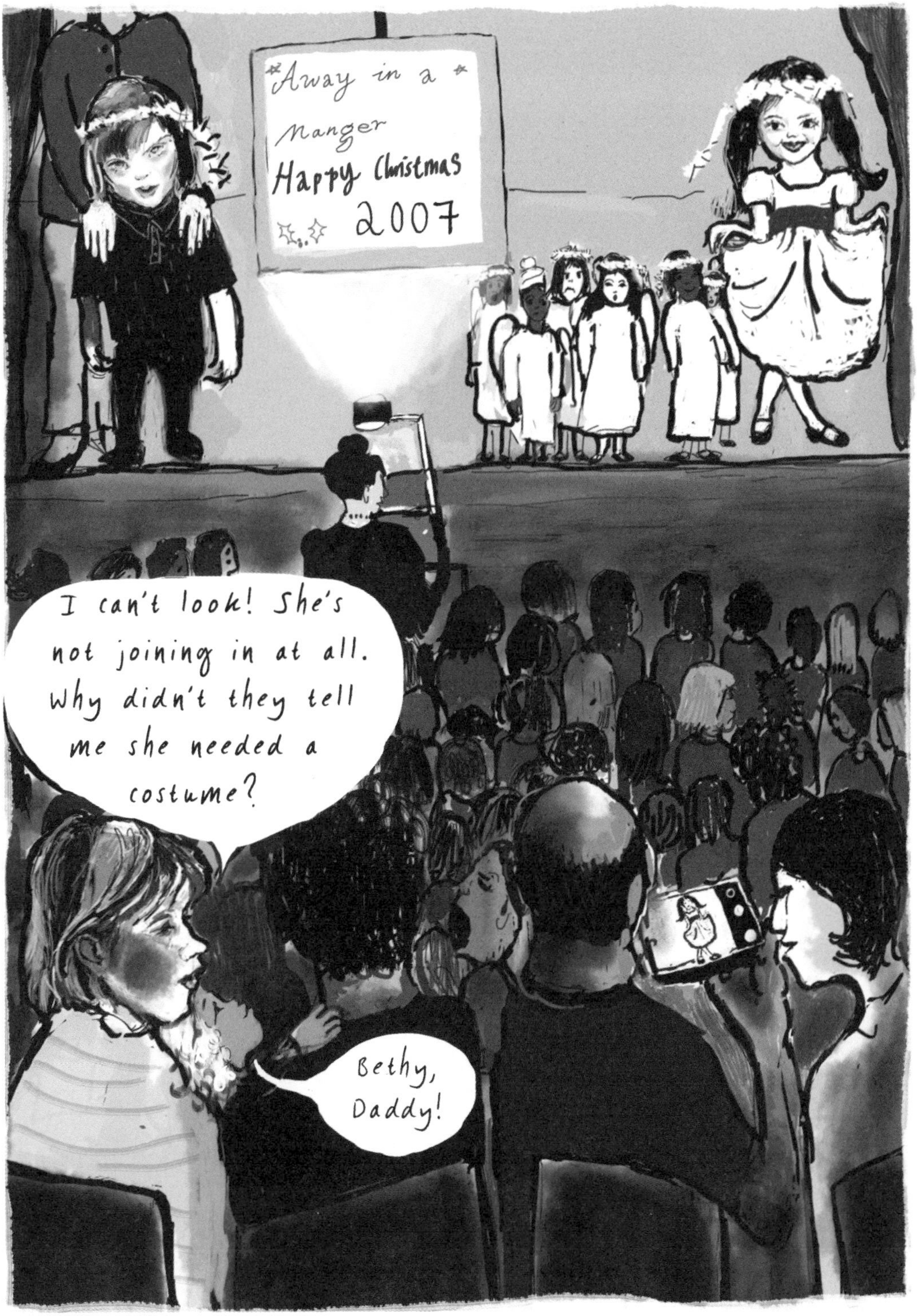
Away in a manger
Happy Christmas 2007
I can't look! She's not joining in at all. Why didn't they tell me she needed a costume?
Bethy, Daddy!

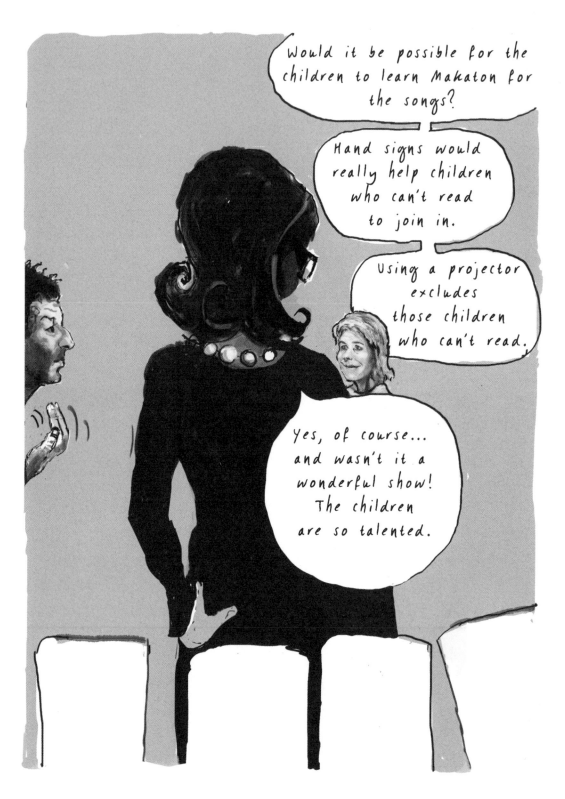

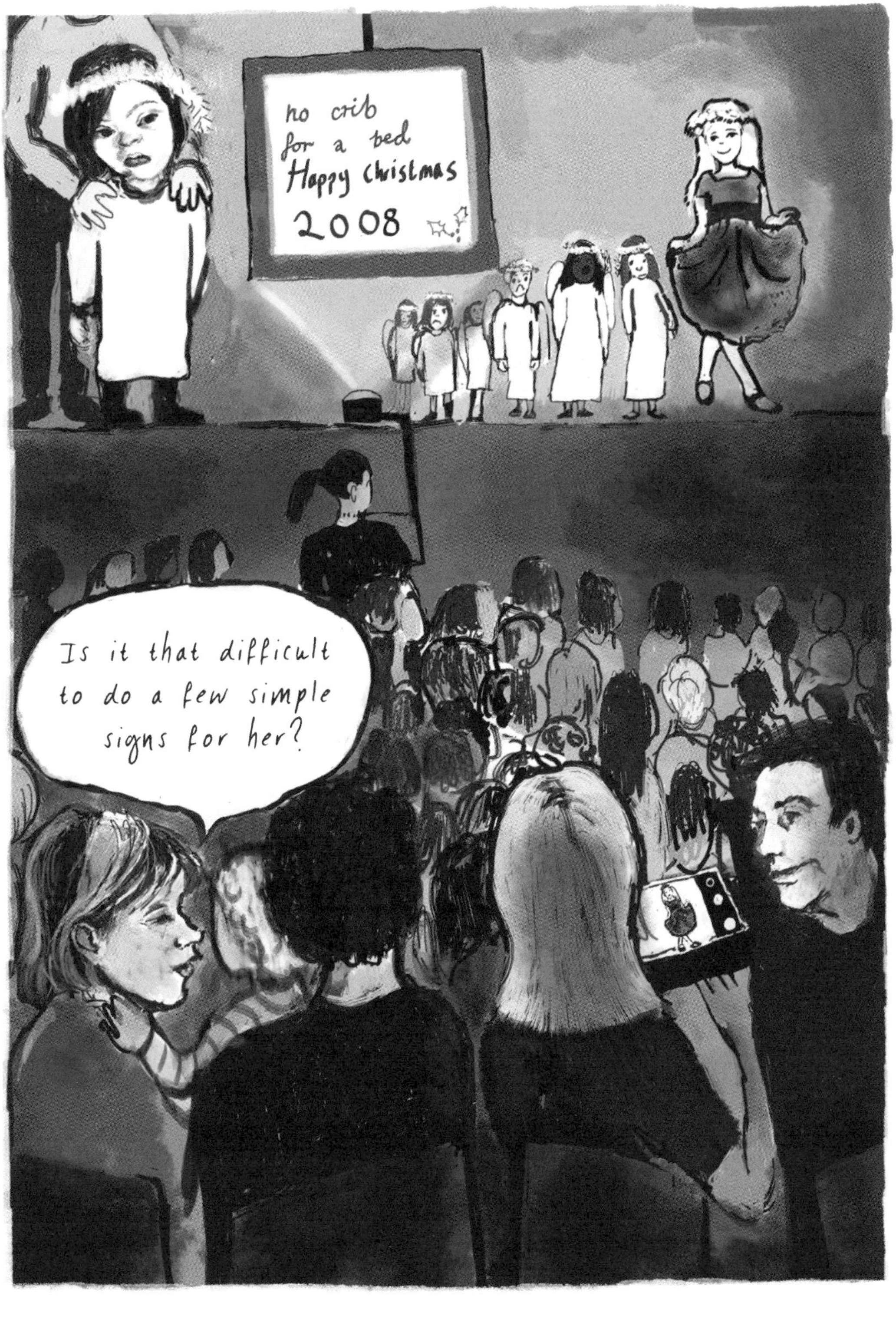
no crib
for a bed
Happy Christmas
2008
Is it that difficult to do a few simple signs for her?

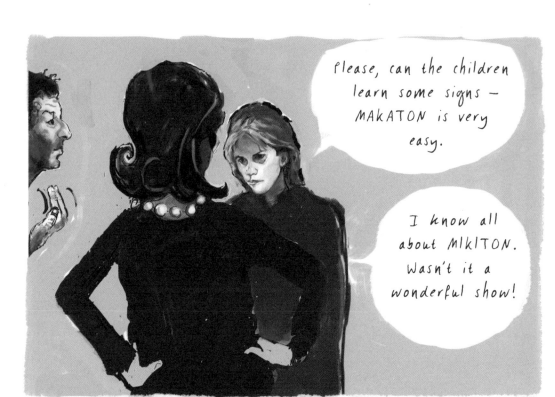

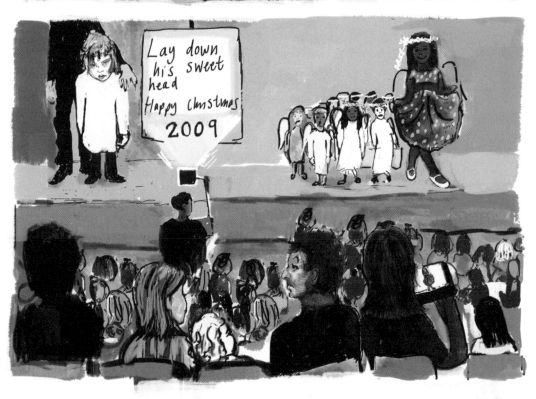

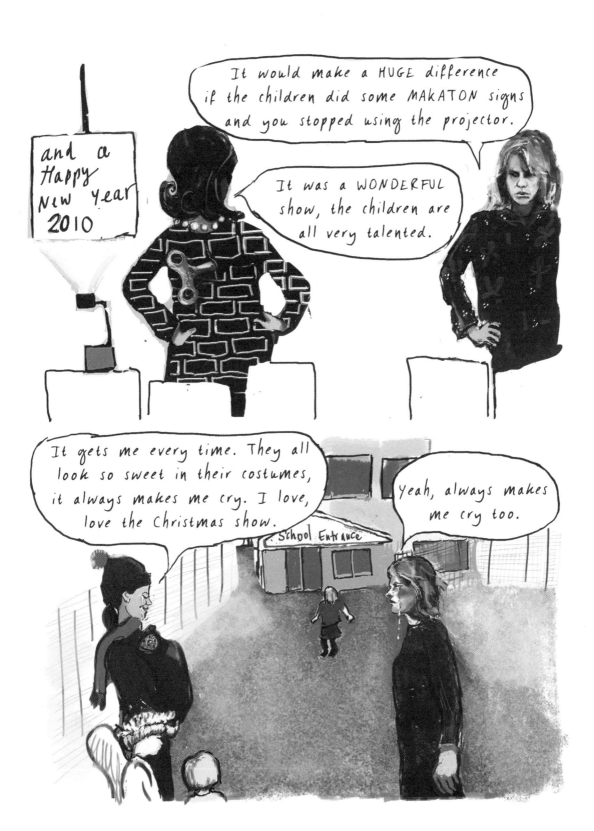

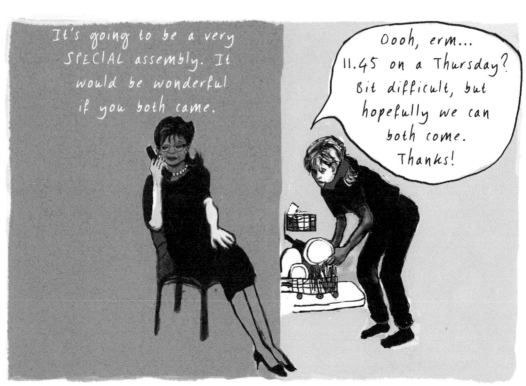

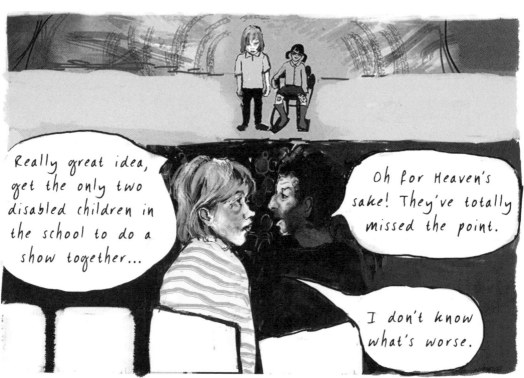

June 2011

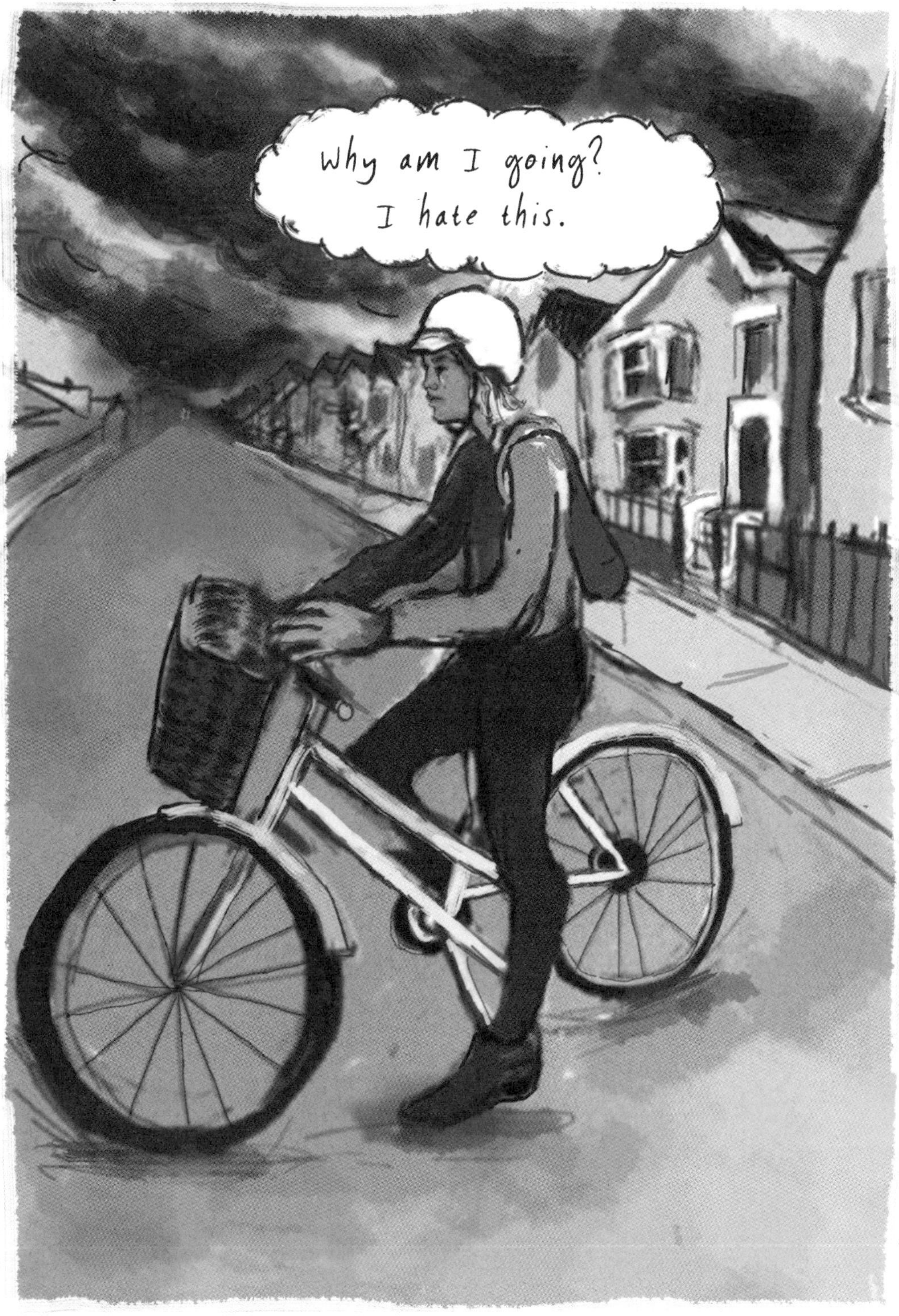
Why am I going?
I hate this.

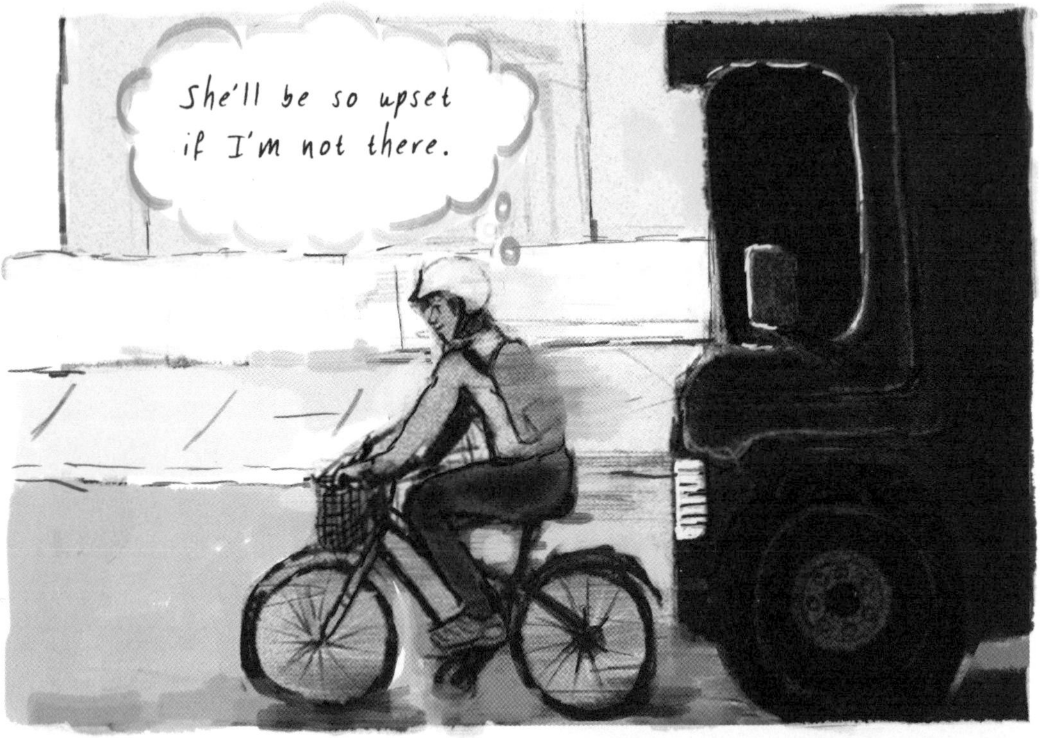
She'll be so upset if I'm not there.

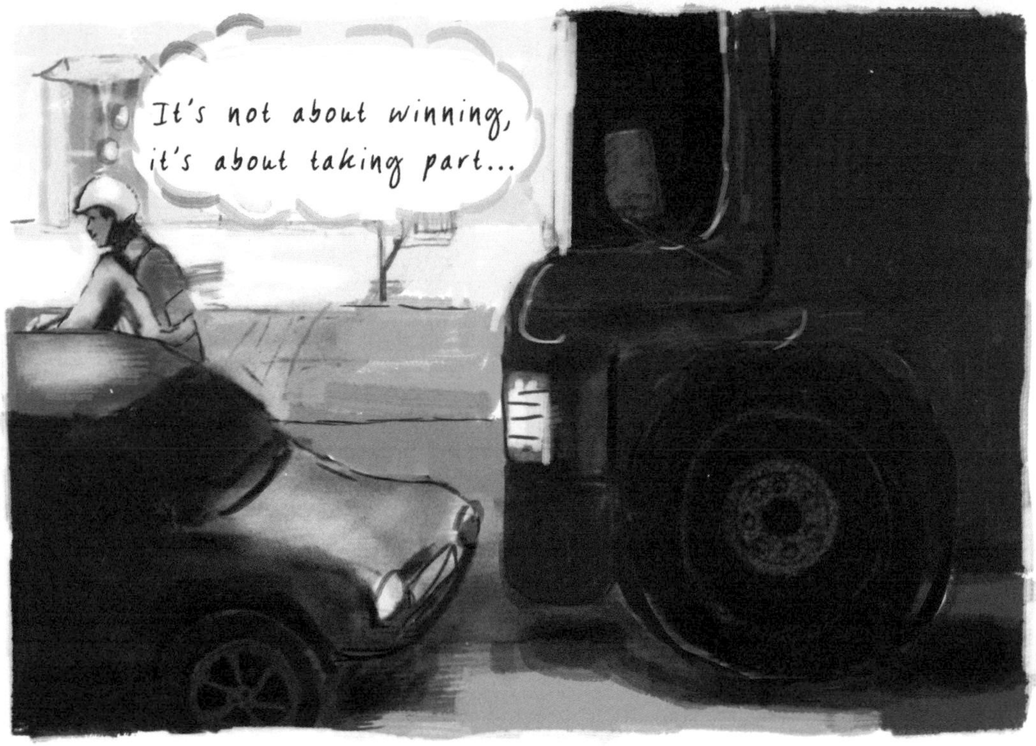
It's not about winning, it's about taking part...

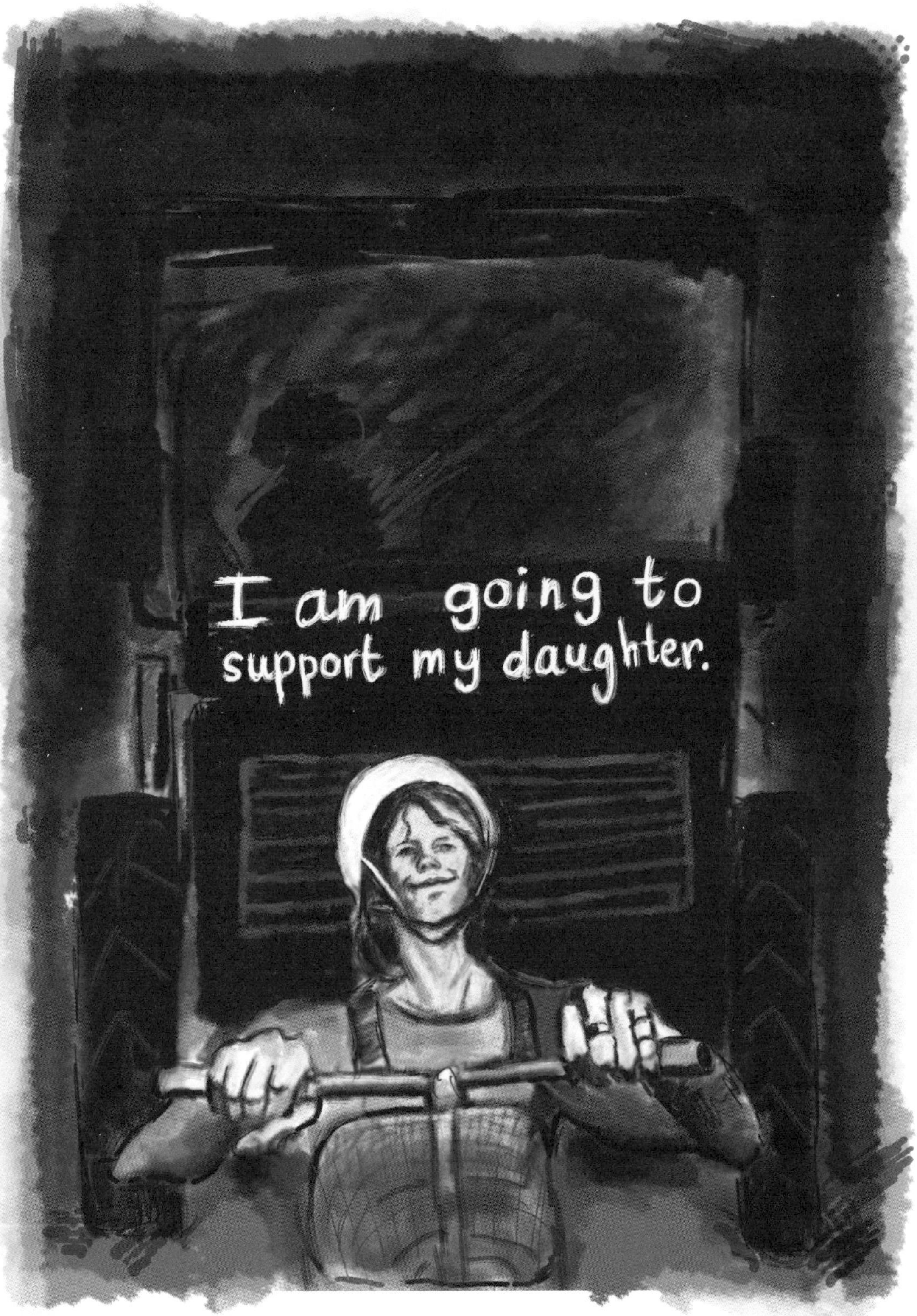
I am going to support my daughter.

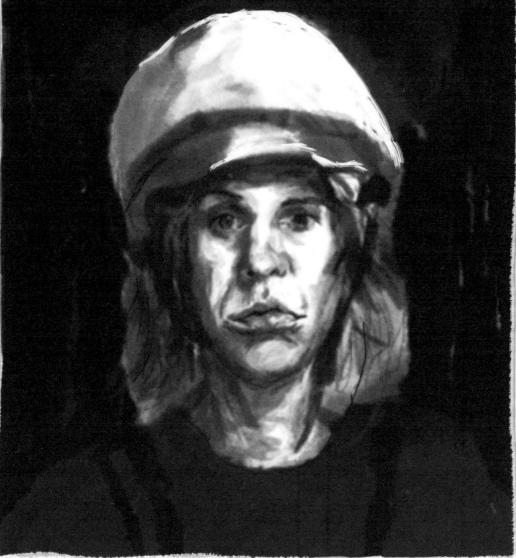

Come last in all her races...

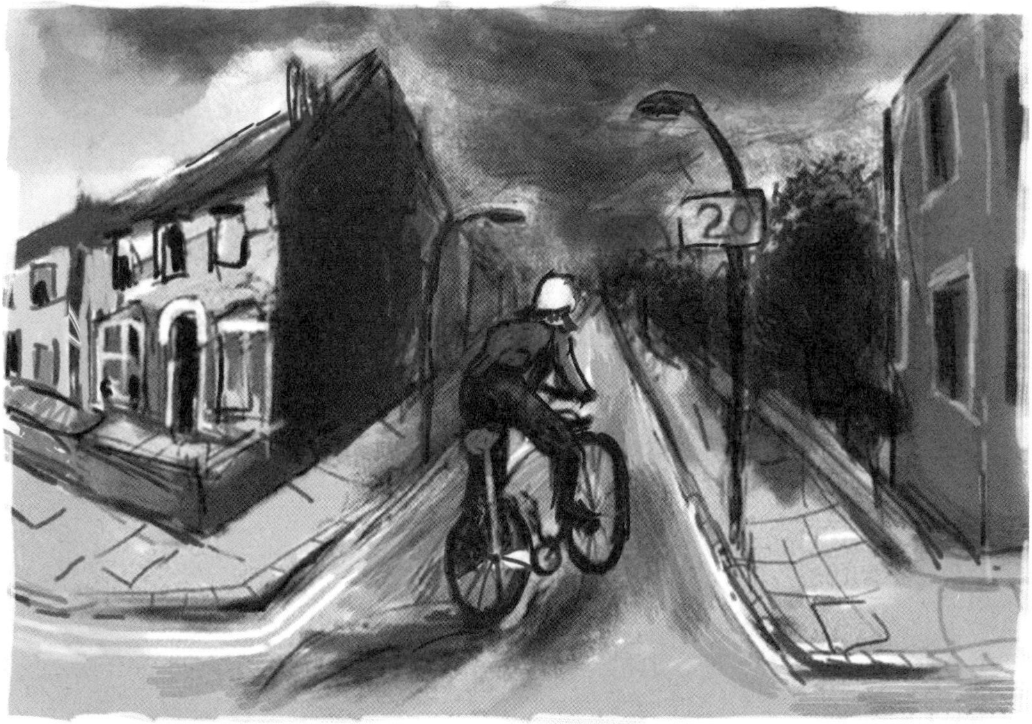
20

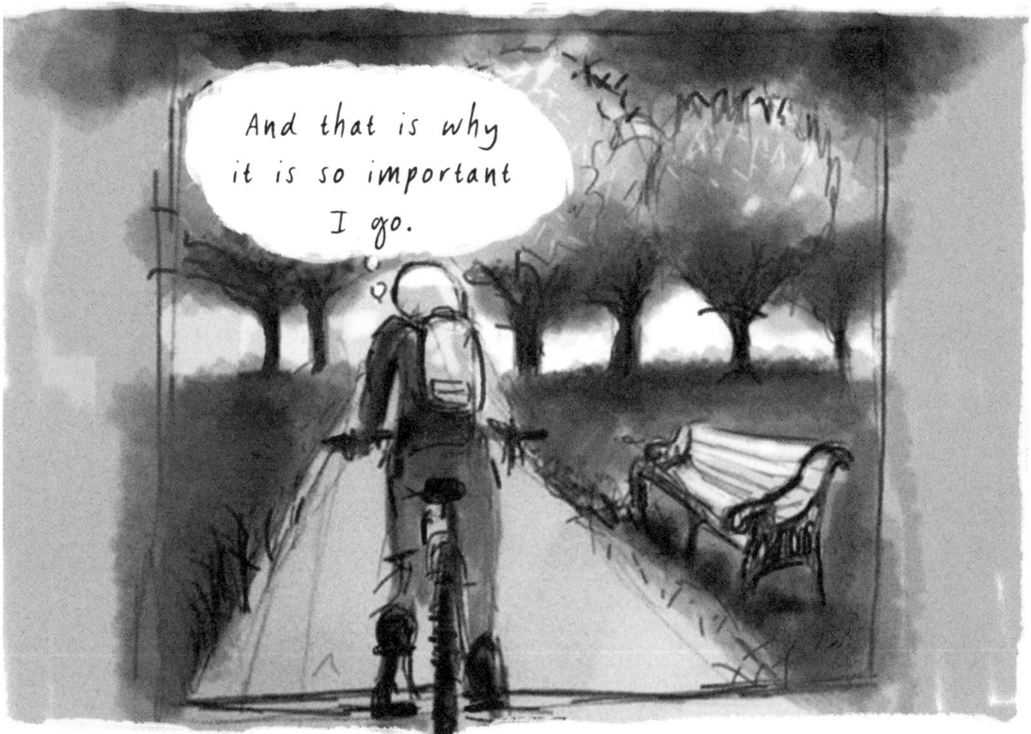
And that is why it is so important I go.

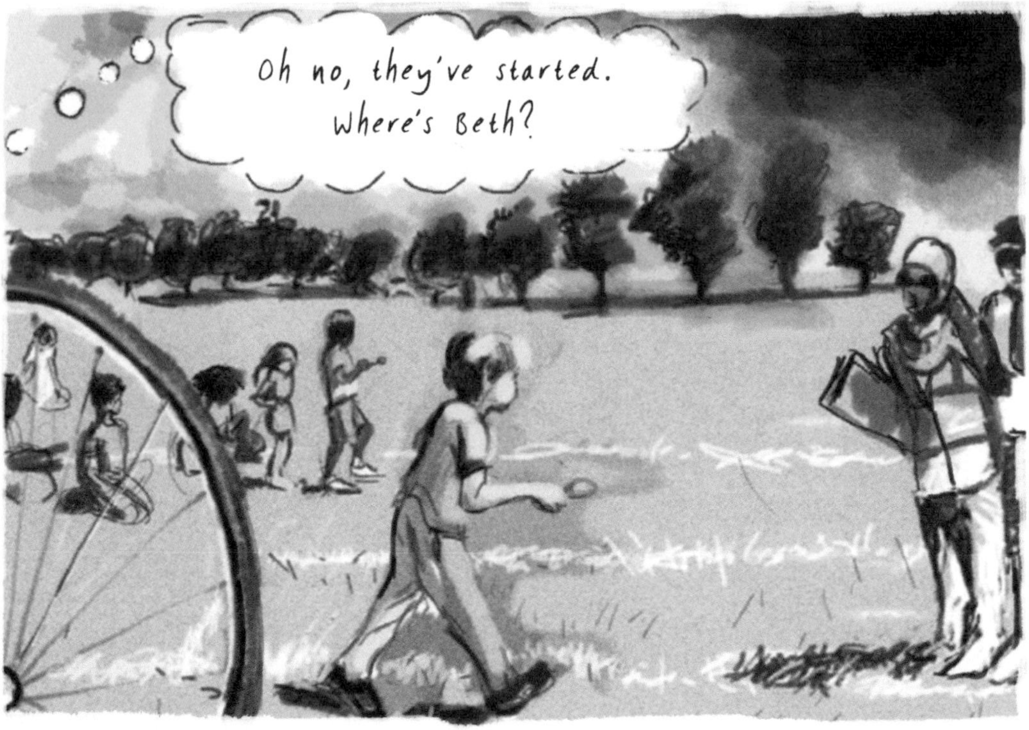
Oh no, they've started.
Where's Beth?

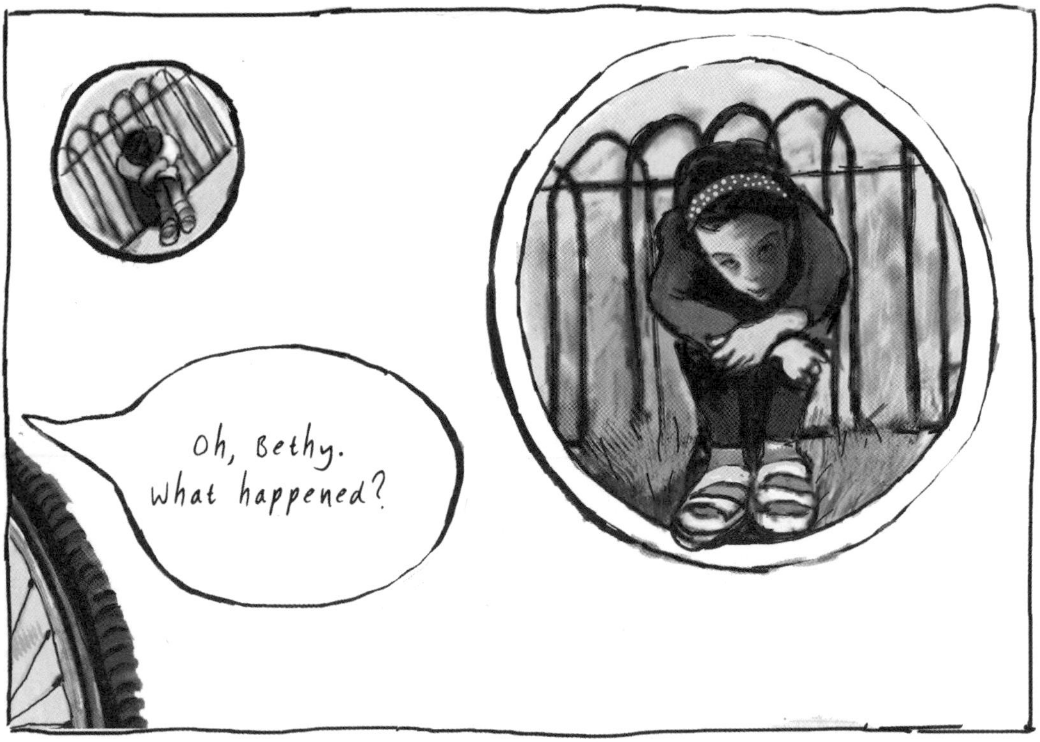
Oh, Bethy.
What happened?

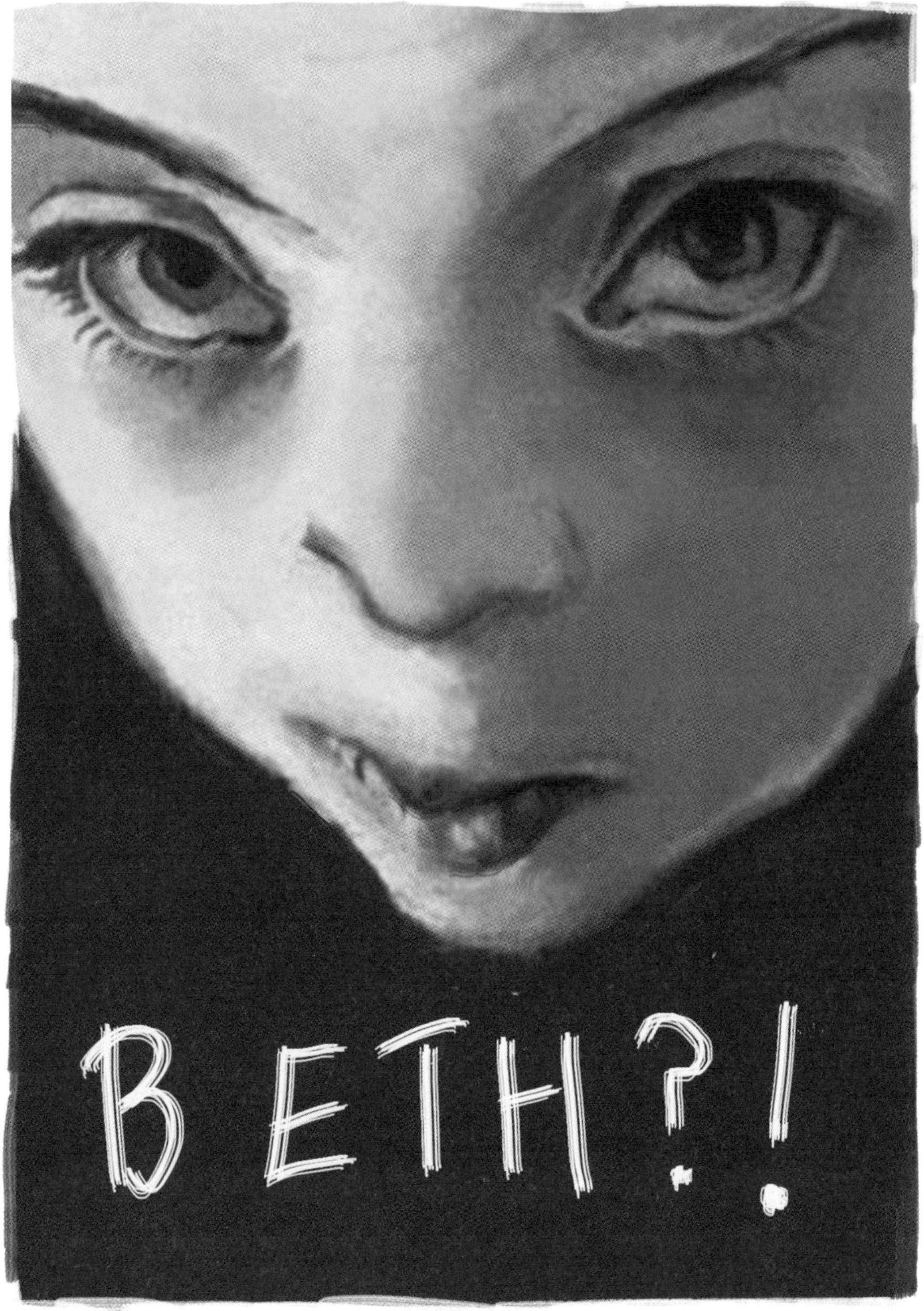
BETH?!

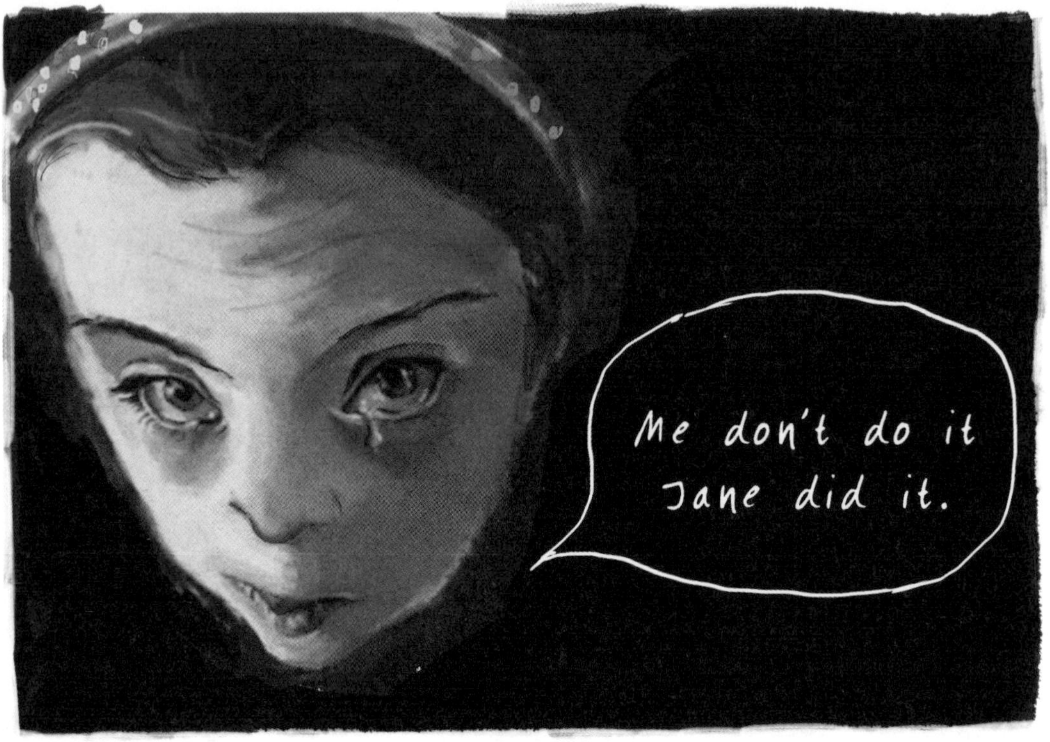
Me don't do it Jane did it.

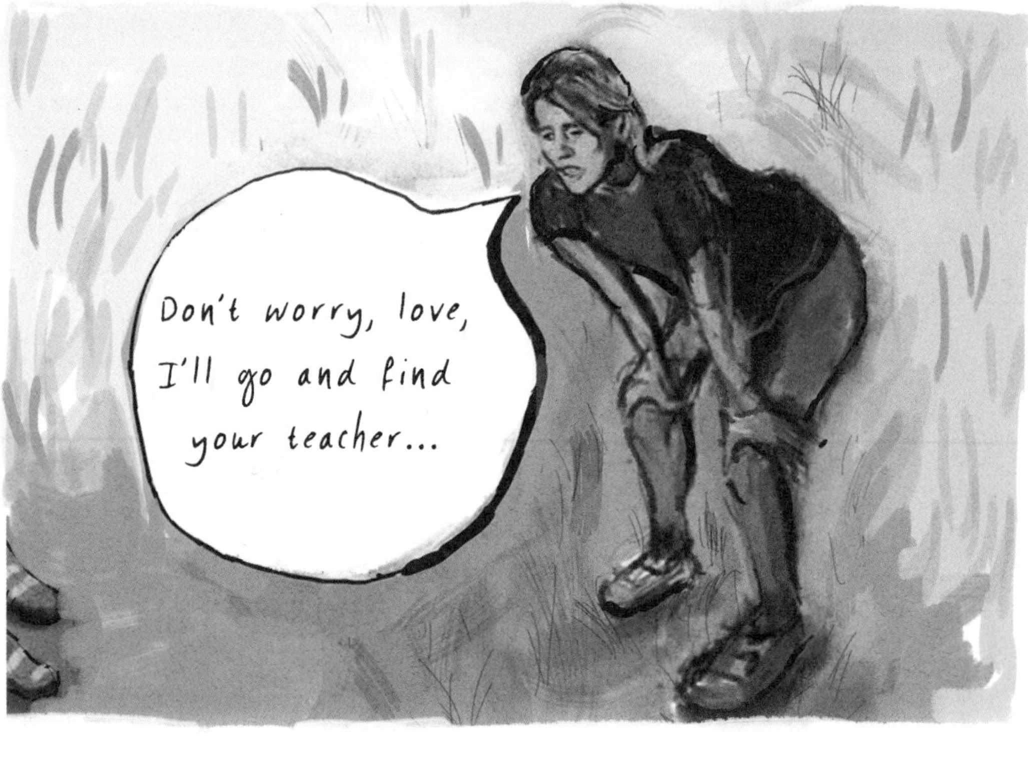
Don't worry, love, I'll go and find your teacher...

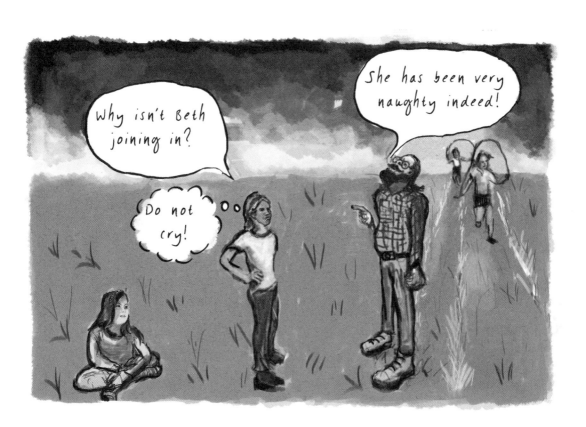

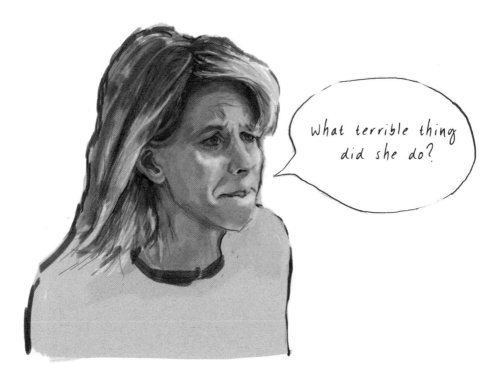

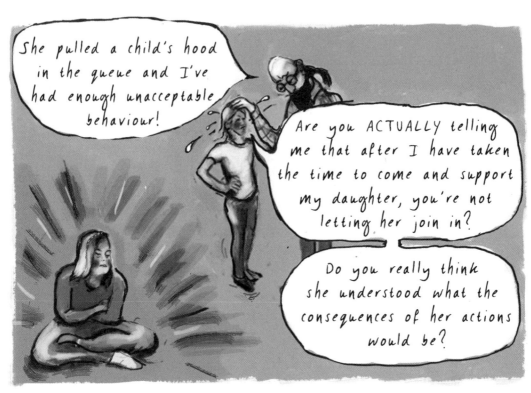

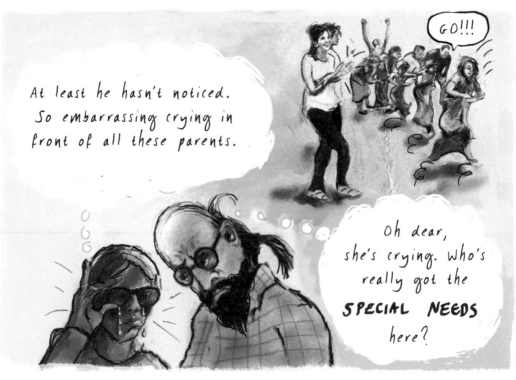

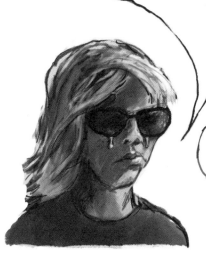

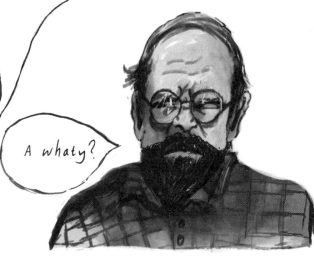

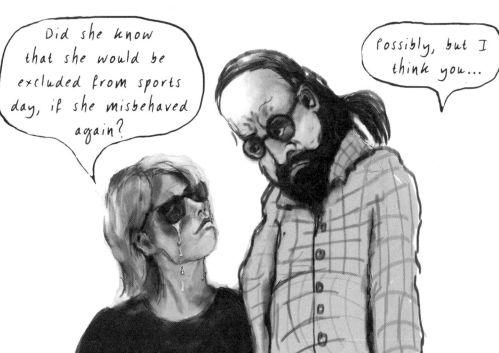

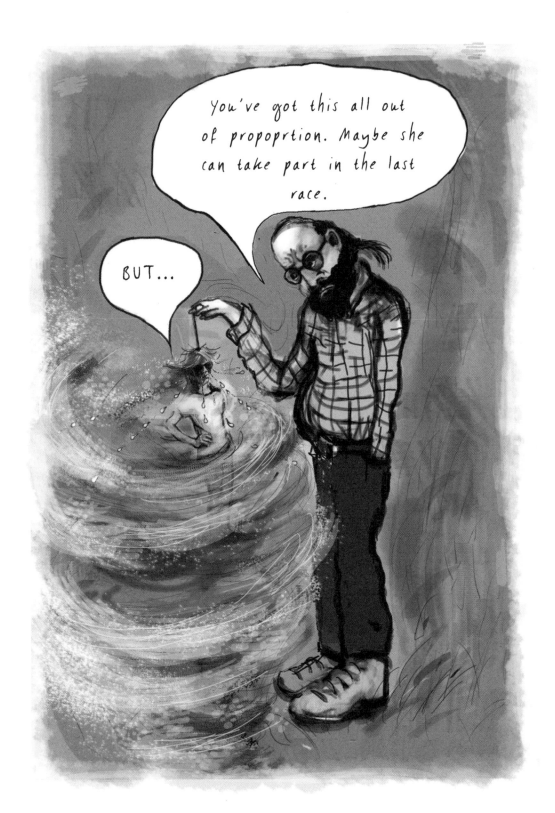

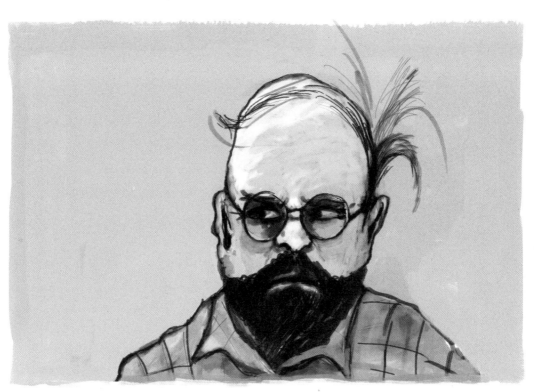

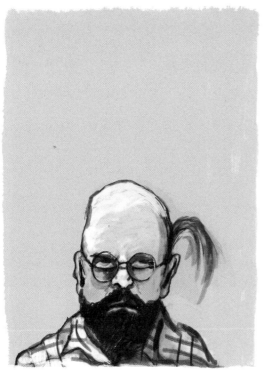

I'm sorry, but there are OTHER children I need to attend to. It is SPORTS DAY!

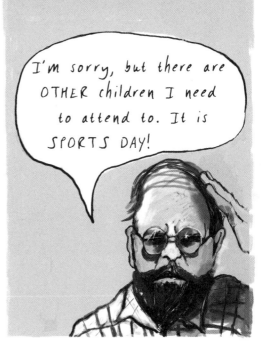

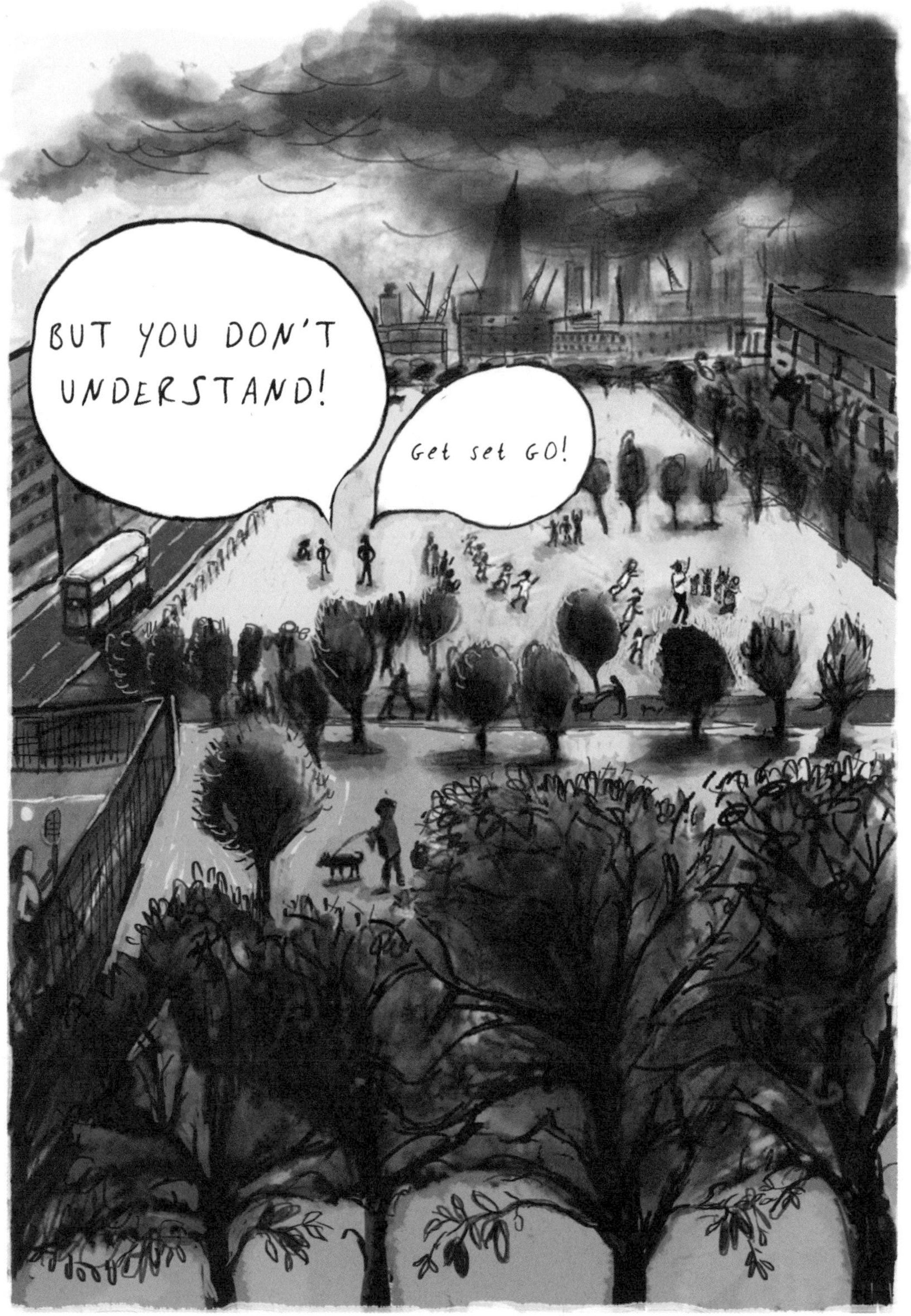
BUT YOU DON'T UNDERSTAND!
Get set GO!

Why don't they get it?

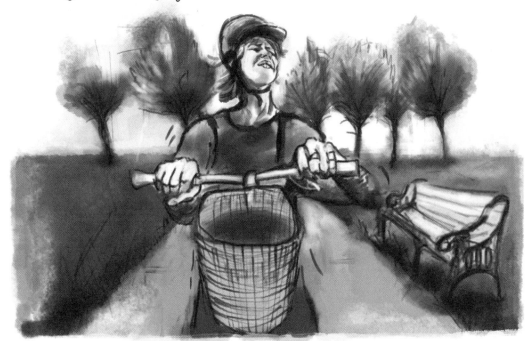

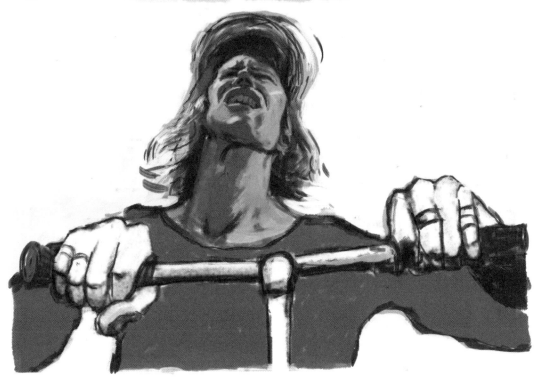

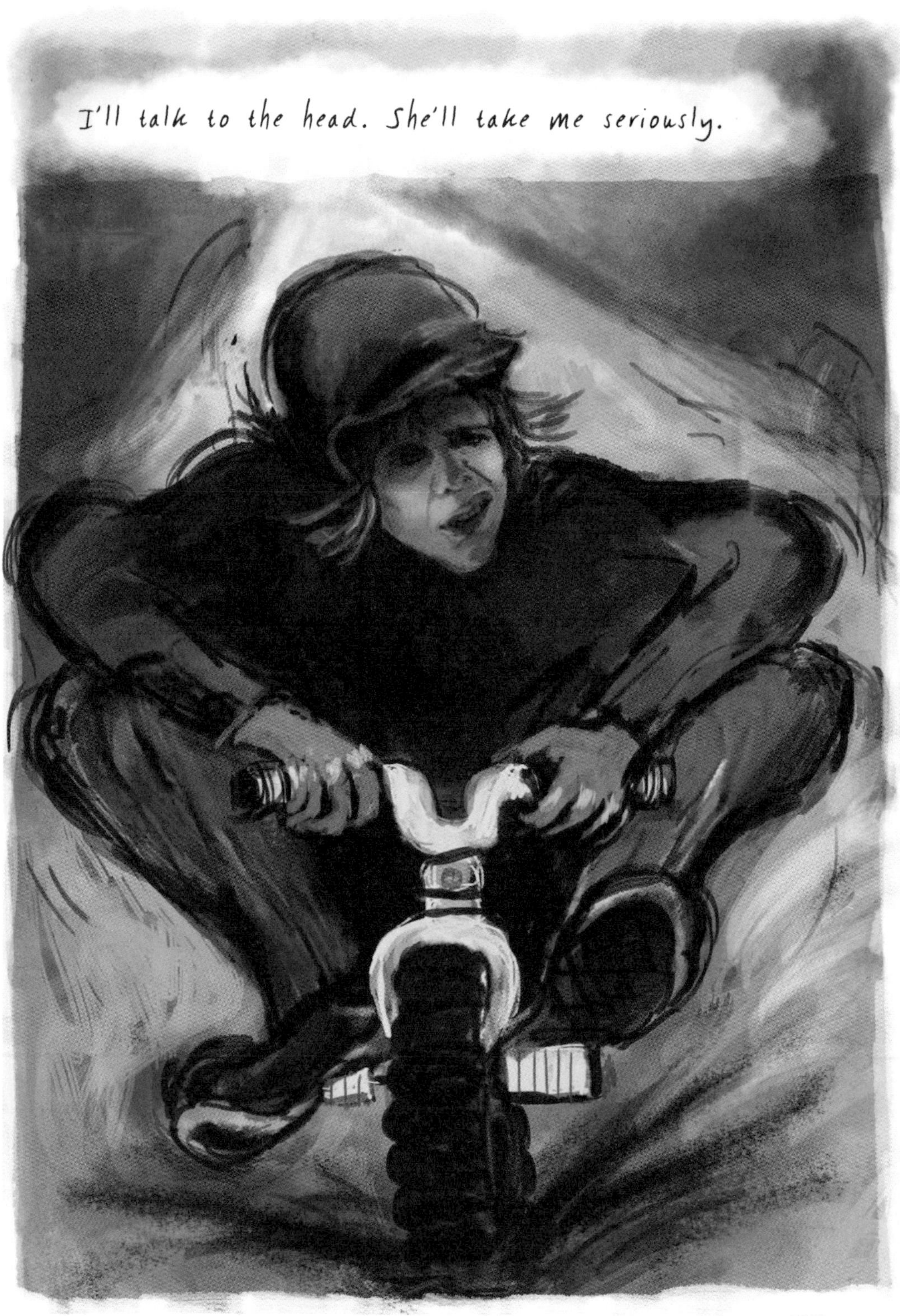
I'll talk to the head. She'll take me seriously.

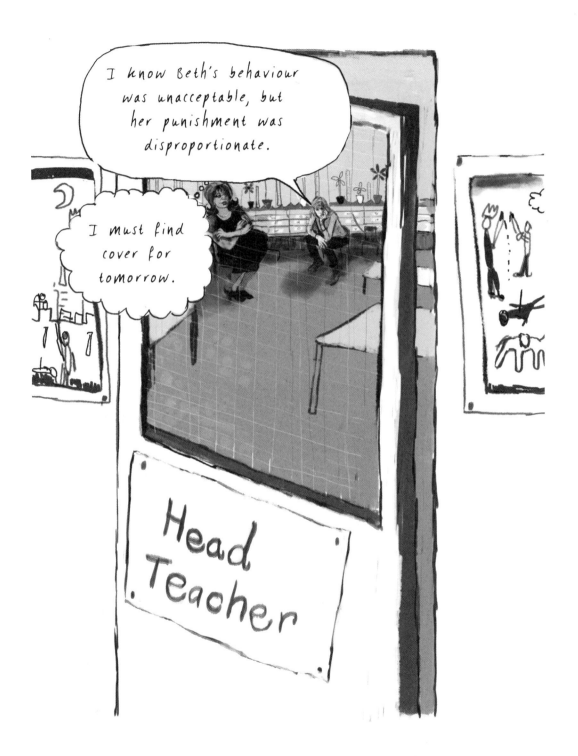

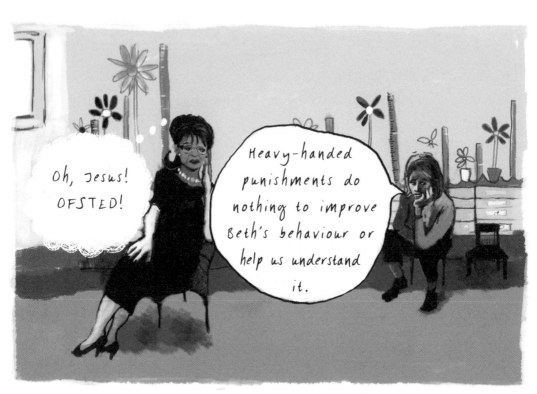

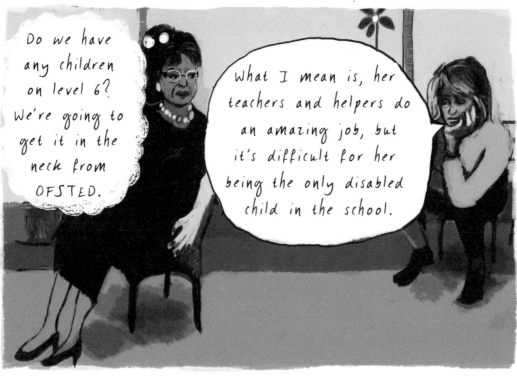

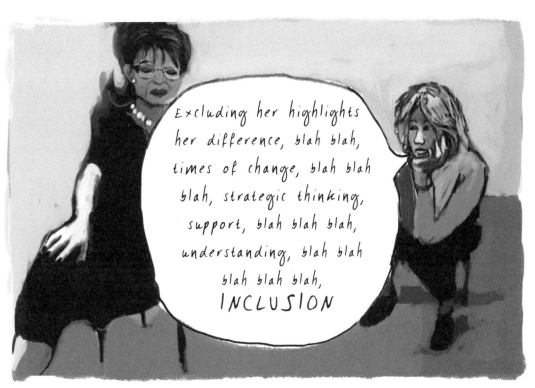

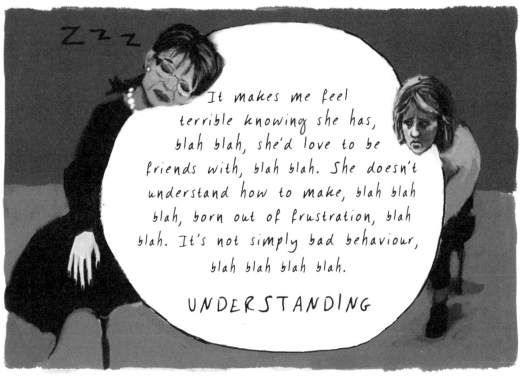

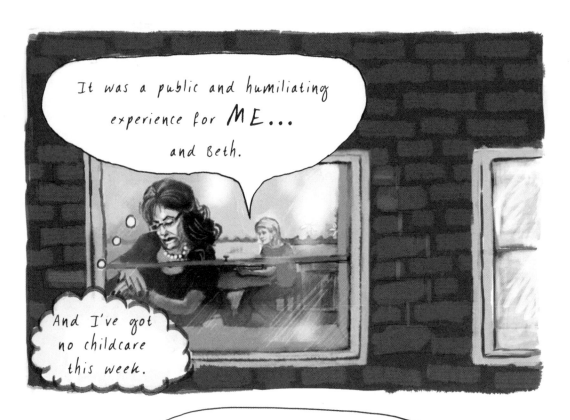

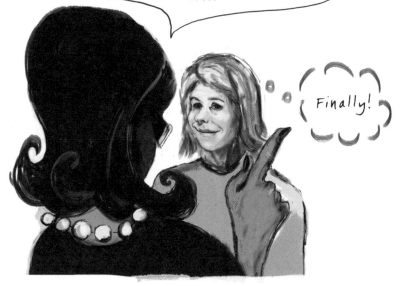

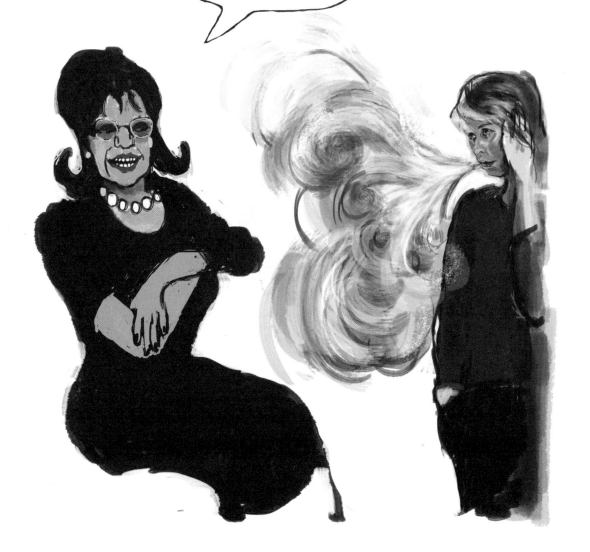

...is how wonderfully kind and TOLERANT all the other children have been with Beth. It's so lovely to see them interact with her.

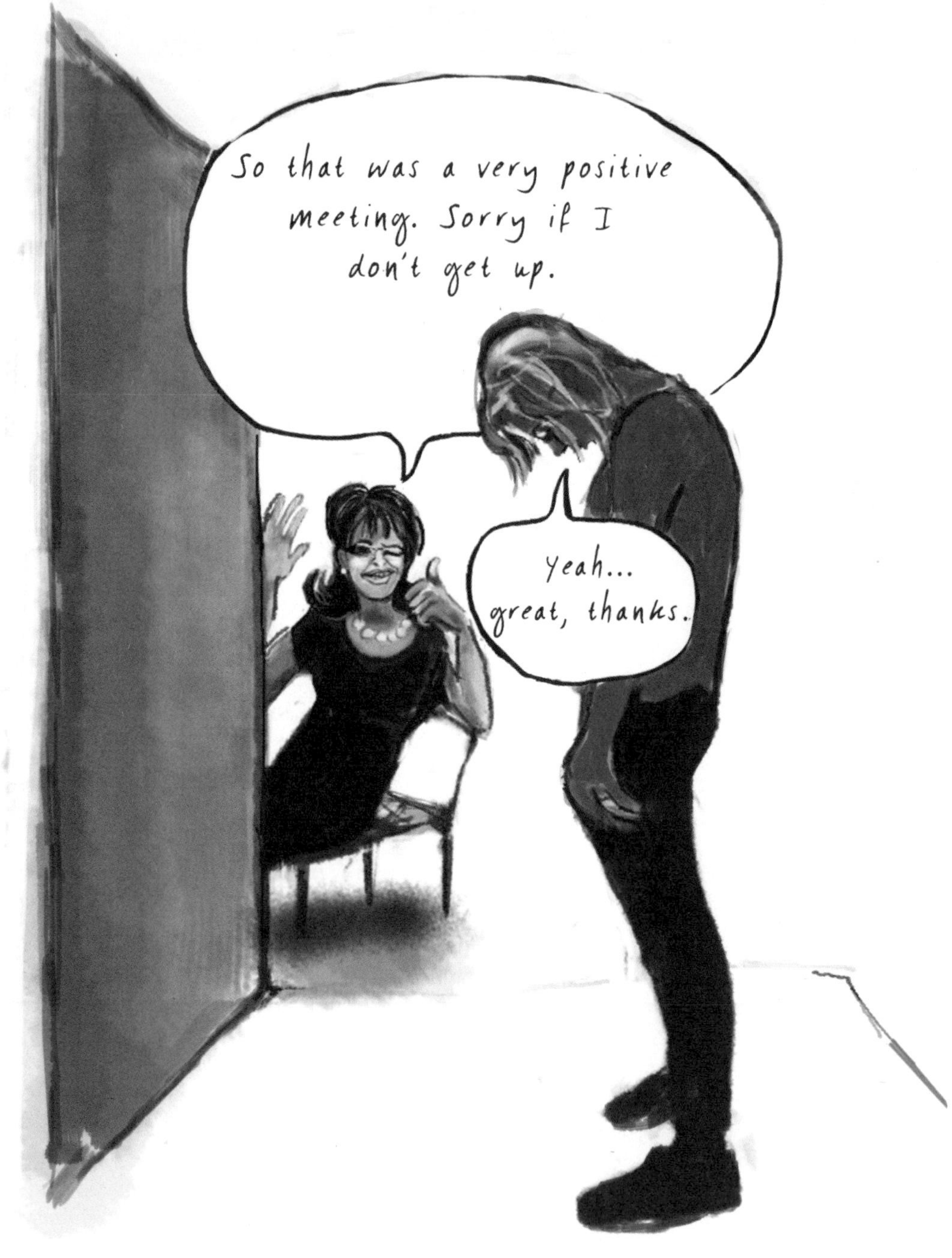
So that was a very positive meeting. Sorry if I don't get up.
Yeah... great, thanks..

Part Four

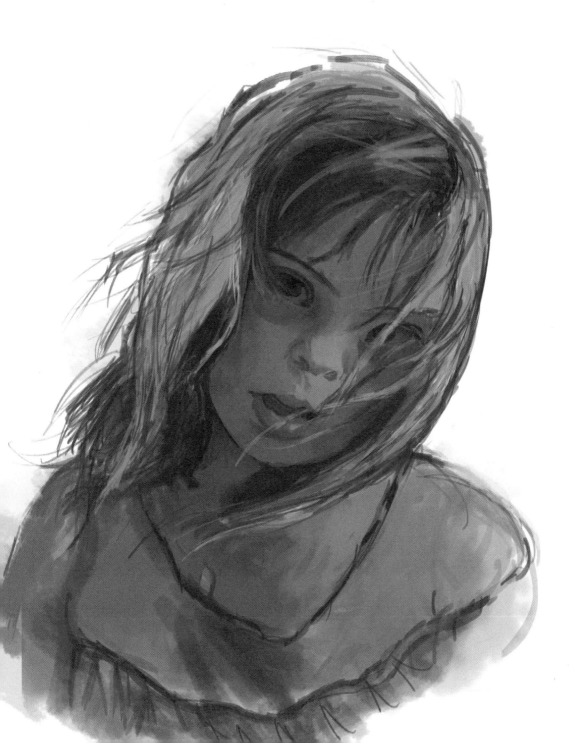

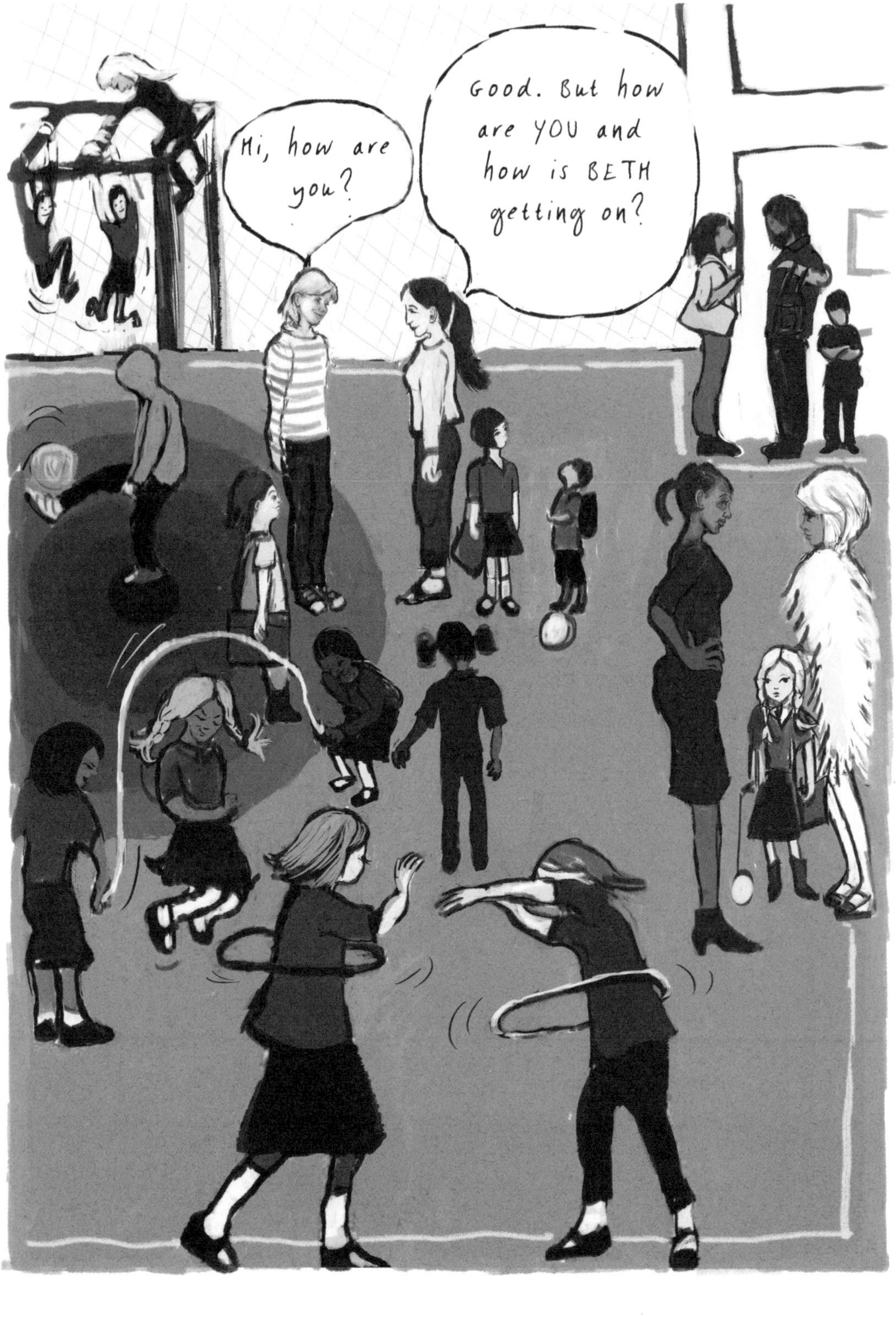
Hi, how are you?
Good. But how are YOU and how is BETH getting on?

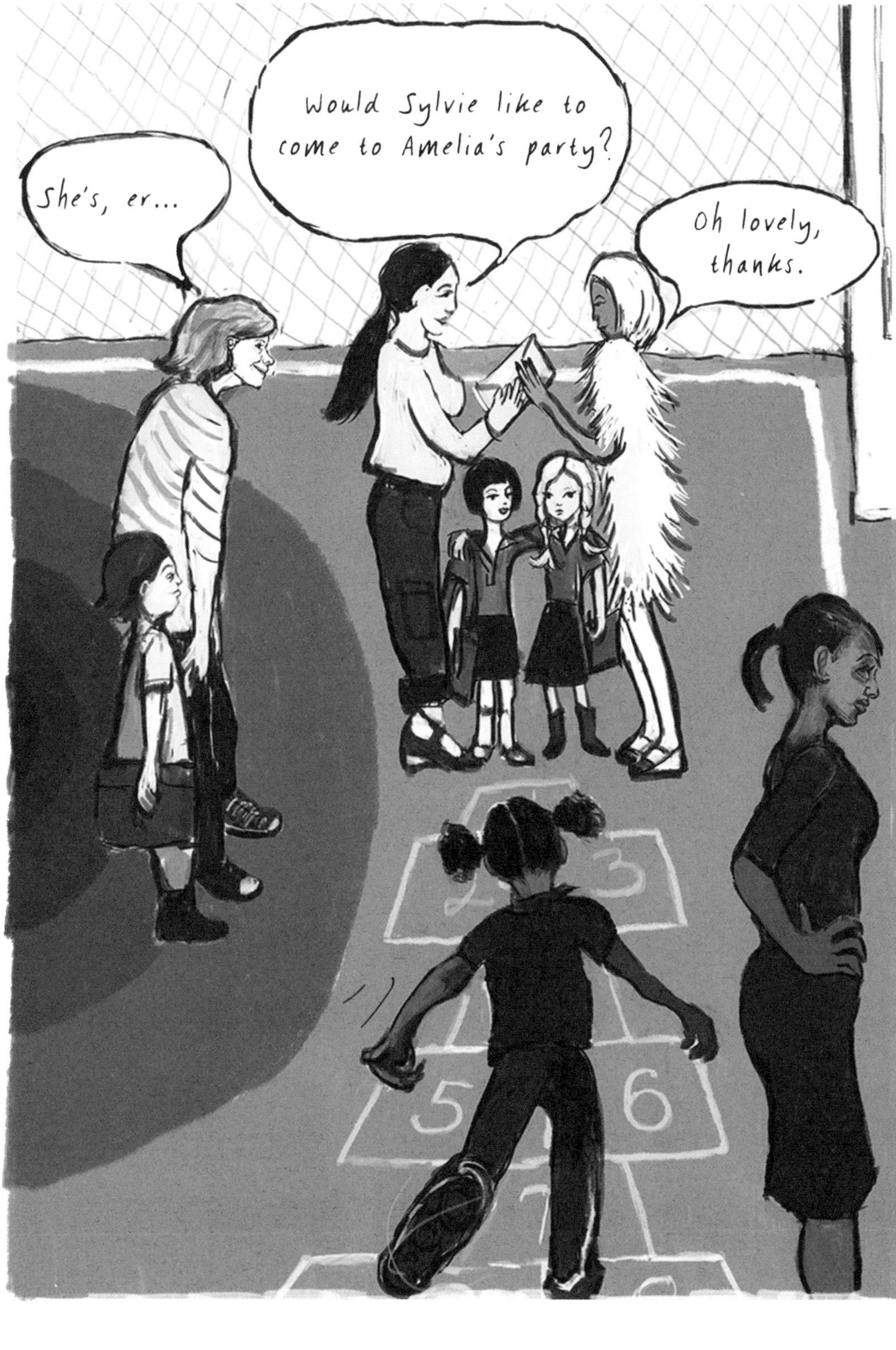
She's, er...
Would Sylvie like to come to Amelia's party?
Oh lovely, thanks.

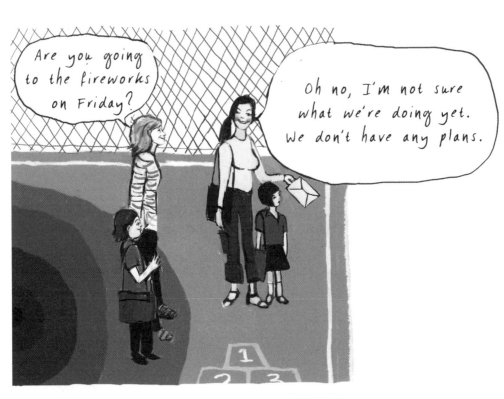

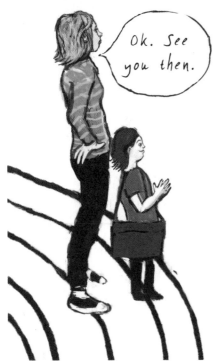

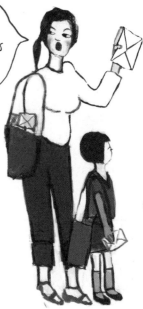

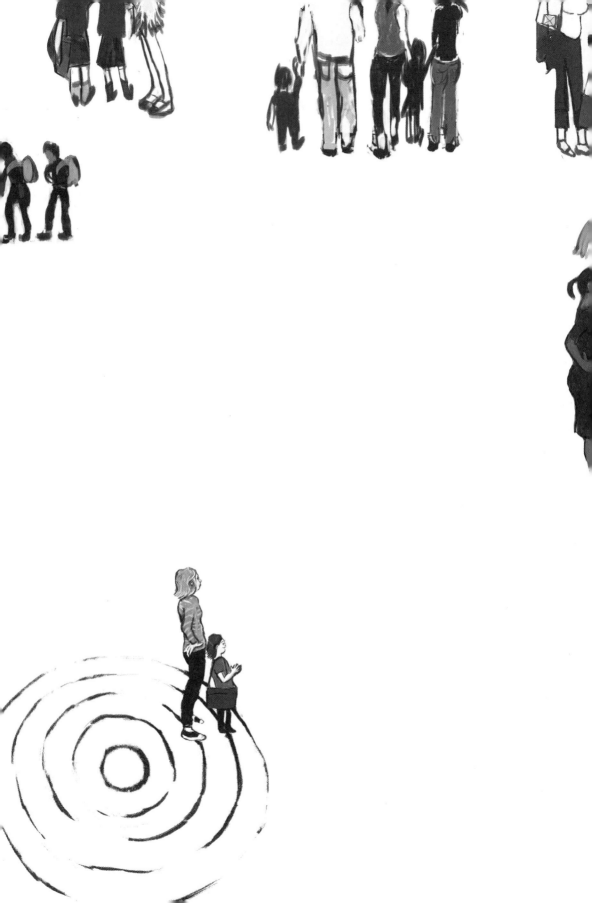

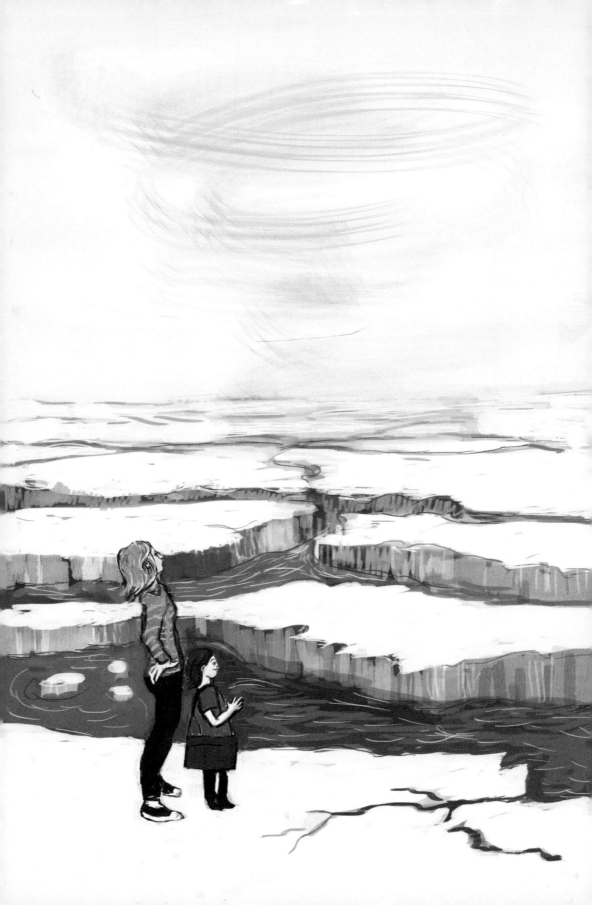

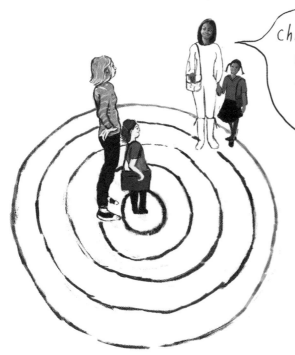

Charlotte wants to know if Beth would like to come to tea? What day would be good for you?

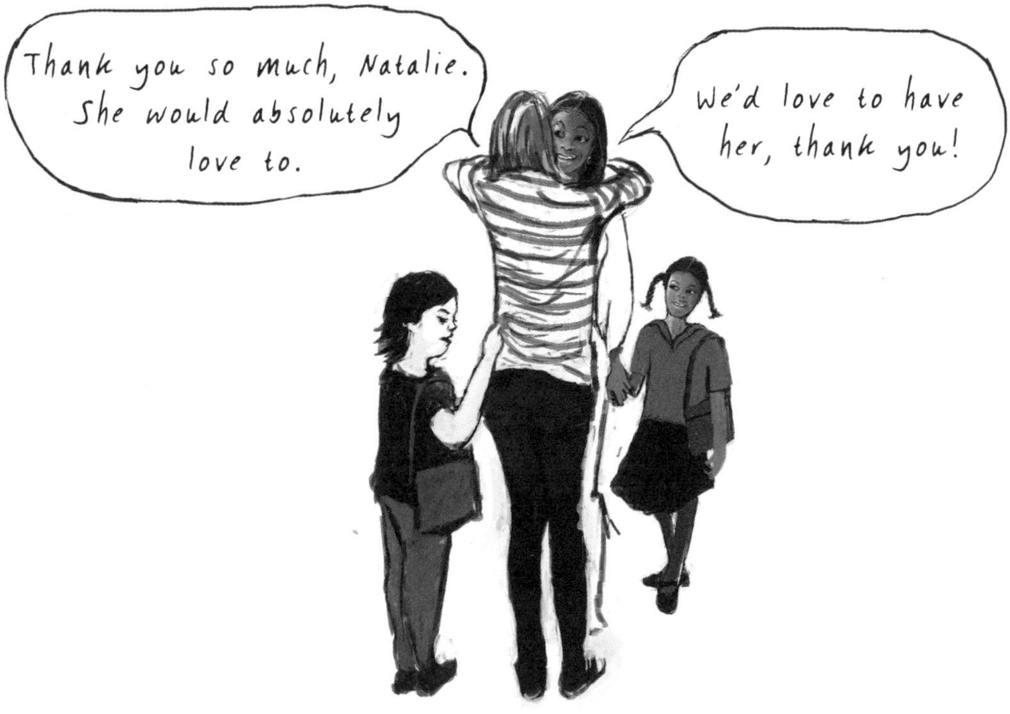

Thank you so much, Natalie. She would absolutely love to.

We'd love to have her, thank you!

November 2011

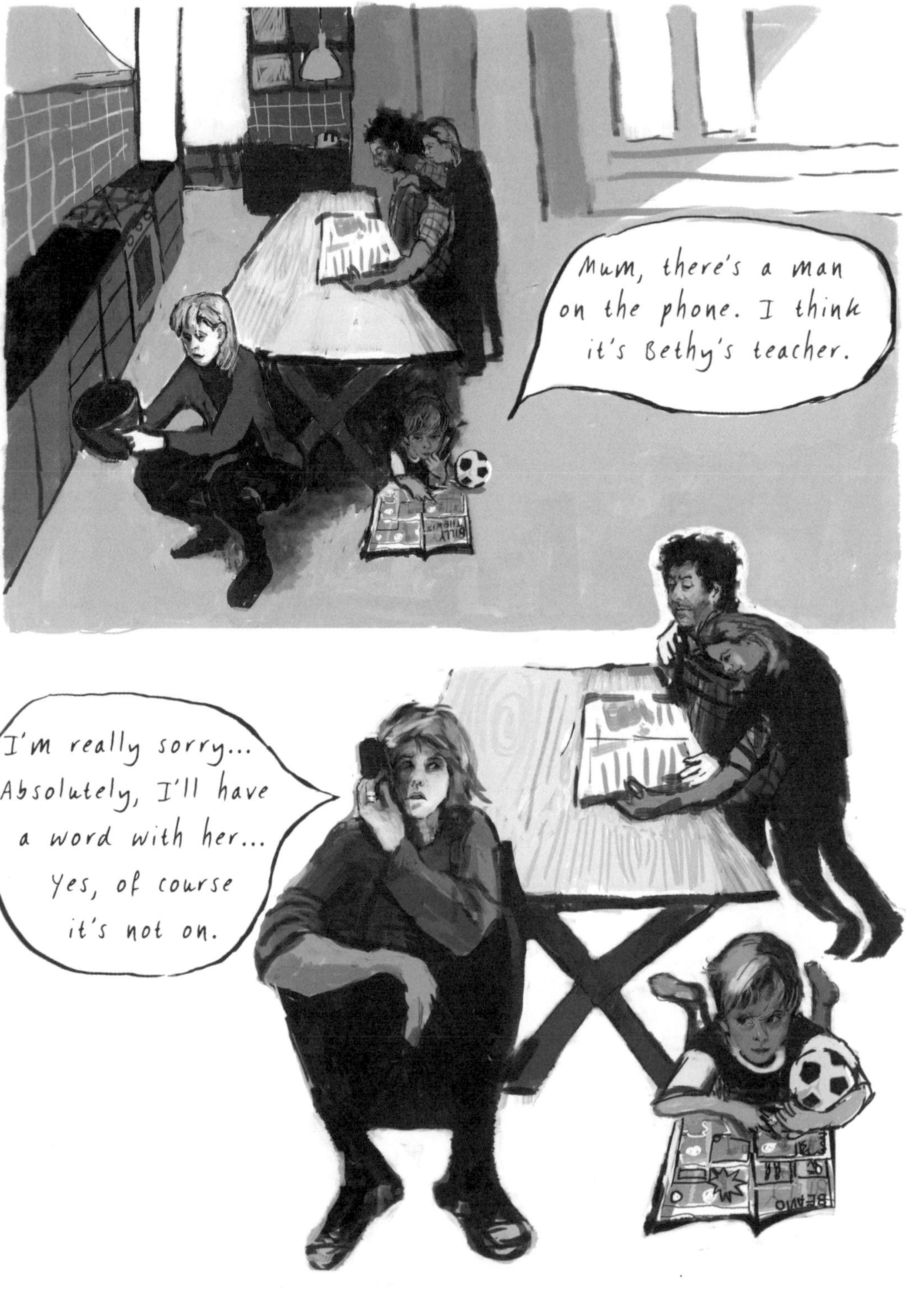
Mum, there's a man on the phone. I think it's Bethy's teacher.
I'm really sorry... Absolutely, I'll have a word with her... Yes, of course it's not on.

December 2011

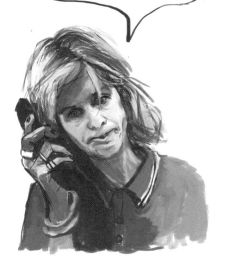

Yes, I'm so sorry she scratched her... Yep, I'll definitely have a word.

February 2012

We thought you'd probably like to know, Beth hit her friend at lunchtime. We have decided that she needs to miss playtime.

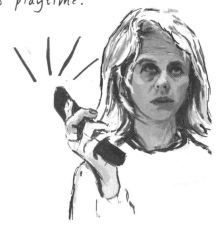

April 2012

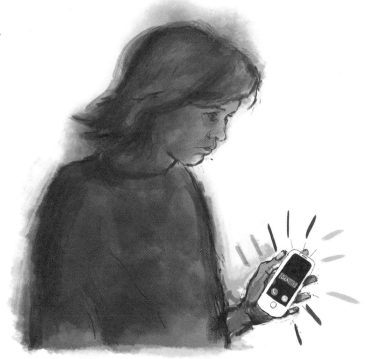

June 2012

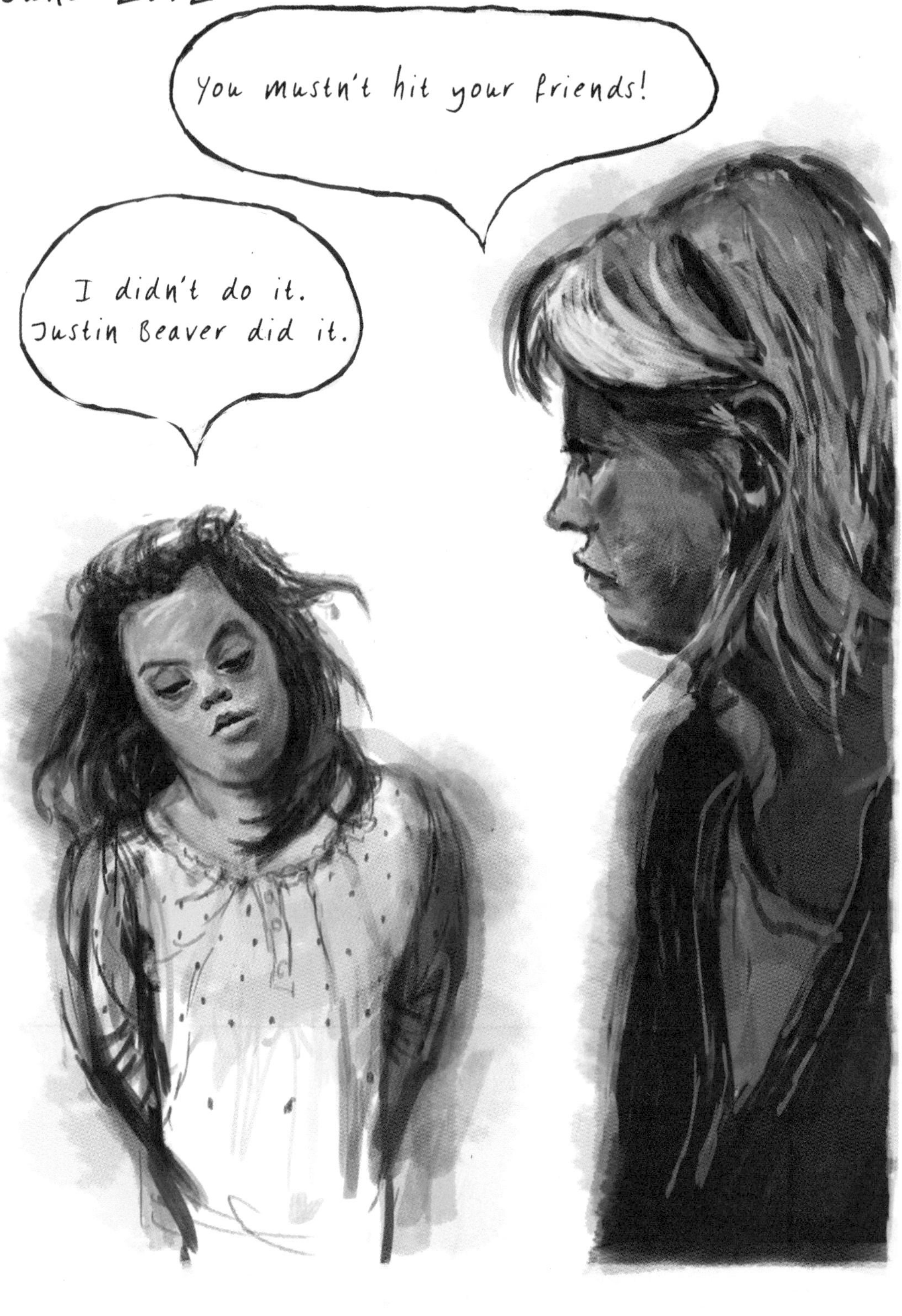
You mustn't hit your friends!
I didn't do it. Justin Beaver did it.

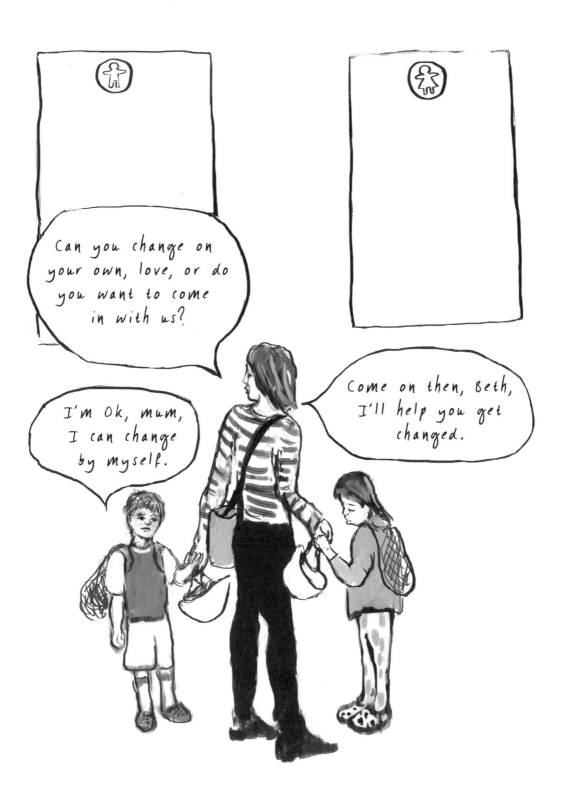

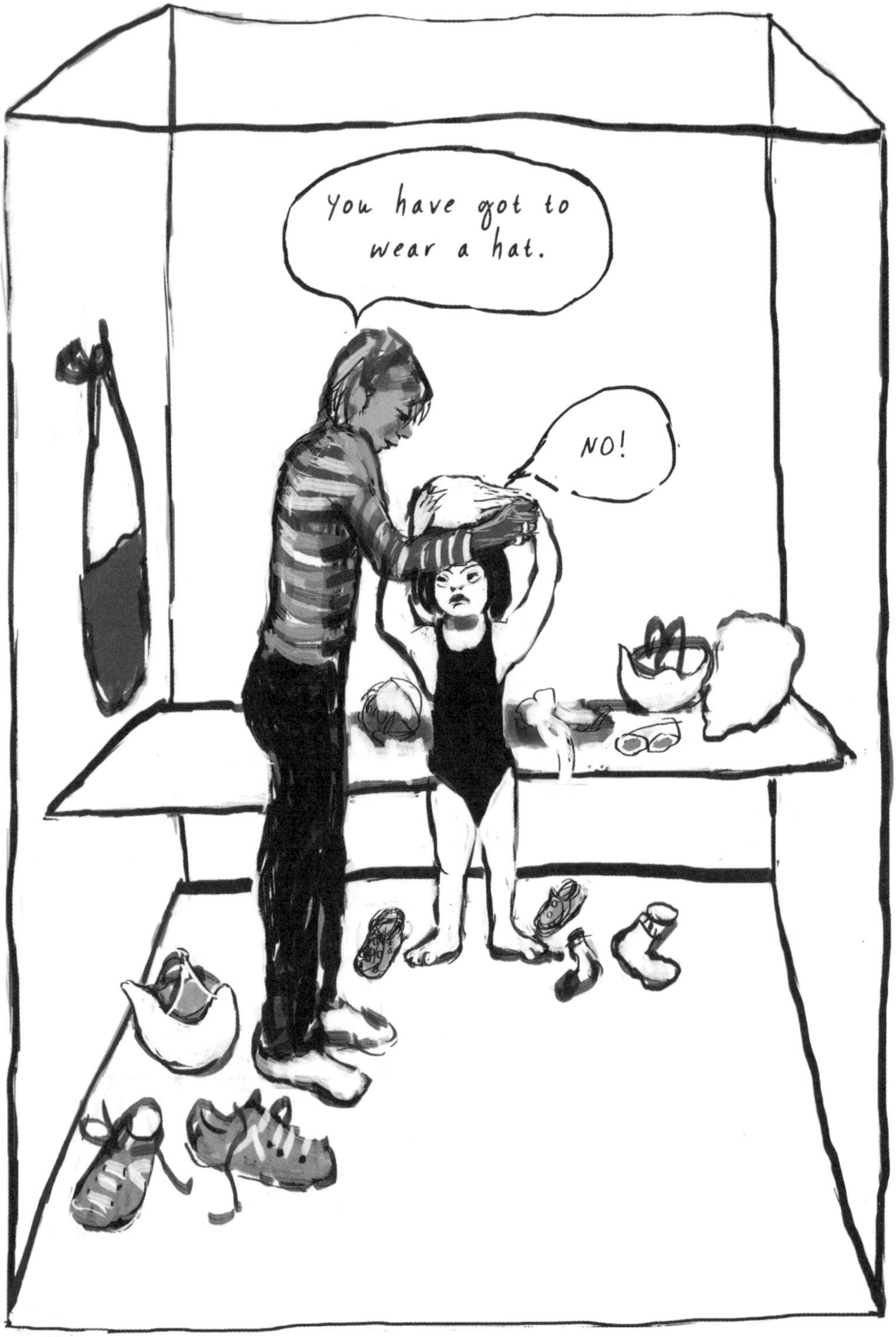
You have got to wear a hat.
NO!

NO!

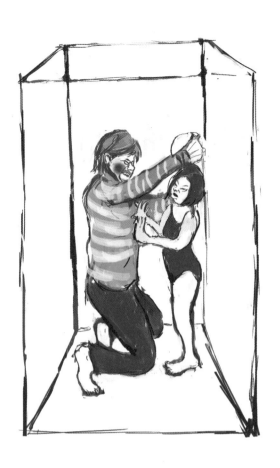

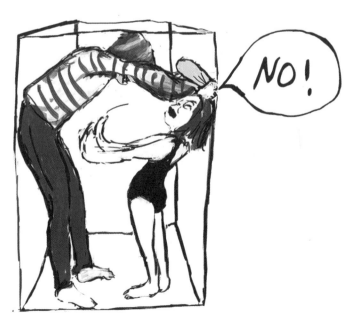

BETH, I AM WARNING YOU
DO NOT TOUCH THAT HAT!

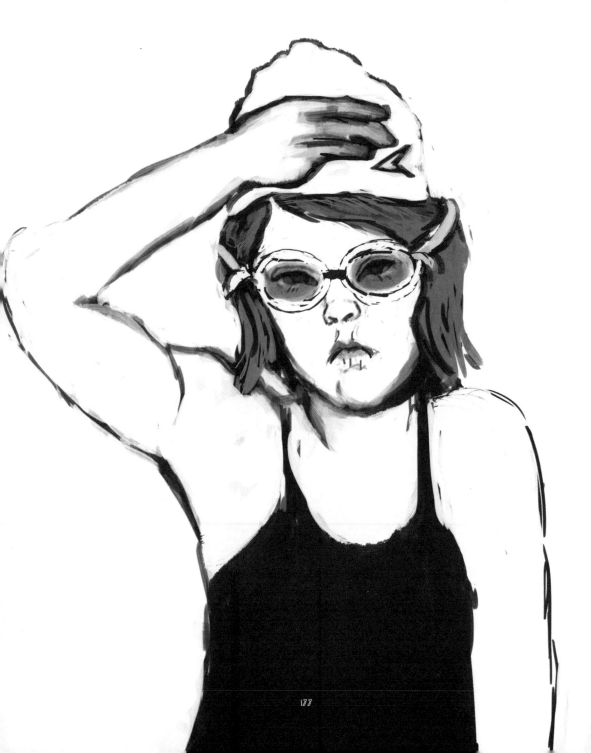

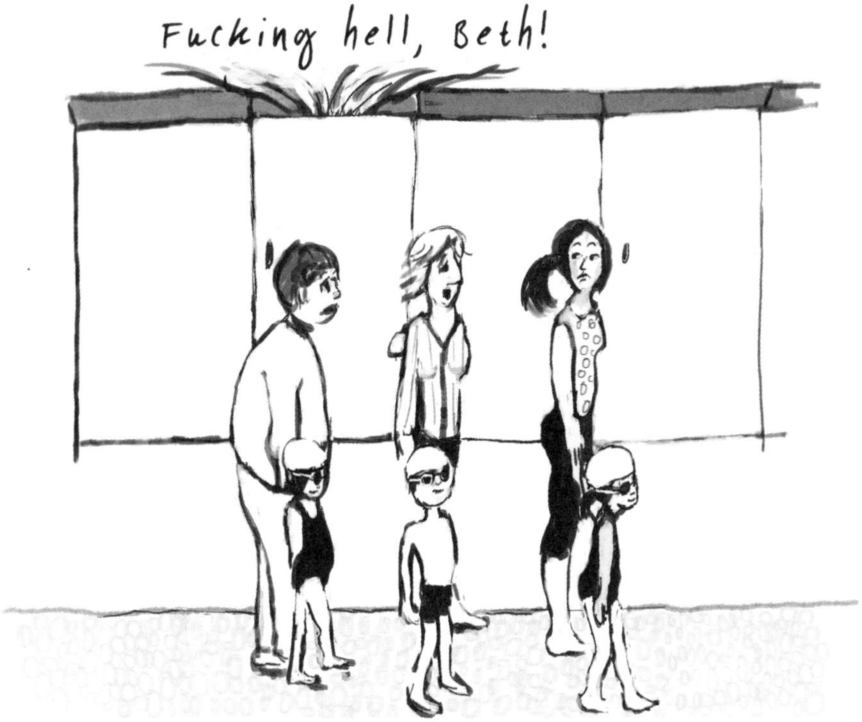
Fucking hell, Beth!

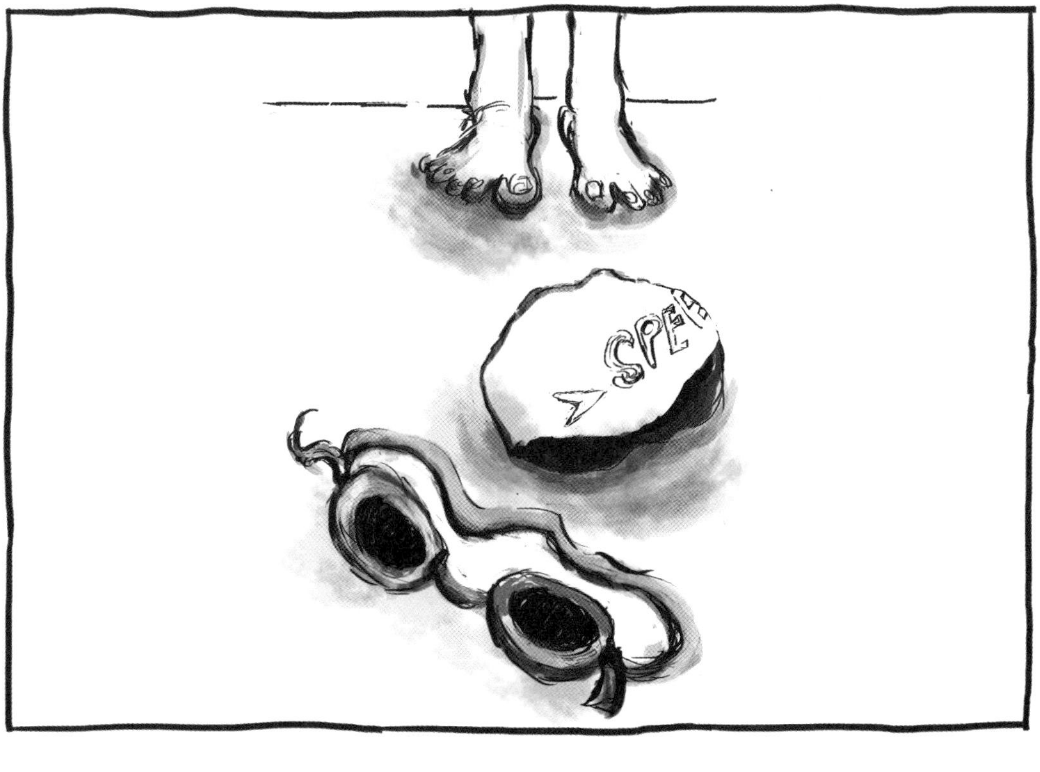
SPE

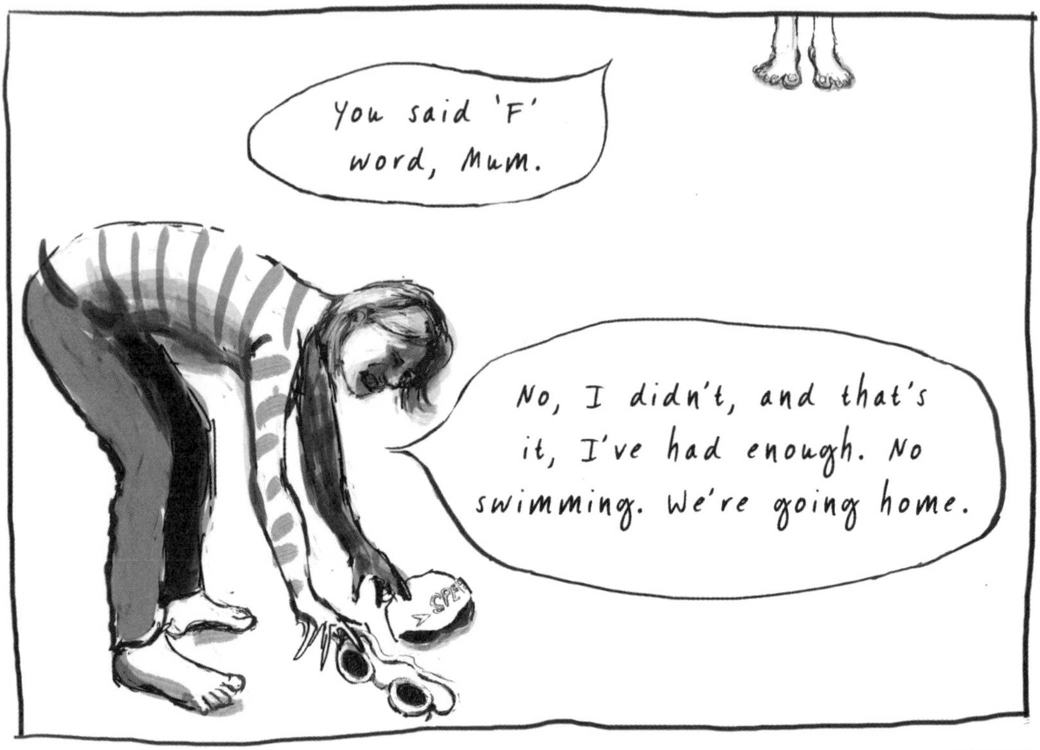
You said 'F' word, Mum.
No, I didn't, and that's it, I've had enough. No swimming. We're going home.

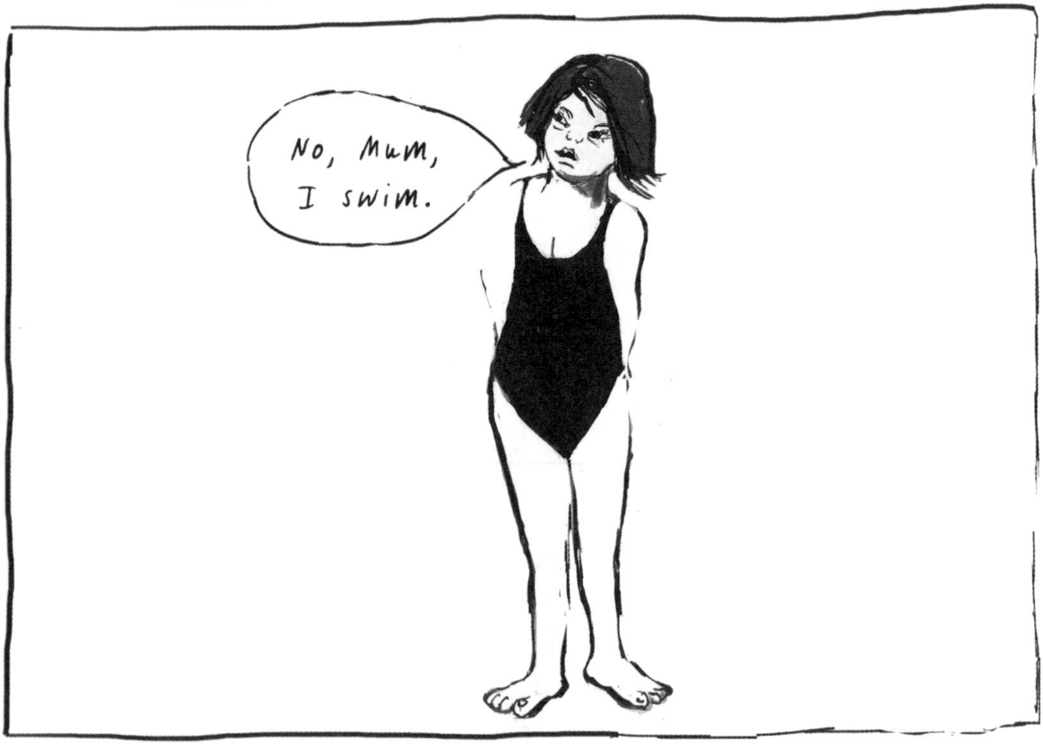
No, Mum, I swim.

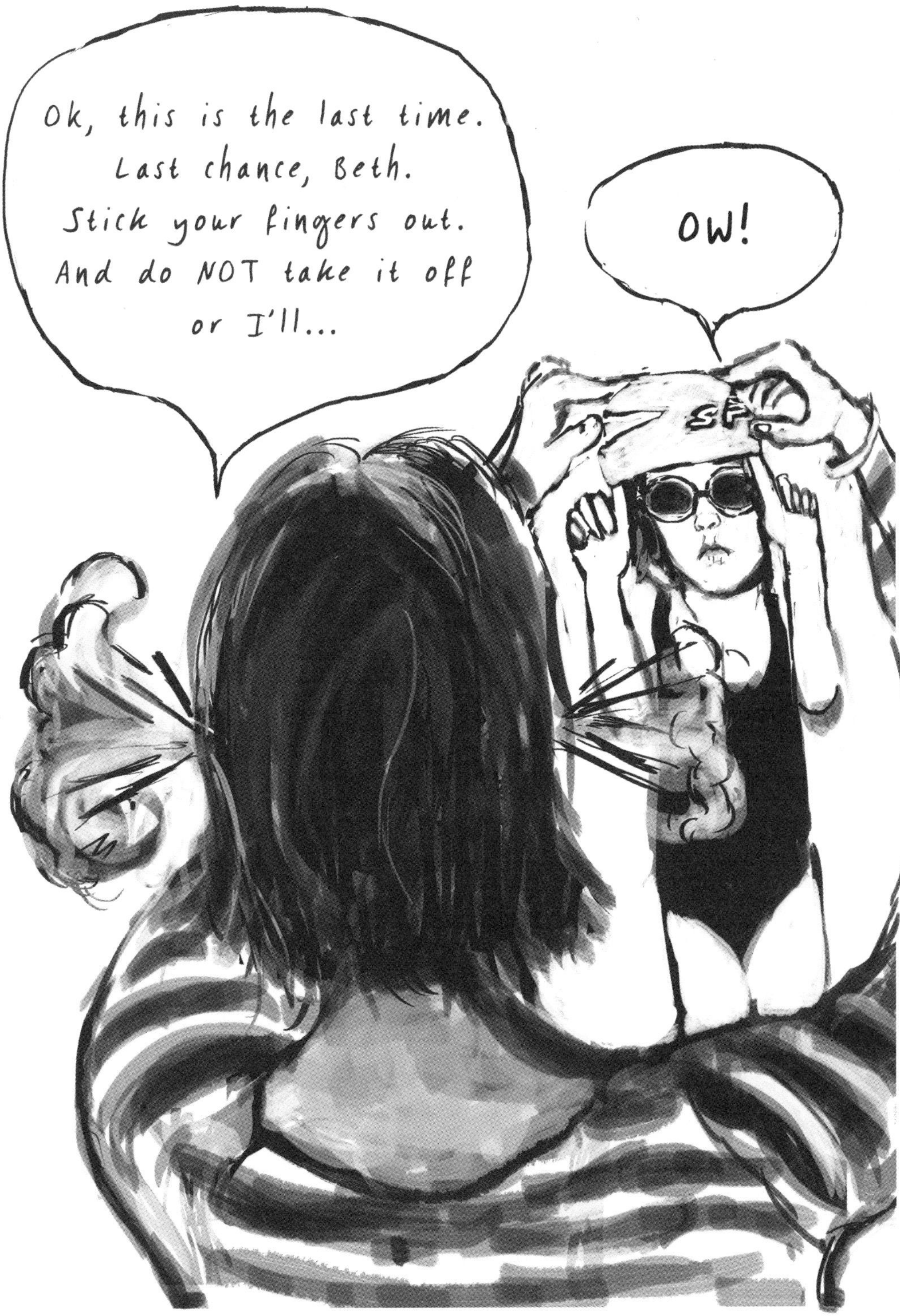
Ok, this is the last time. Last chance, Beth. Stick your fingers out. And do NOT take it off or I'll...
OW!

...be very angry. You must keep your hat on in the pool and you're going to behave yourself. Do you understand me?

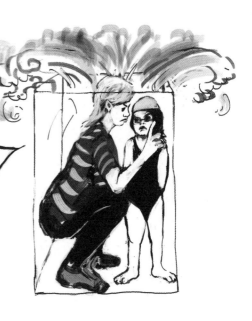

The hat is the least of our problems. What am I going to do if she pushes that child in again?

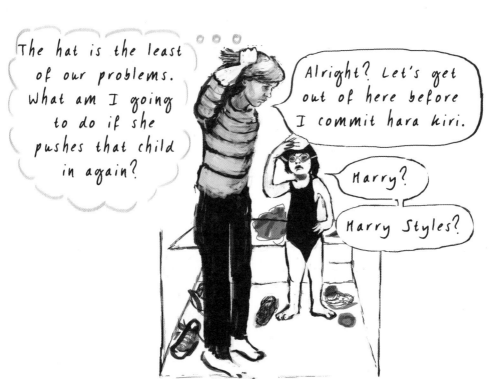

Alright? Let's get out of here before I commit hara kiri.

Harry?

Harry Styles?

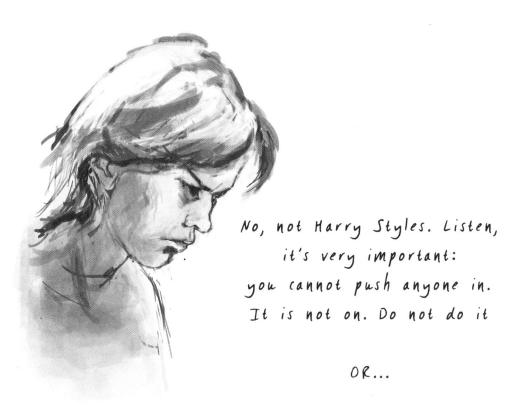

No, not Harry Styles. Listen,
it's very important:
you cannot push anyone in.
It is not on. Do not do it

OR...

THERE WILL BE BIG TROUBLE.

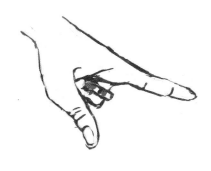

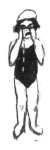

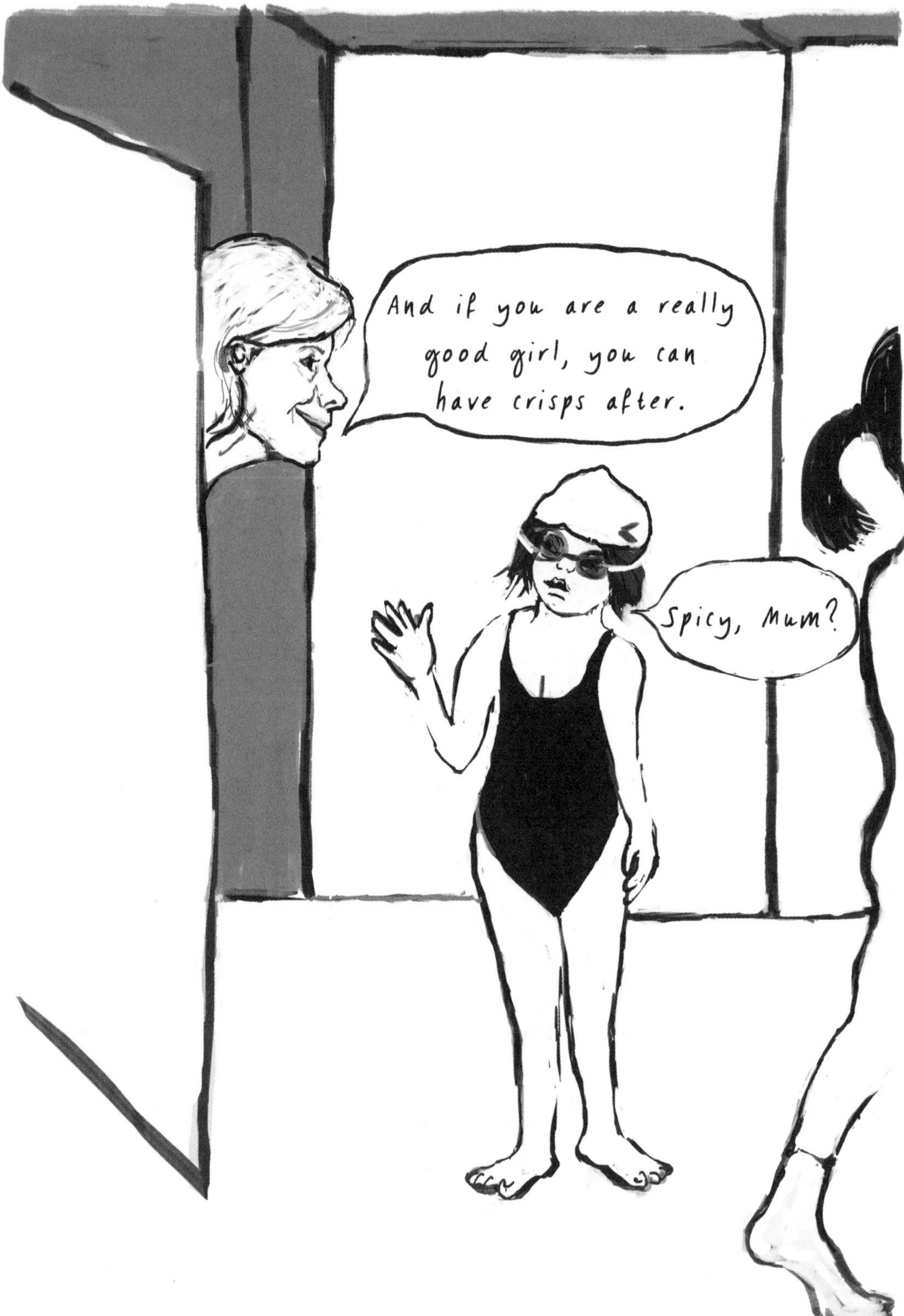
And if you are a really good girl, you can have crisps after.
Spicy, Mum?

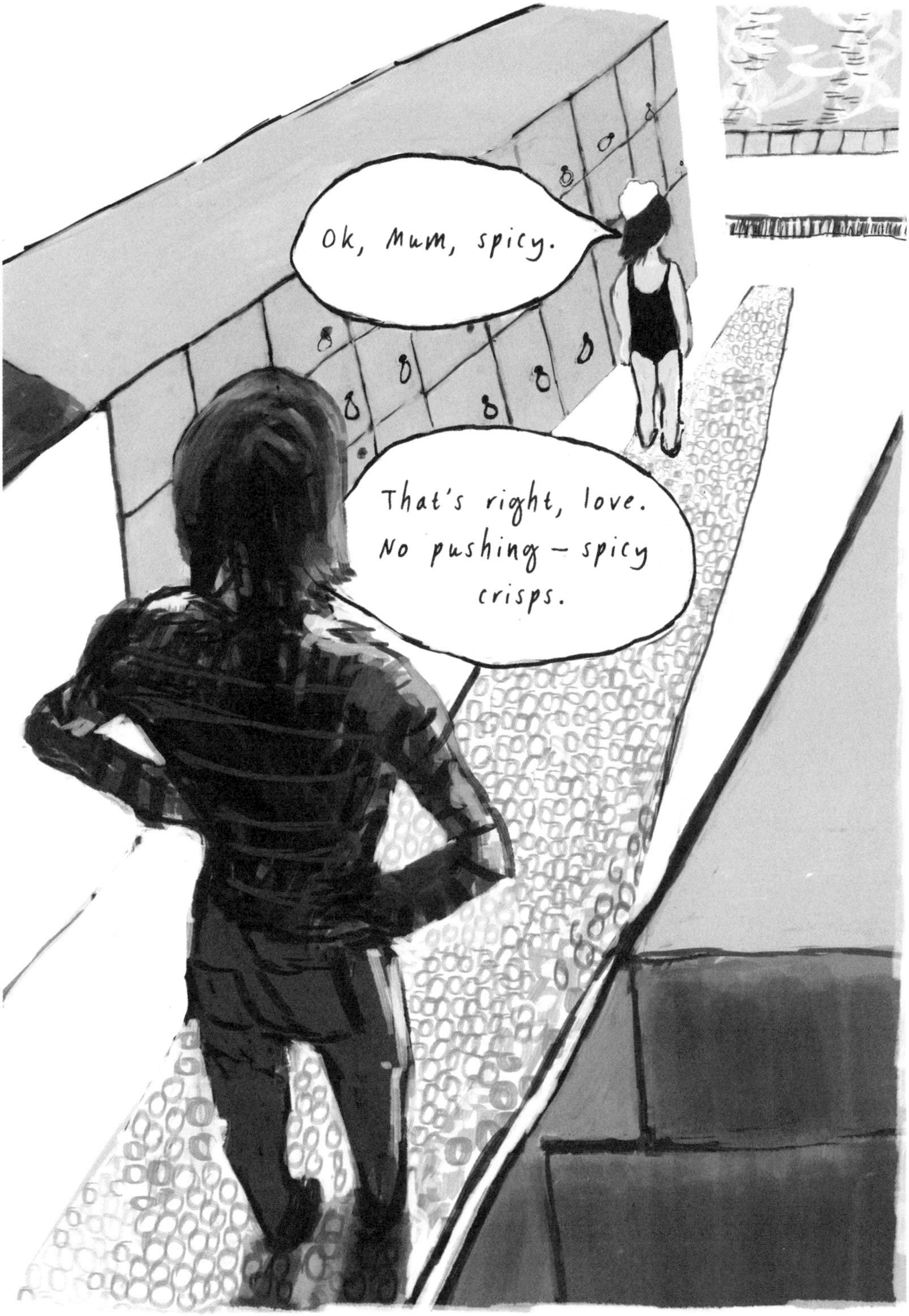
Ok, Mum, spicy.
That's right, love. No pushing – spicy crisps.

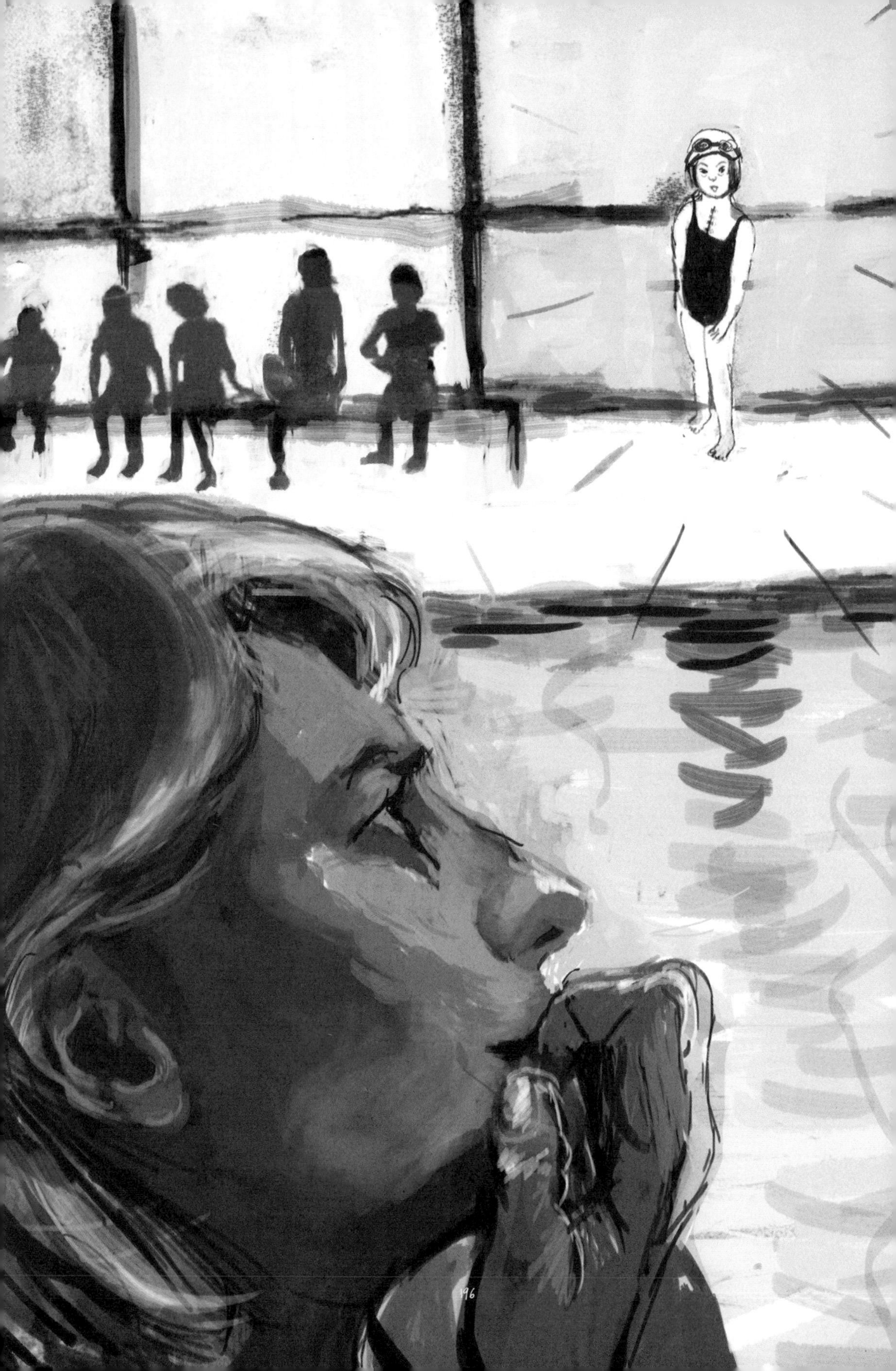

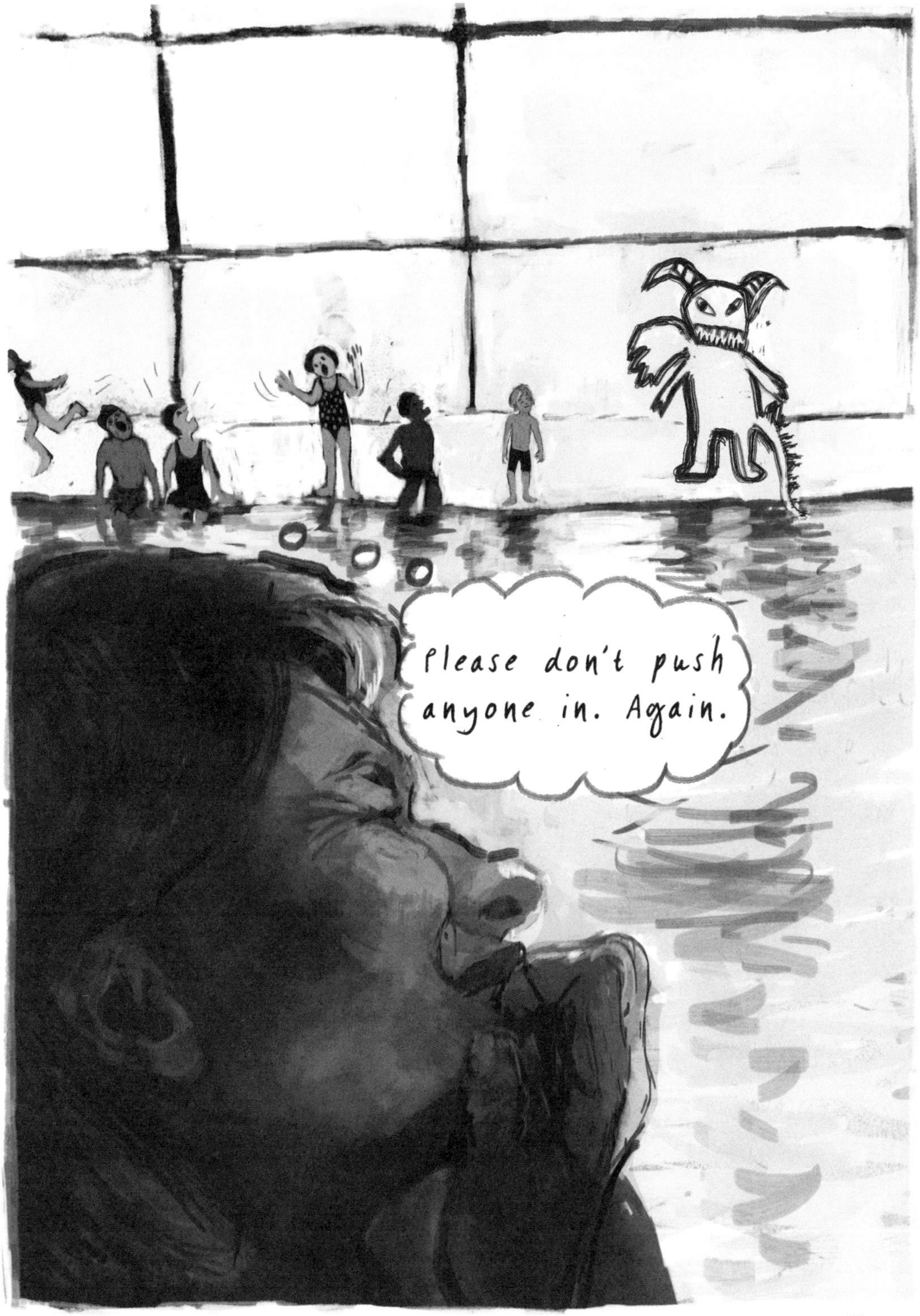
Please don't push anyone in. Again.

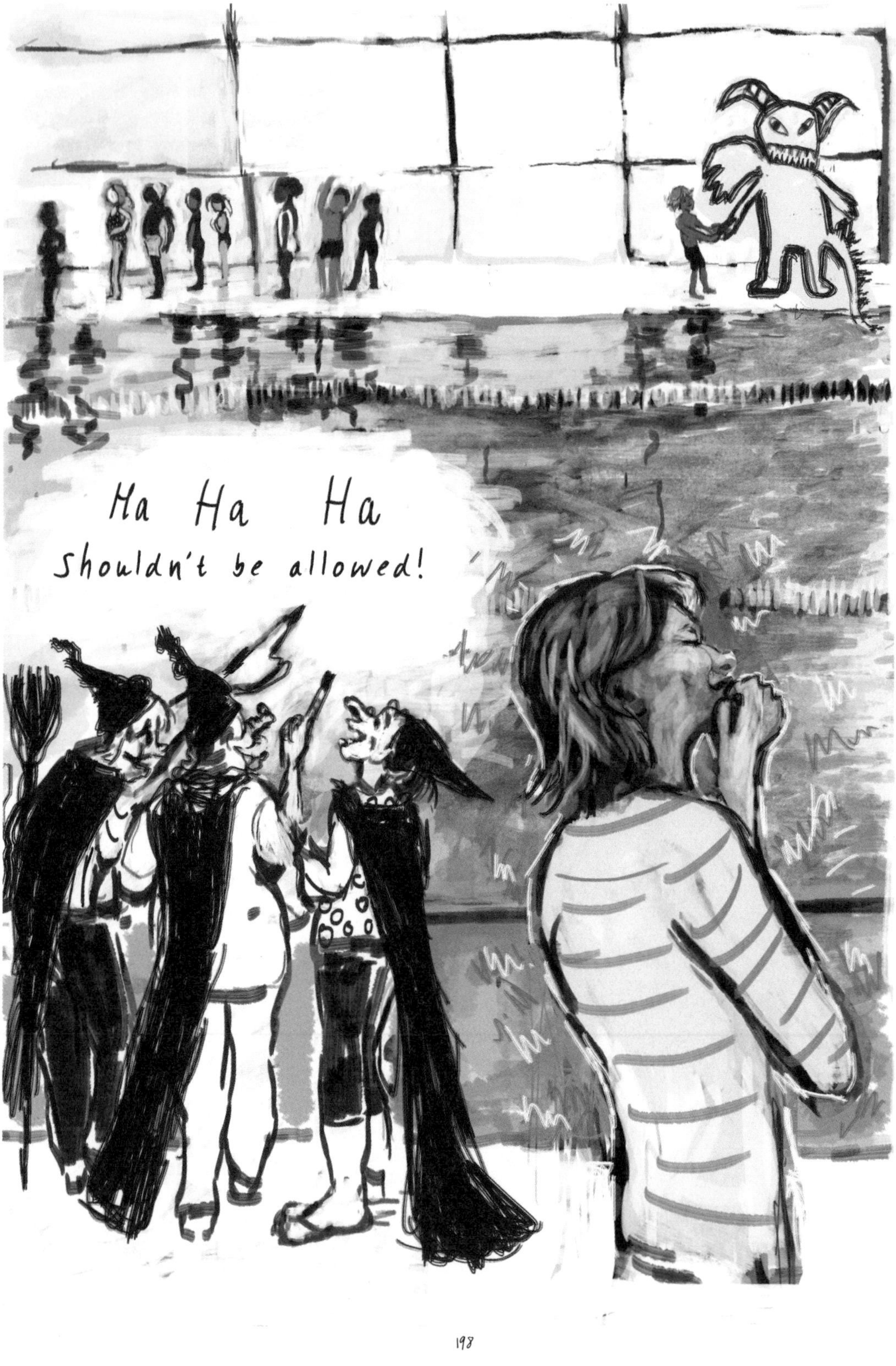
Ha Ha Ha
Shouldn't be allowed!

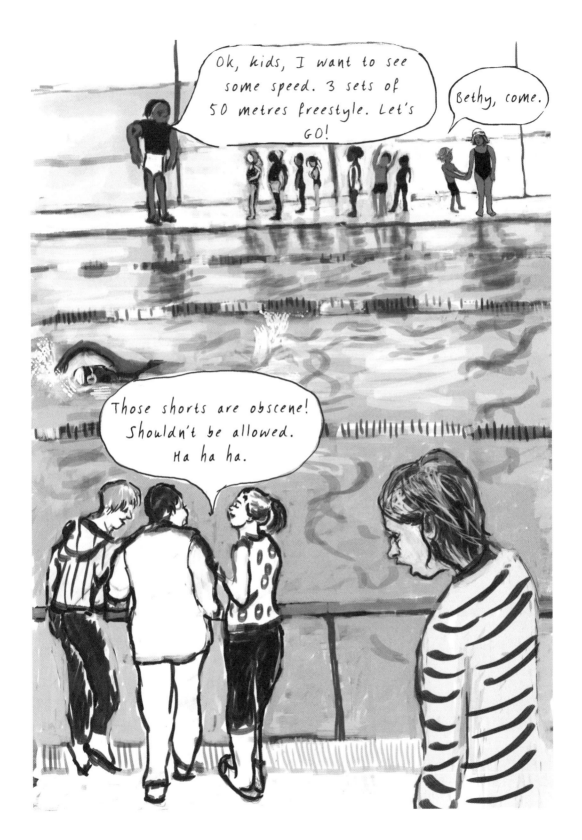

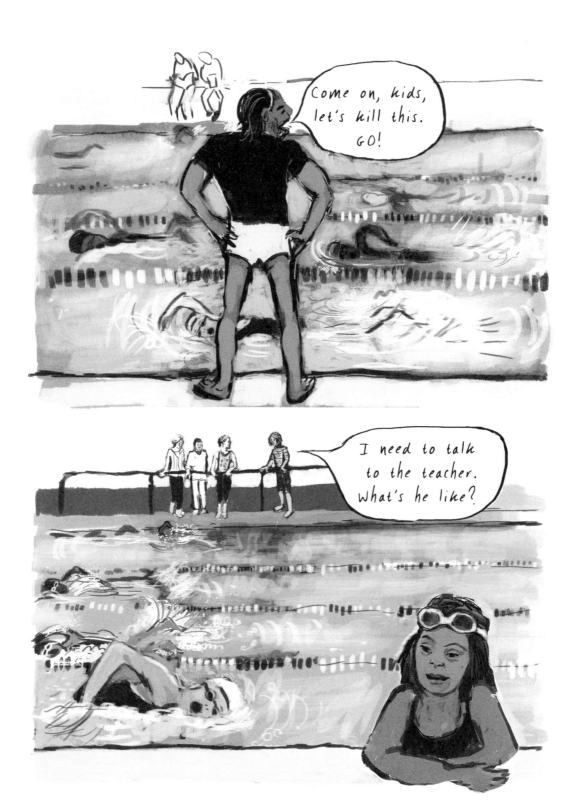

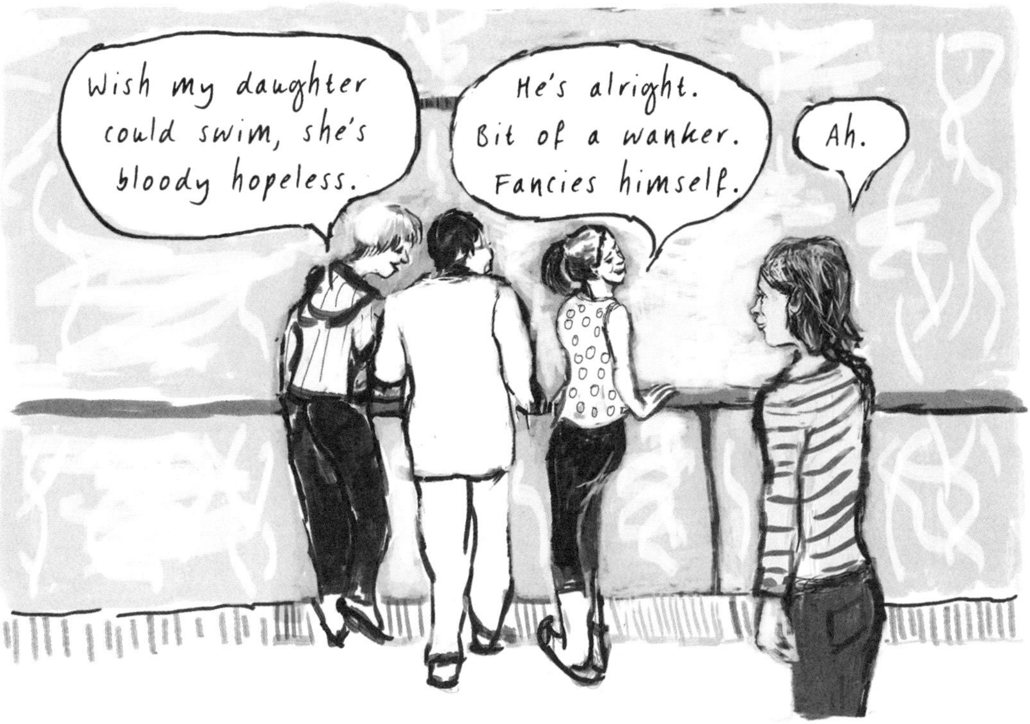
Wish my daughter could swim, she's bloody hopeless.
He's alright. Bit of a wanker. Fancies himself.
Ah.

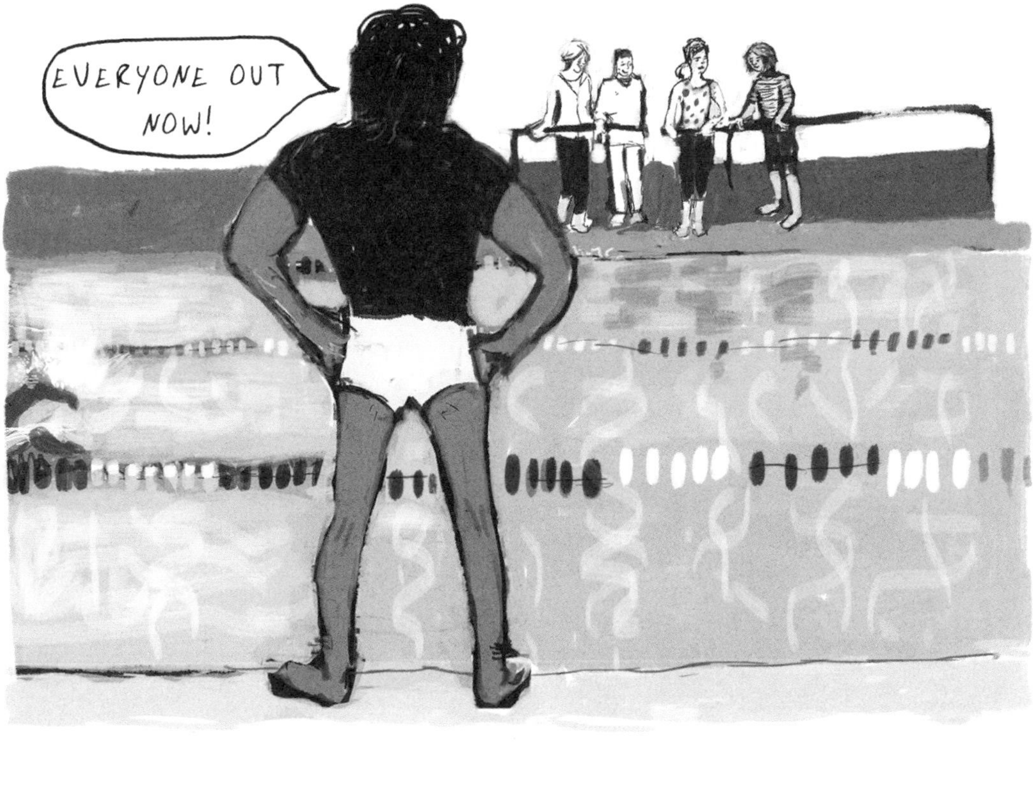
EVERYONE OUT NOW!

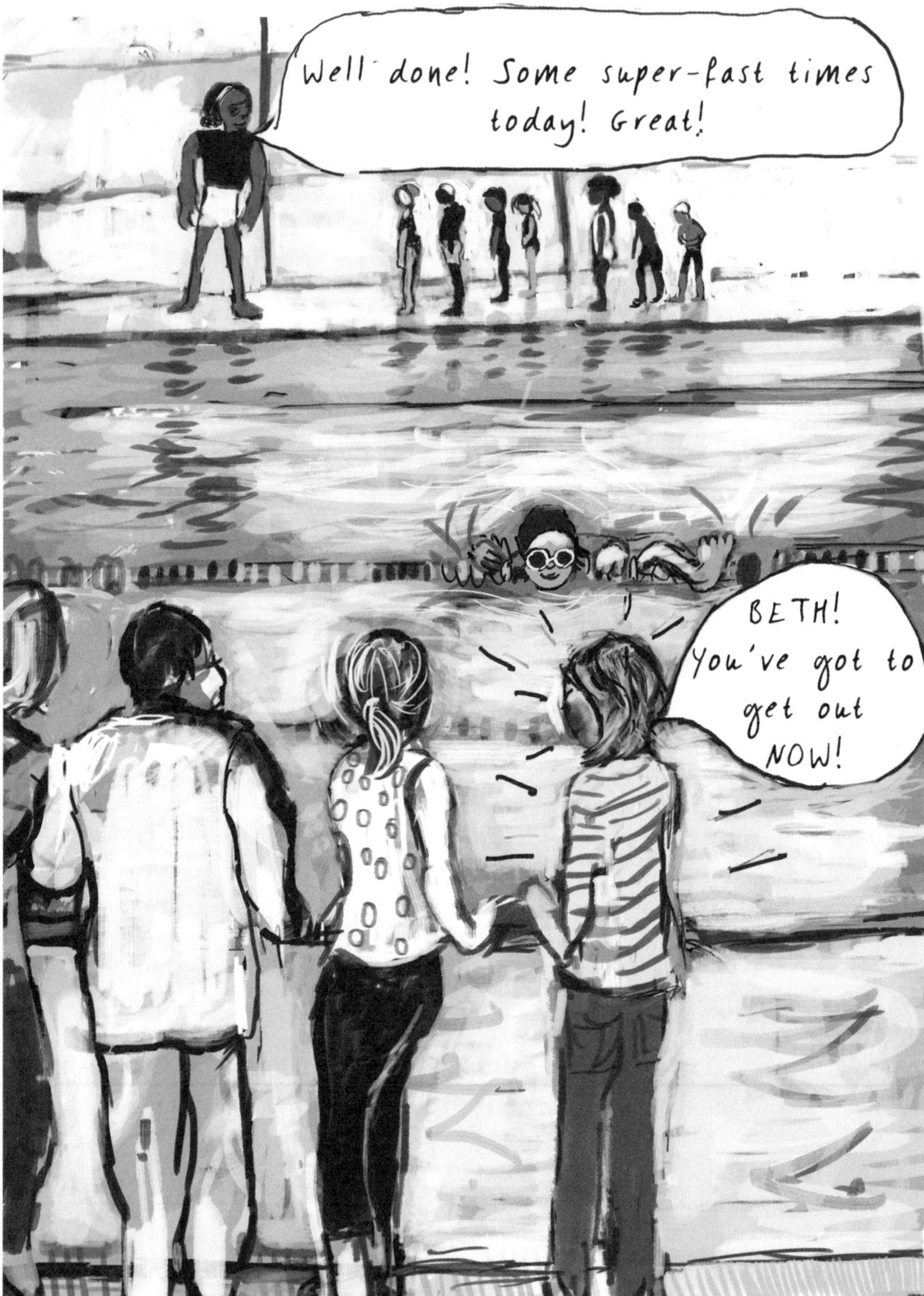
Well done! Some super-fast times today! Great!
BETH! You've got to get out NOW!

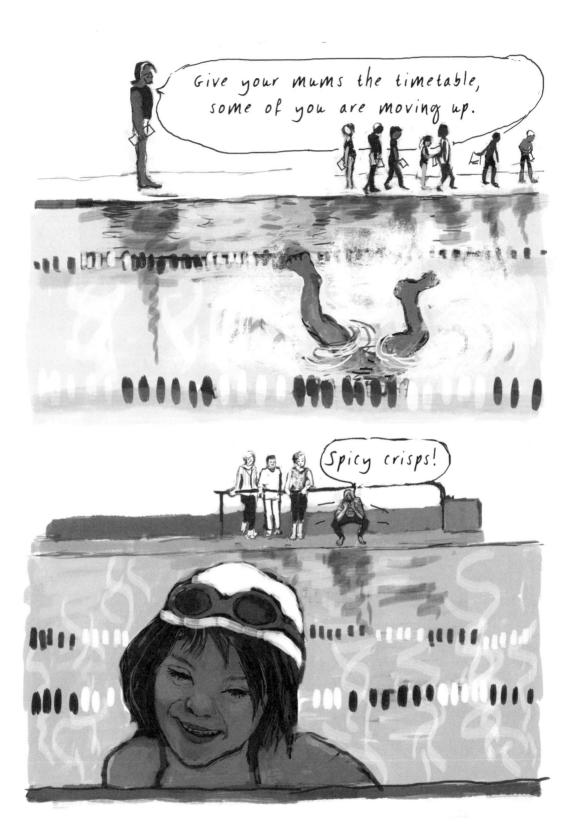

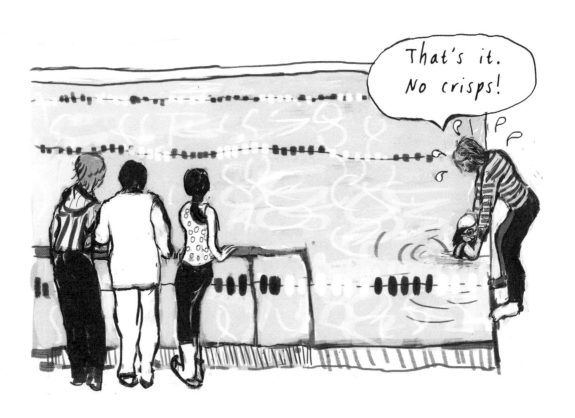

That's it. No crisps!

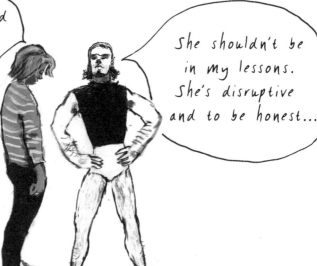

Sorry, can I have a word with you about Beth? She didn't get a timetable.

She finds it difficult to follow your instructions.

She shouldn't be in my lessons. She's disruptive and to be honest...

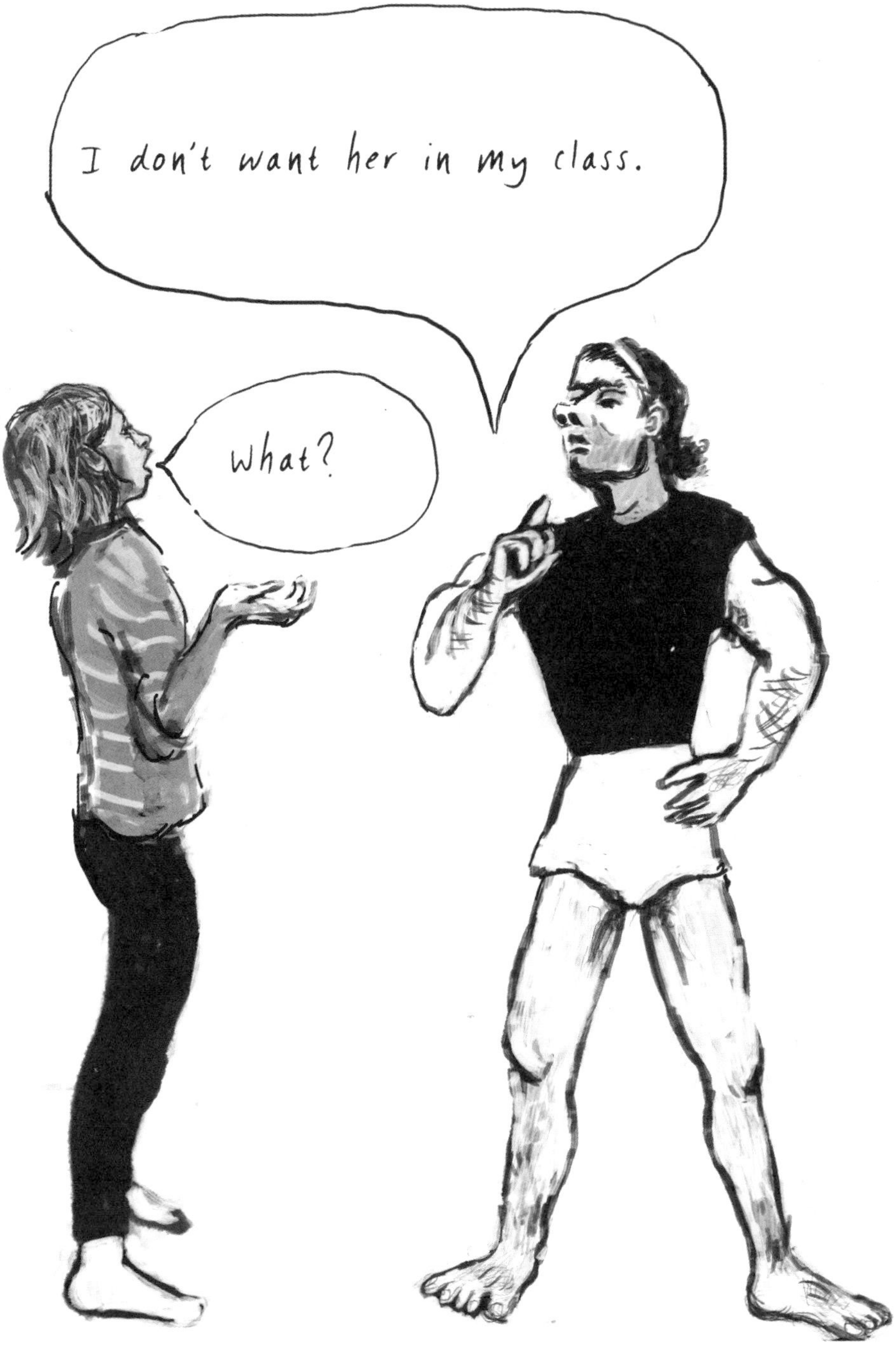
I don't want her in my class.
What?

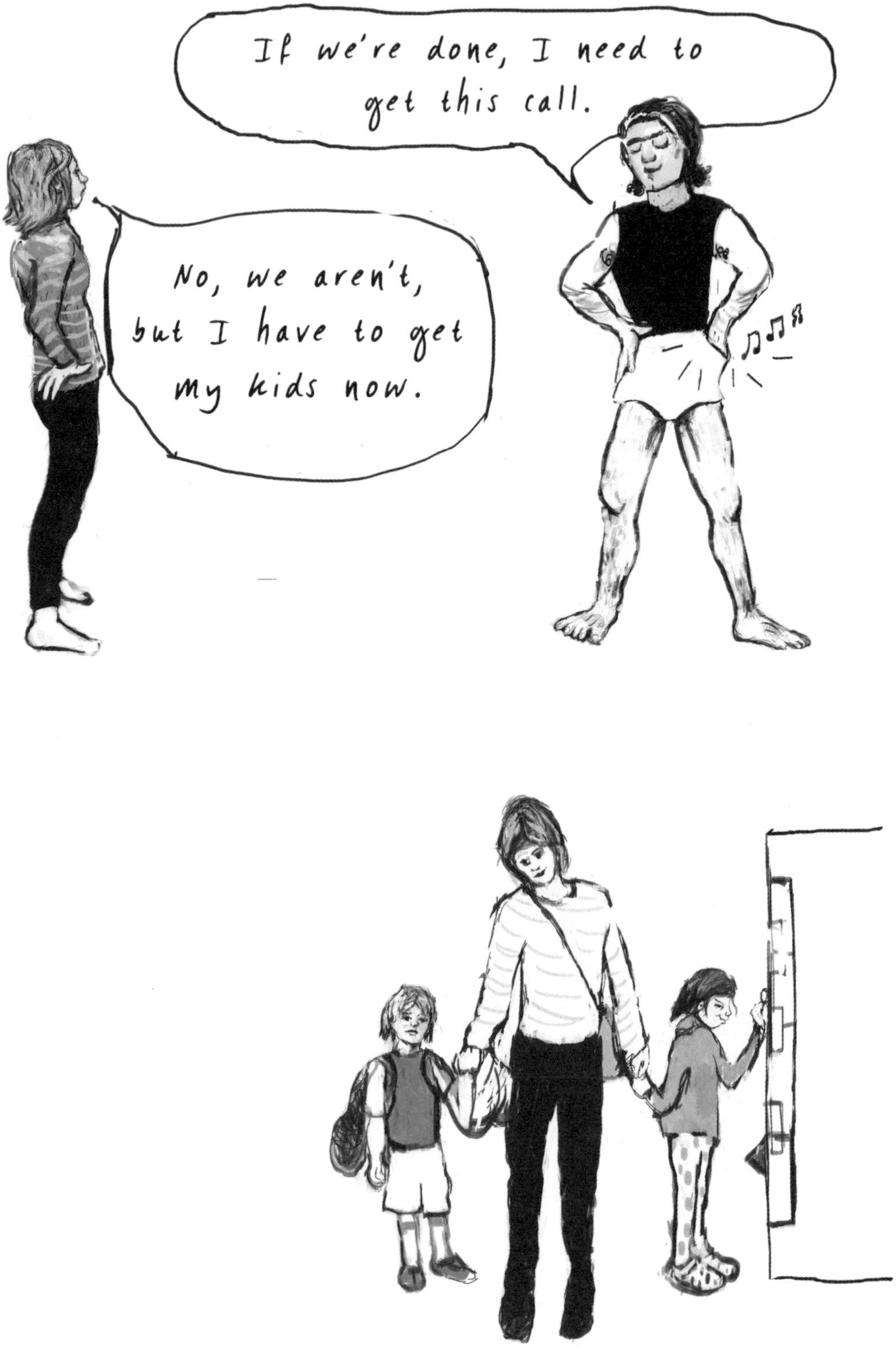
If we're done, I need to get this call.
No, we aren't, but I have to get my kids now.

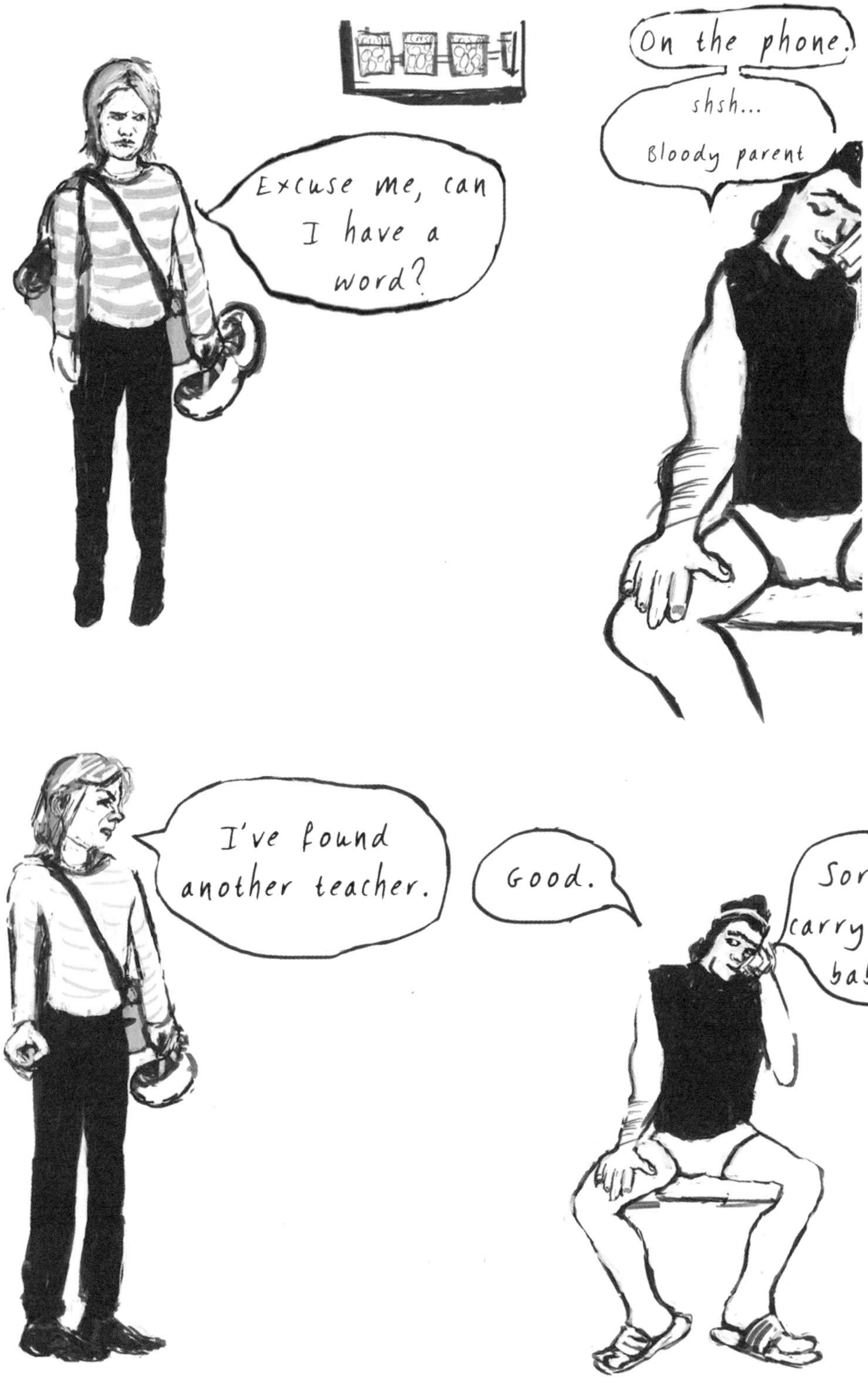
Excuse me, can I have a word?
On the phone.
shsh... Bloody parent
I've found another teacher.
Good.
Sorry, carry on, babe.

SPICY
HOT
HOT

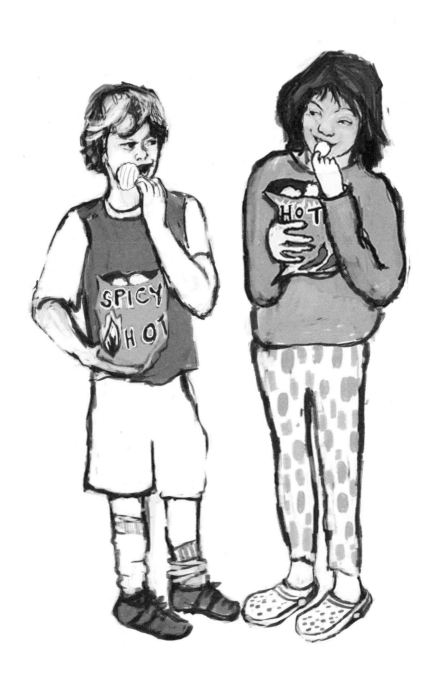

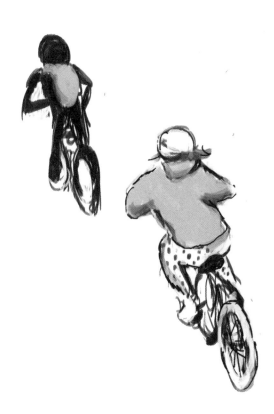
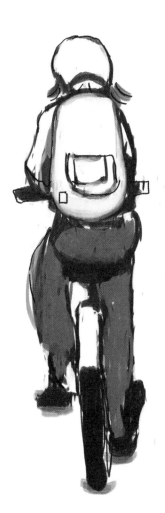

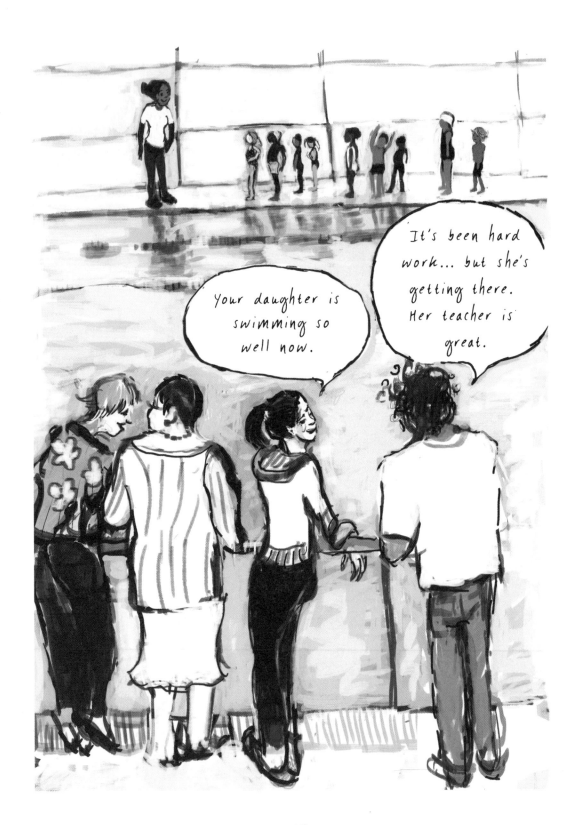

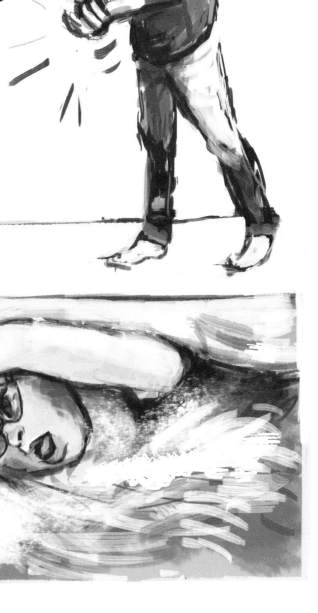

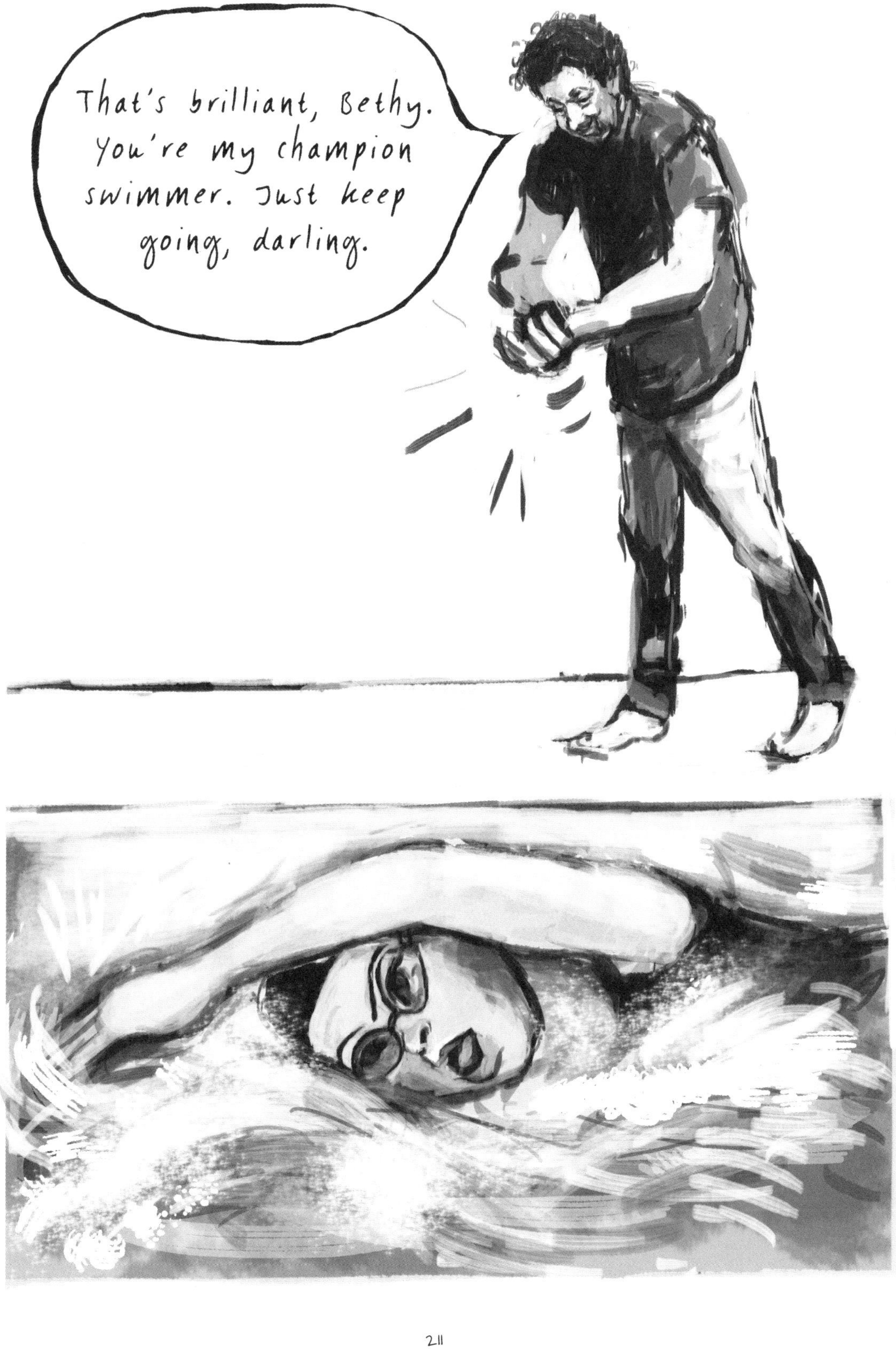
That's brilliant, Bethy. You're my champion swimmer. Just keep going, darling.

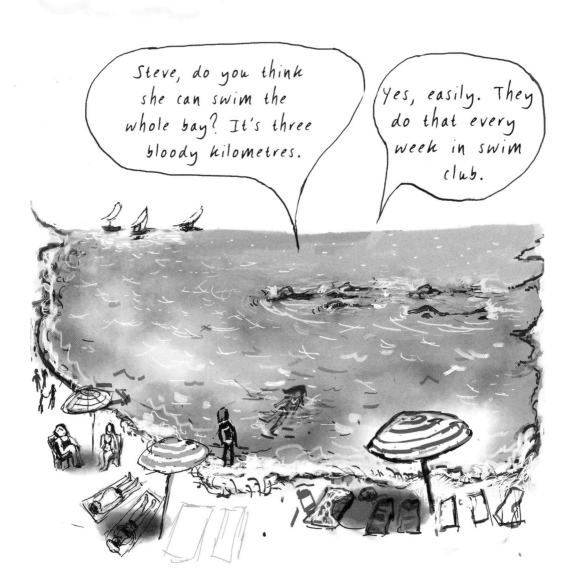

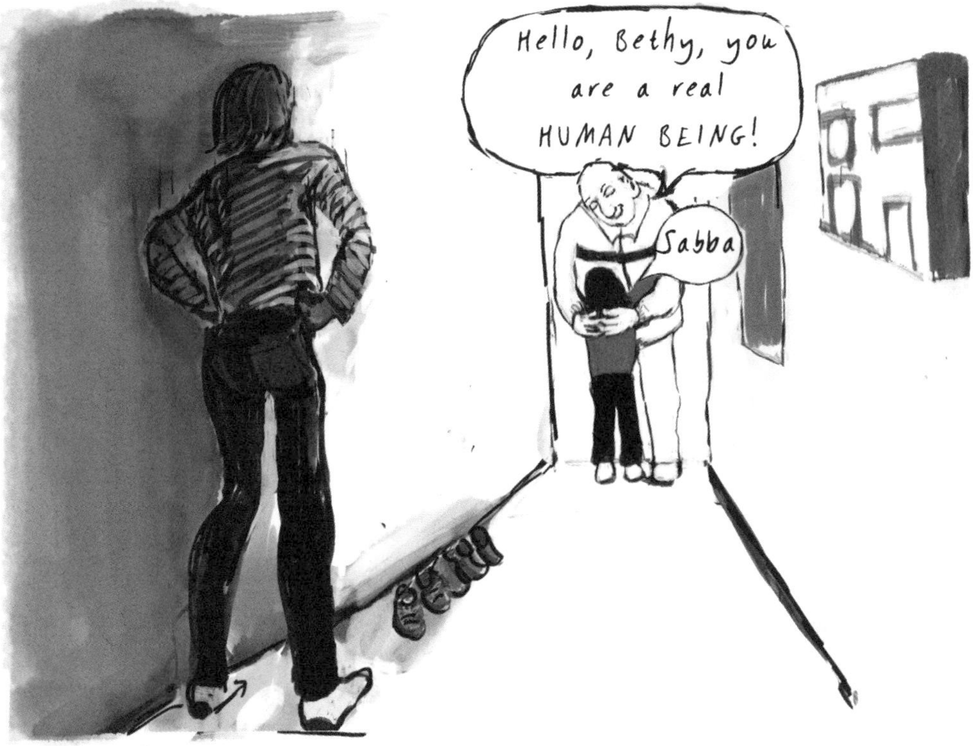
Hello, Bethy, you are a real HUMAN BEING!
Sabba

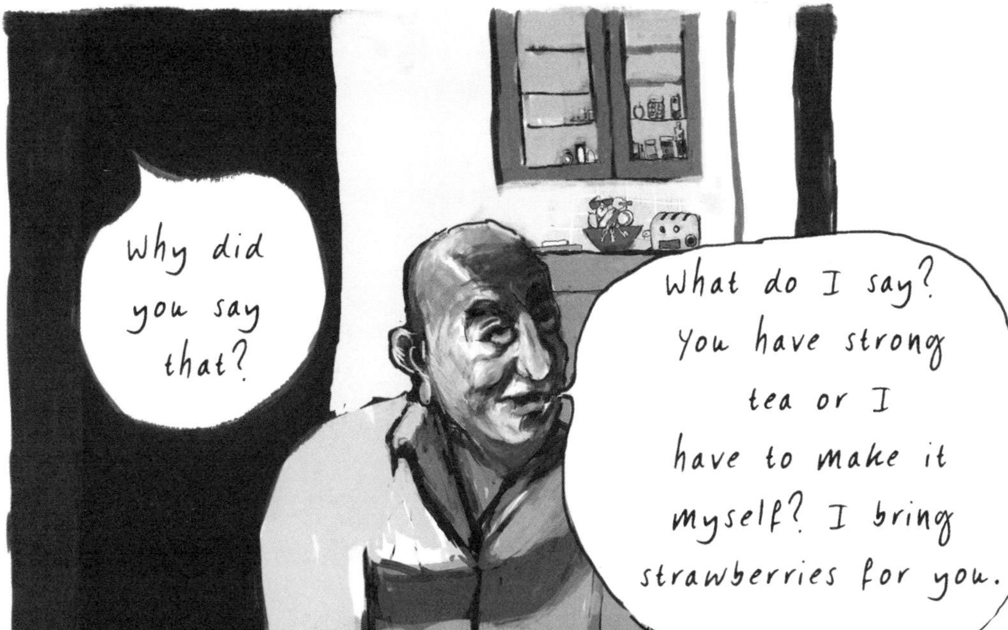
Why did you say that?
What do I say? You have strong tea or I have to make it myself? I bring strawberries for you.

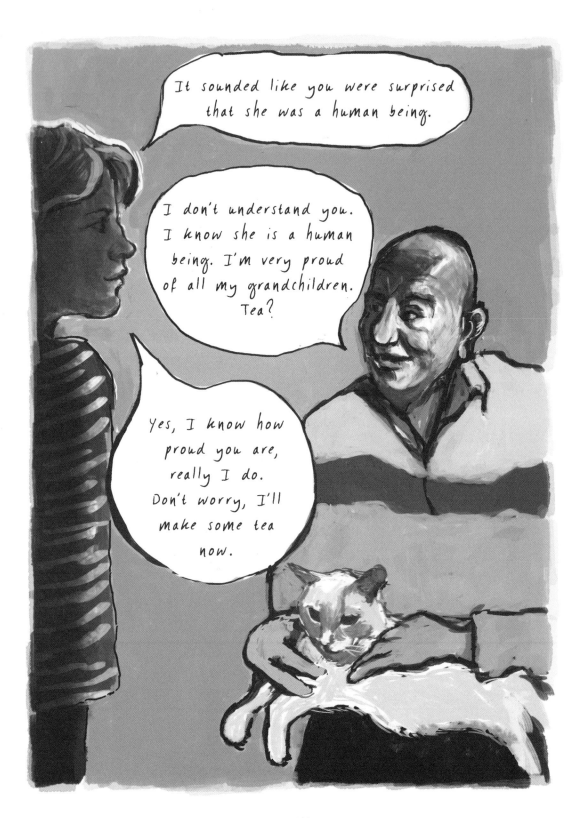

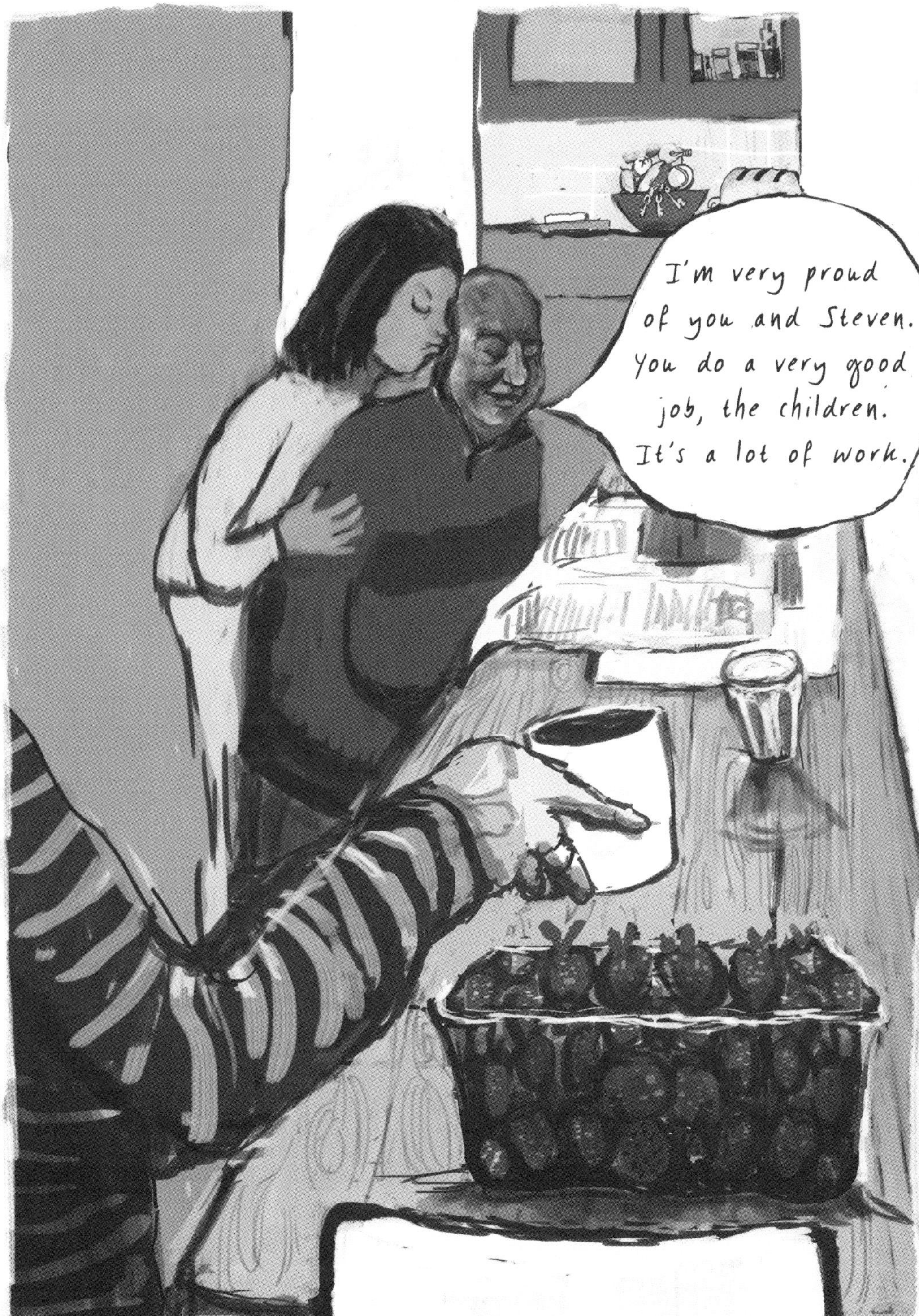
I'm very proud of you and Steven. You do a very good job, the children. It's a lot of work.

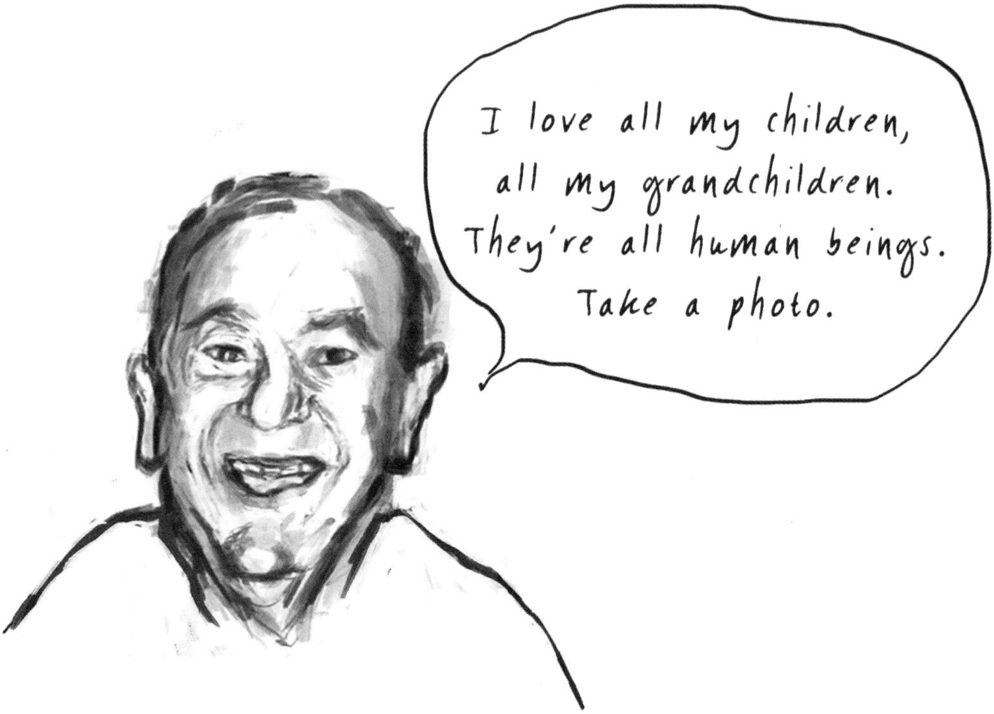

I love all my children, all my grandchildren. They're all human beings. Take a photo.

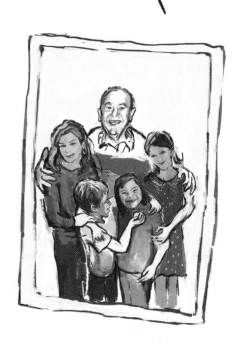

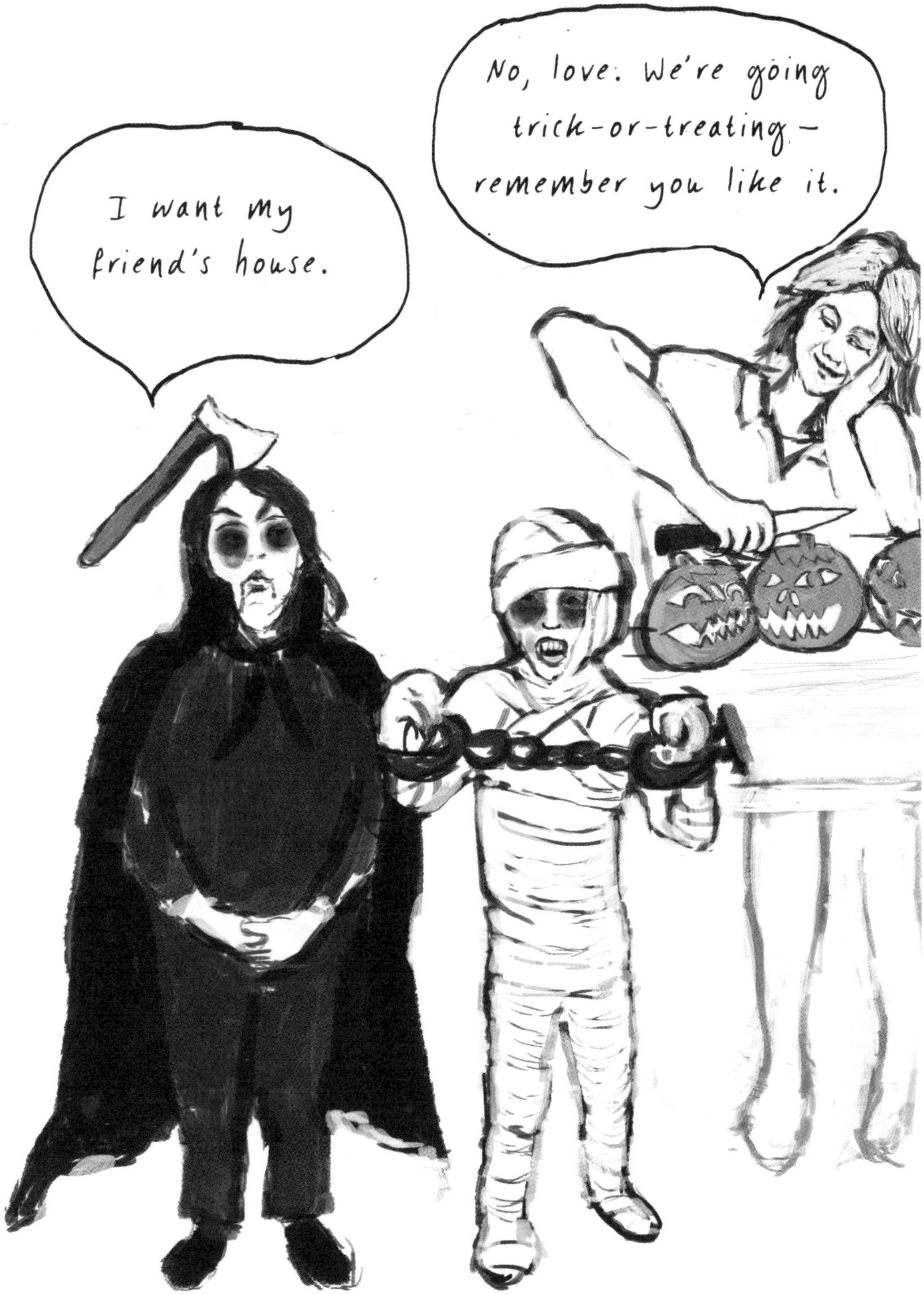
I want my friend's house.
No, love. We're going trick-or-treating – remember you like it.

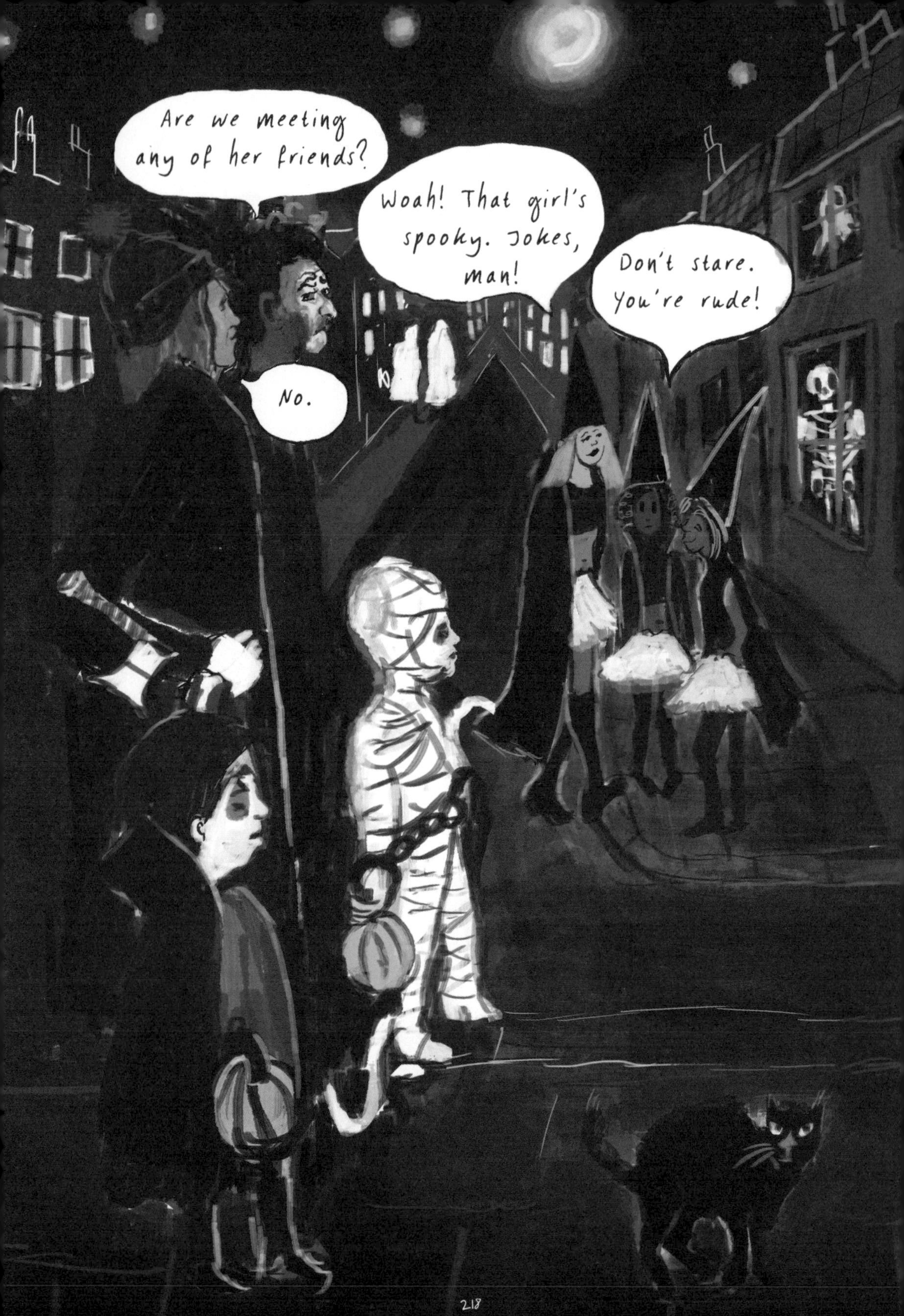
Are we meeting any of her friends?
No.
Woah! That girl's spooky. Jokes, man!
Don't stare. You're rude!

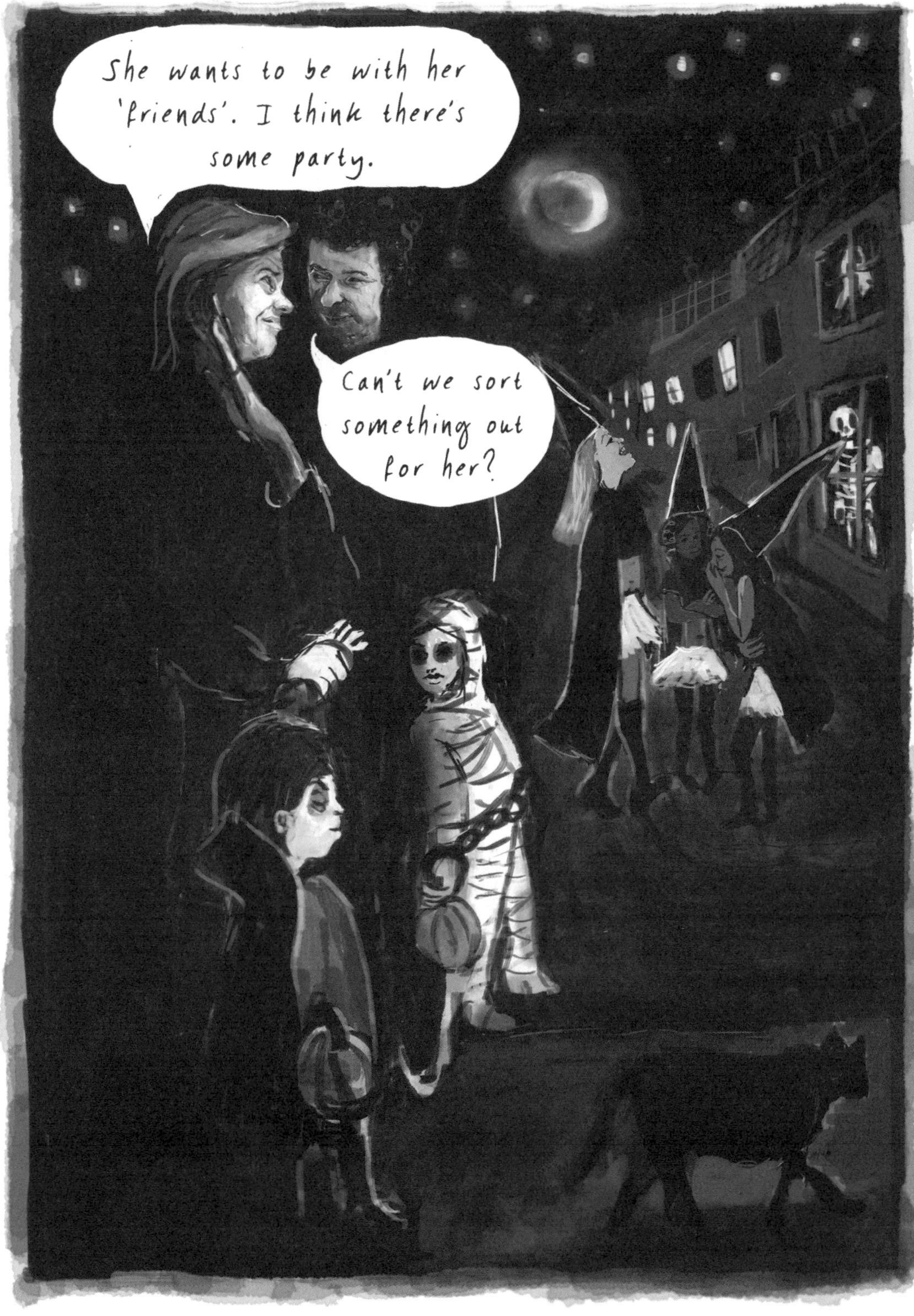
She wants to be with her 'friends'. I think there's some party.
Can't we sort something out for her?

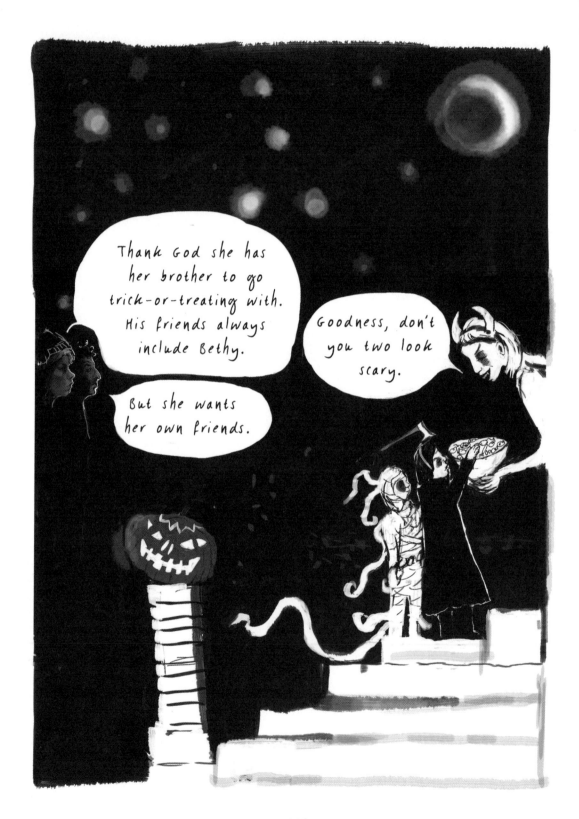

220

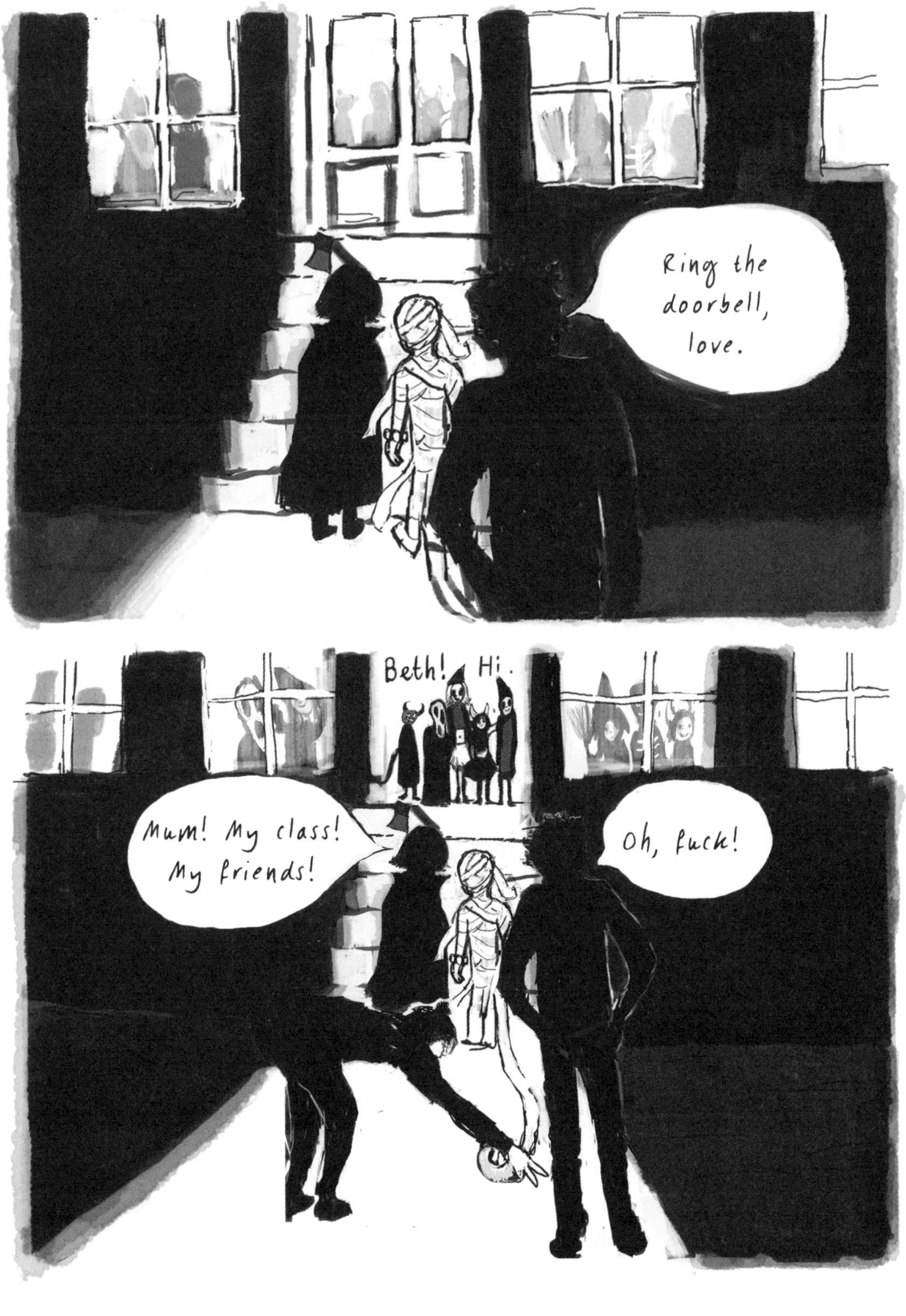
Ring the doorbell, love.
Beth! Hi.
Mum! My class! My friends!
Oh, fuck!

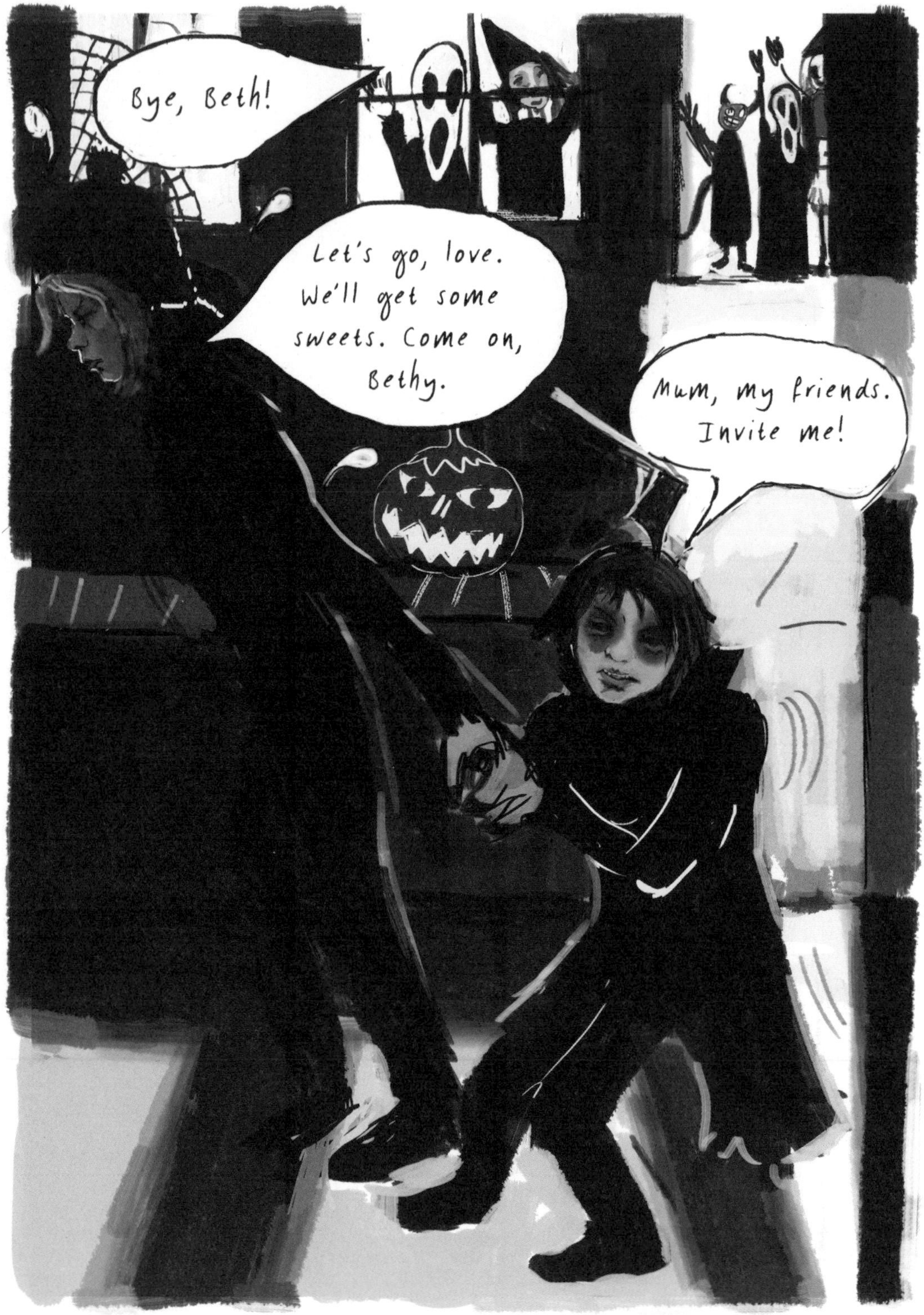
Bye, Beth!
Let's go, love. We'll get some sweets. Come on, Bethy.
Mum, my friends. Invite me!

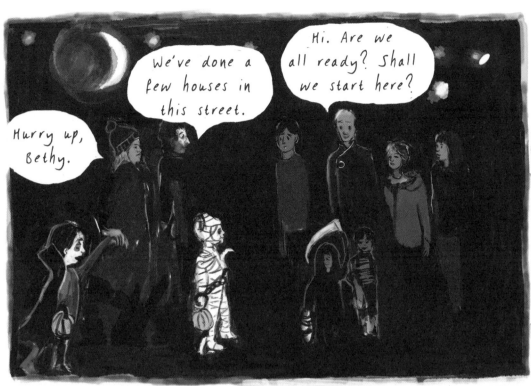

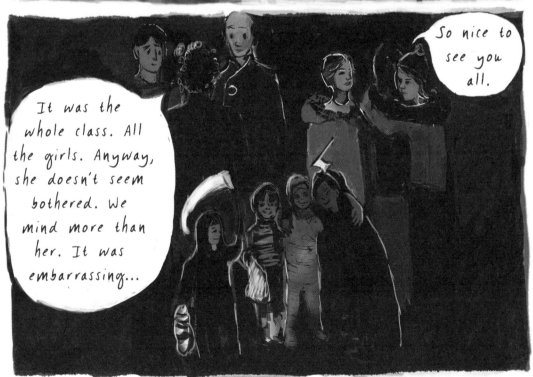

223

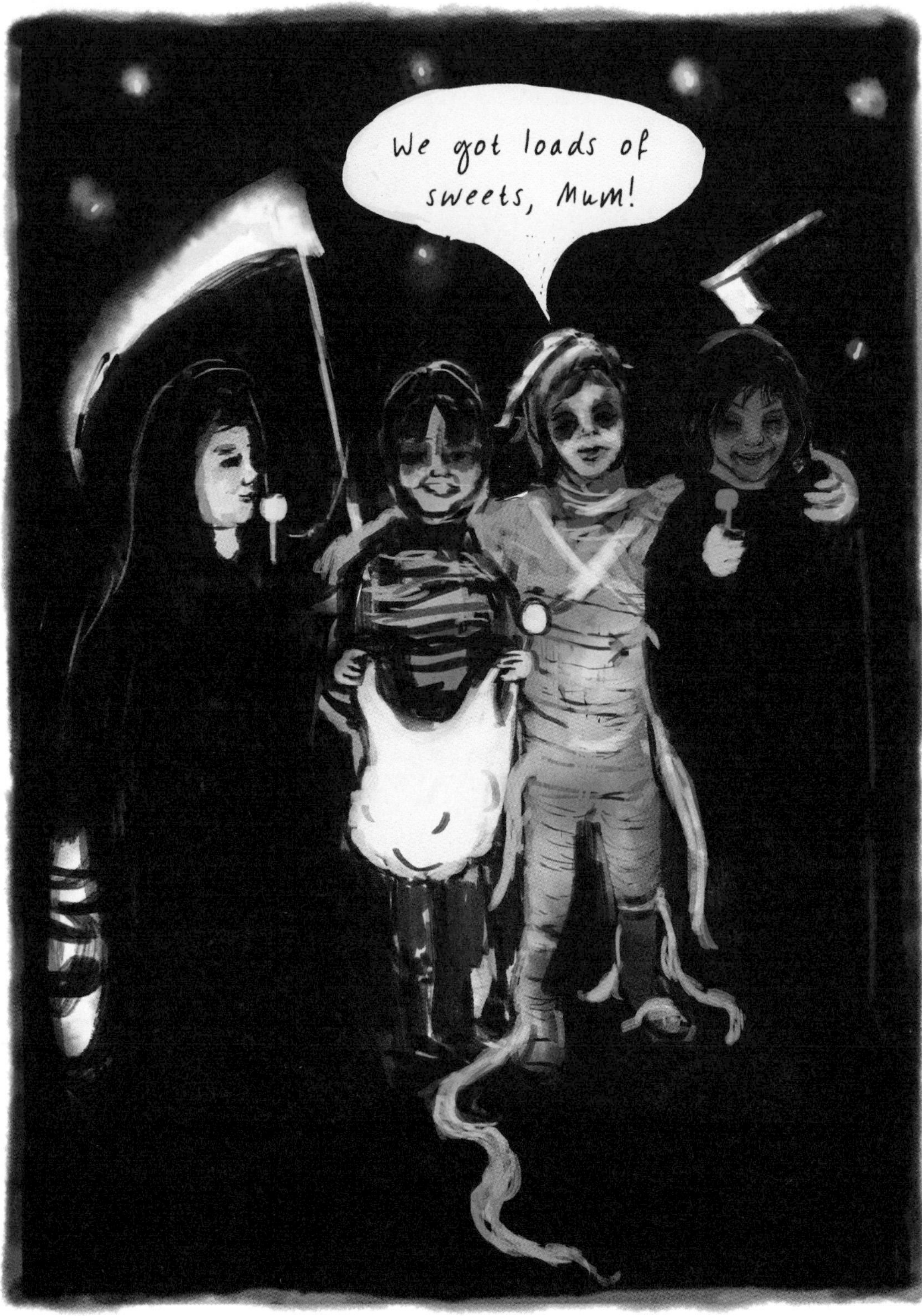
We got loads of sweets, Mum!

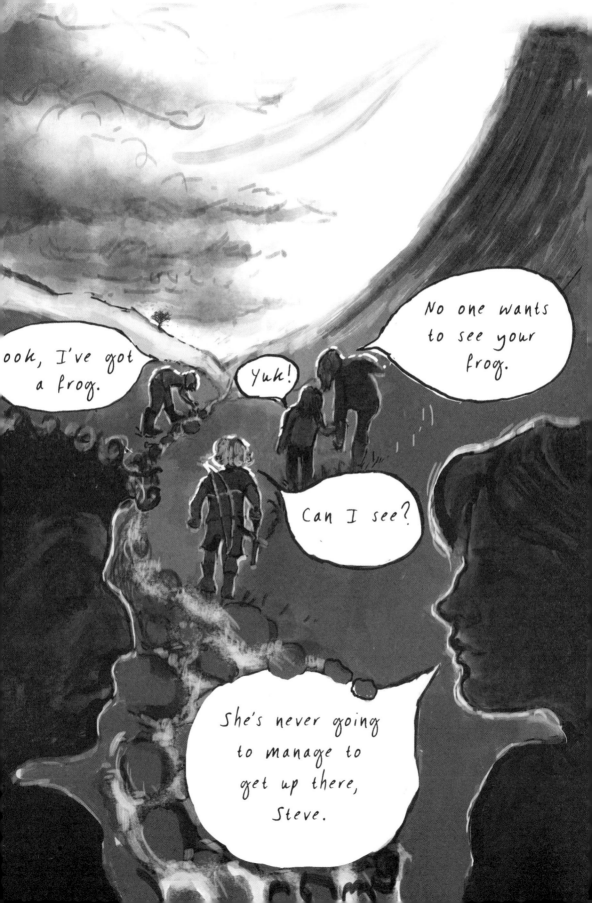

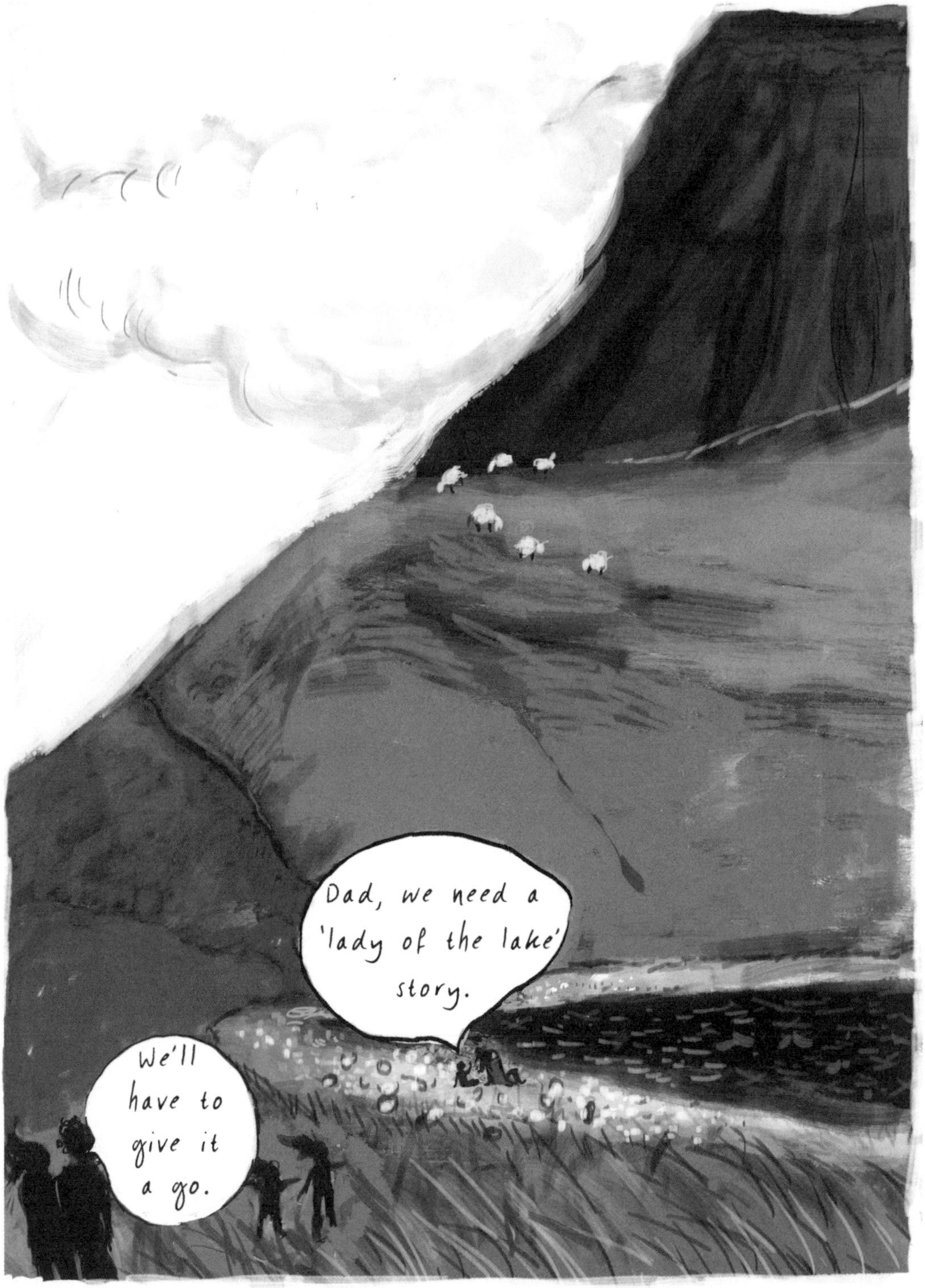
Dad, we need a 'lady of the lake' story.
We'll have to give it a go.

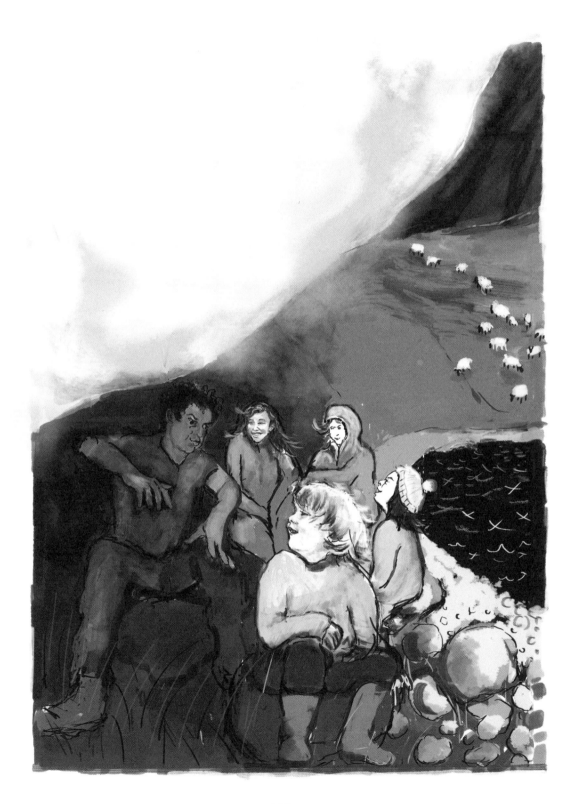

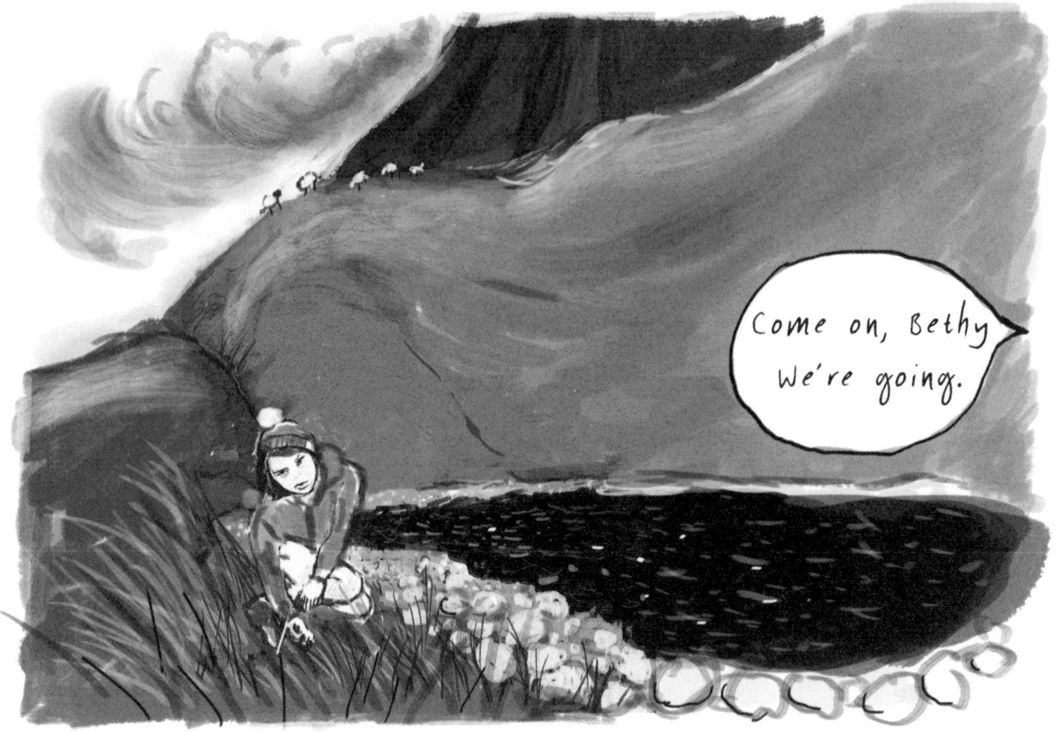
Come on, Bethy
We're going.

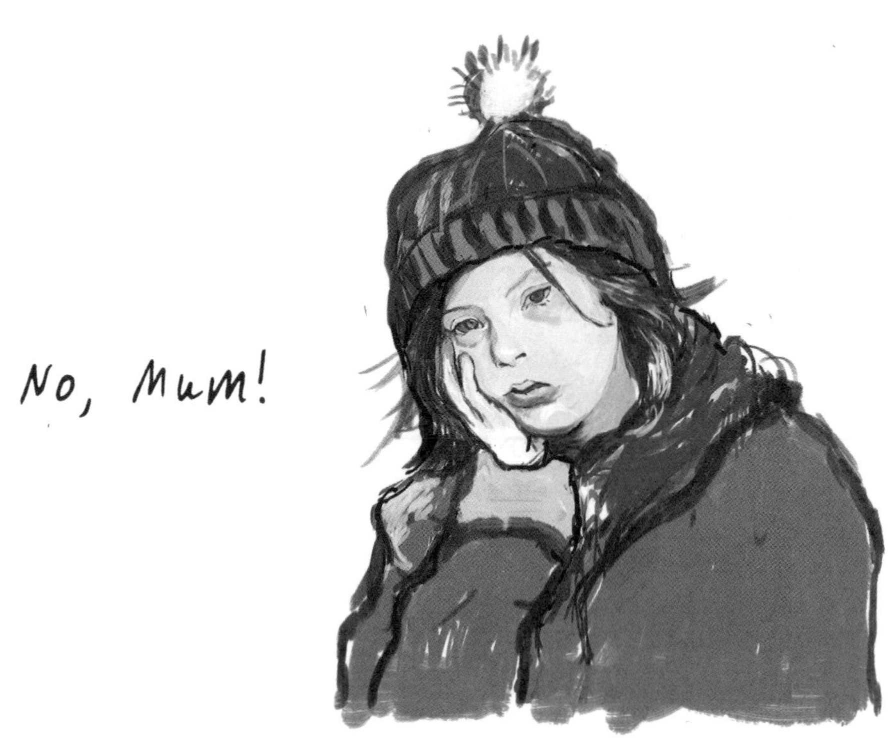
No, Mum!

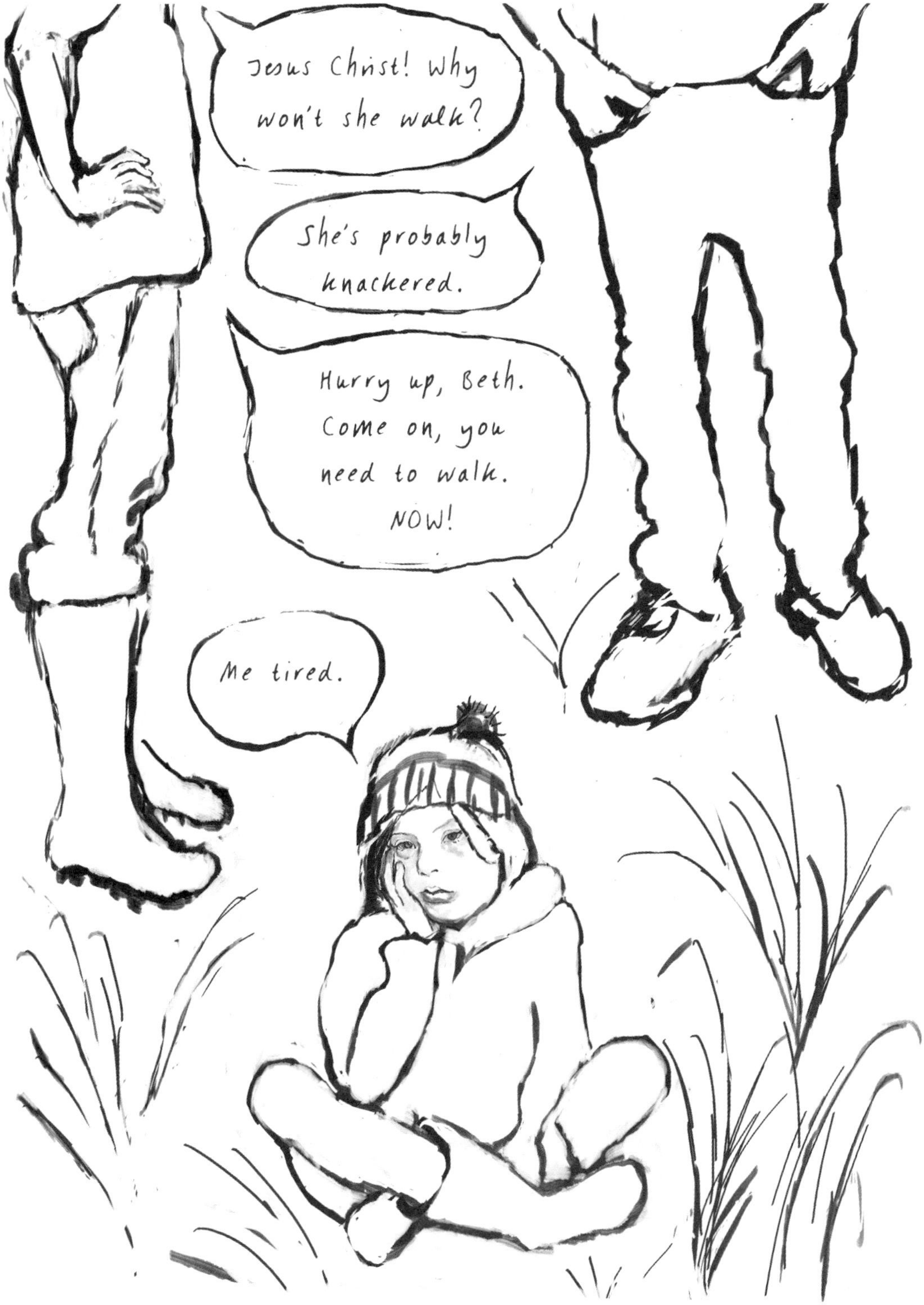
Jesus Christ! Why won't she walk?
She's probably knackered.
Hurry up, Beth. Come on, you need to walk. NOW!
Me tired.

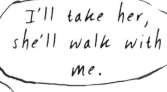

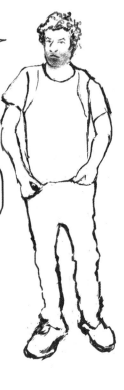

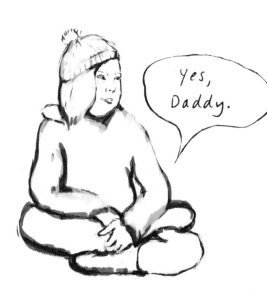

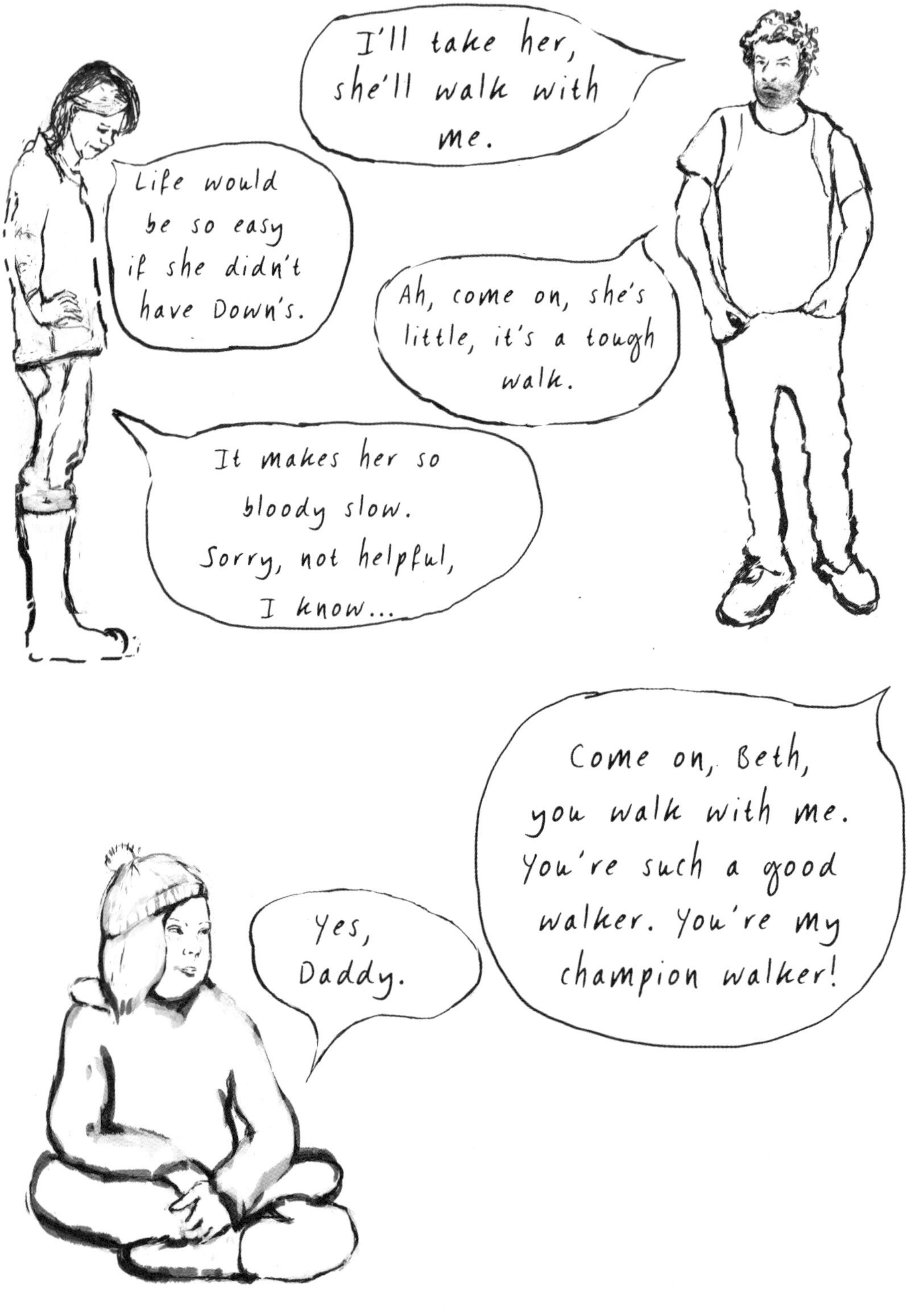

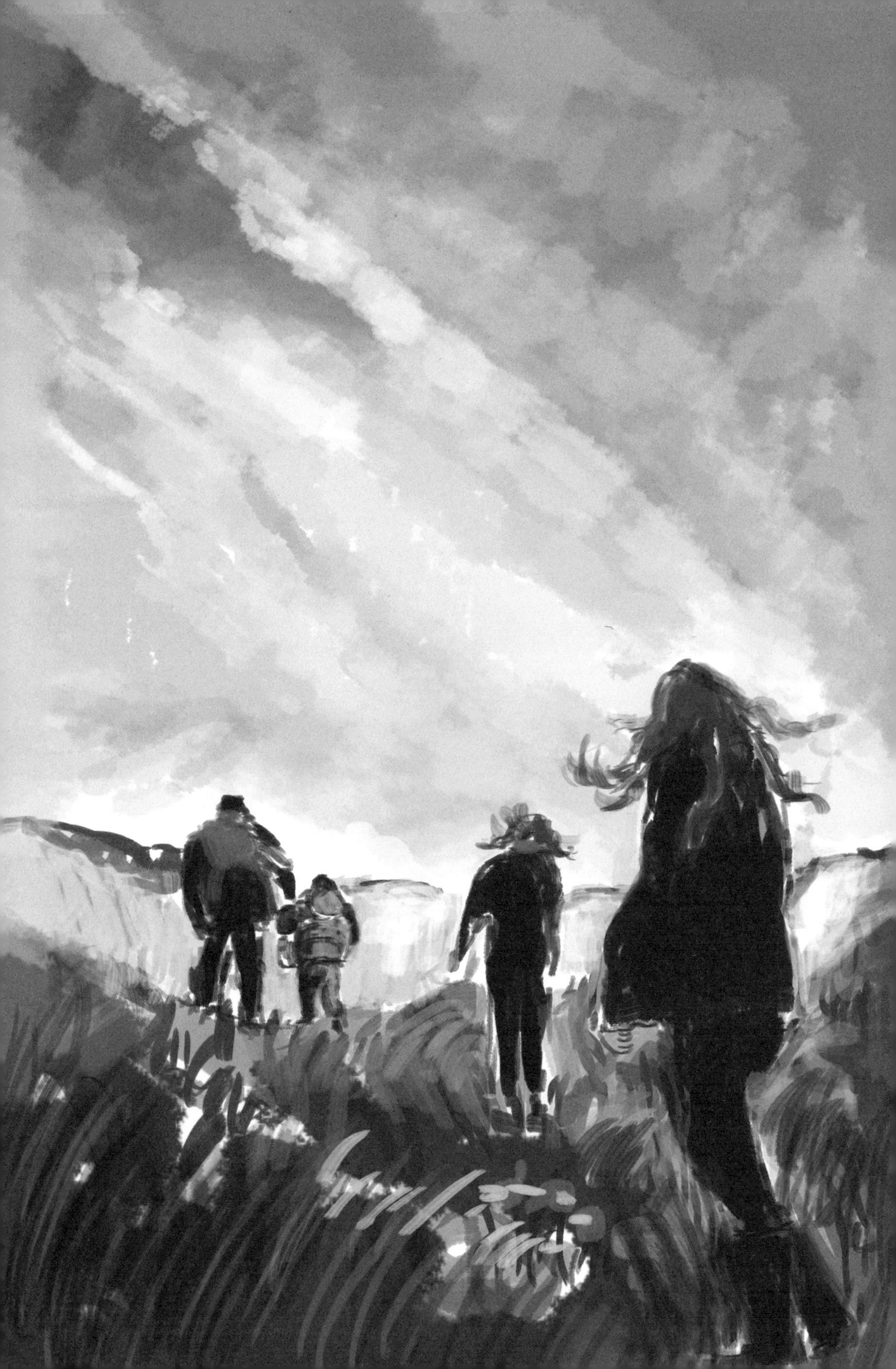

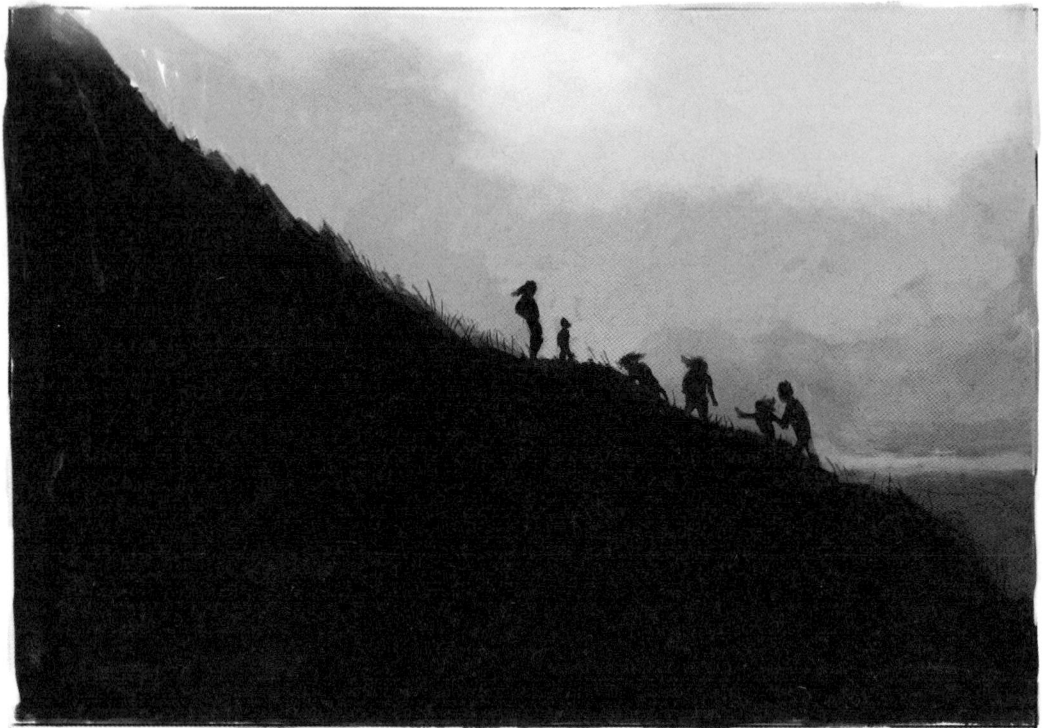

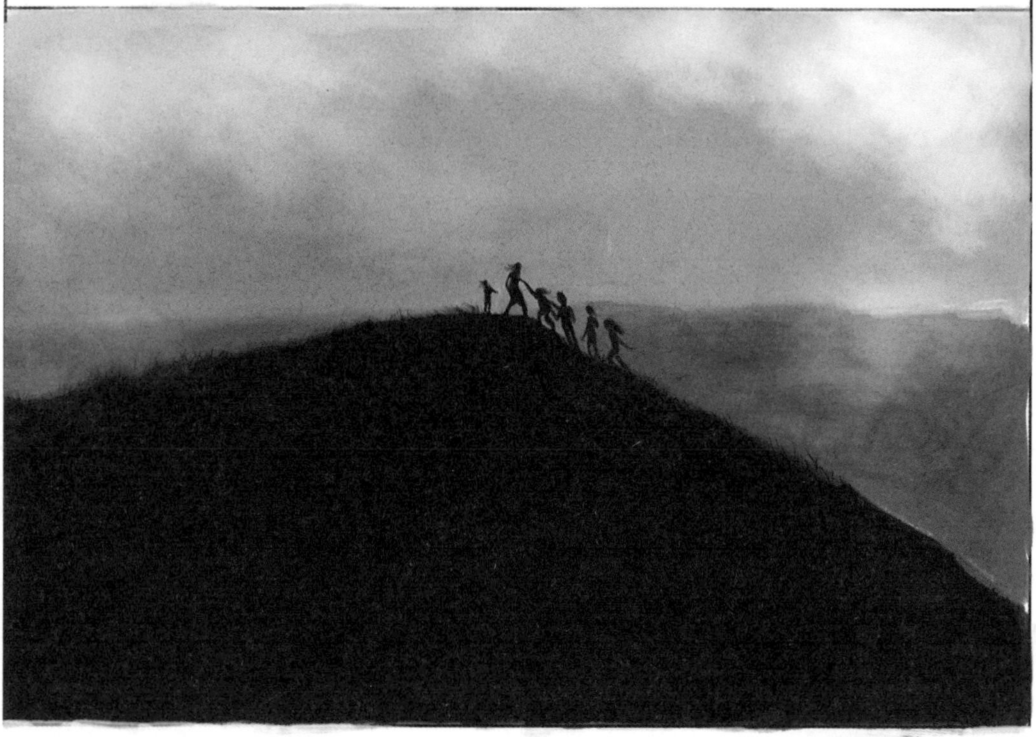

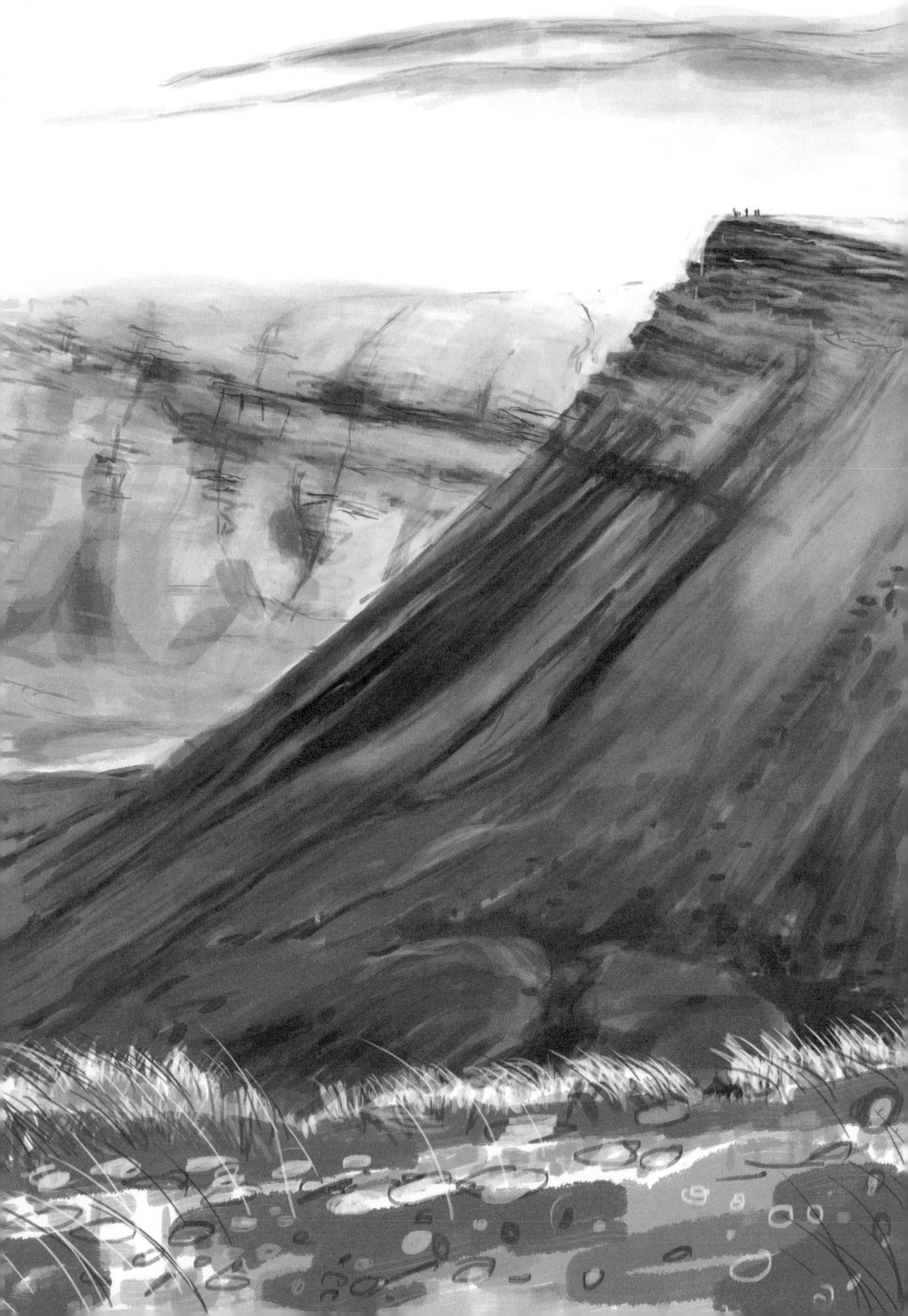

August 2012

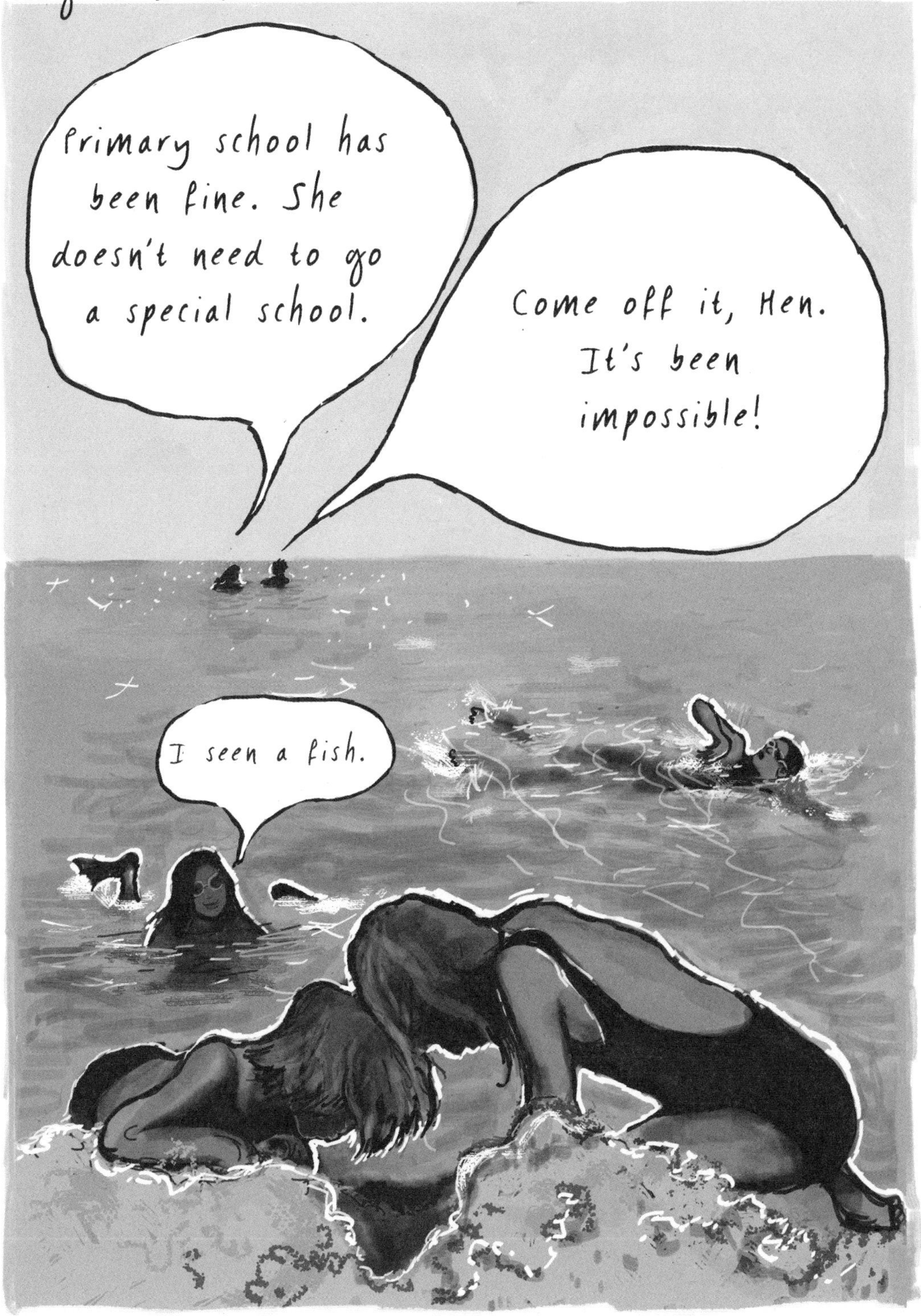
Primary school has been fine. She doesn't need to go a special school.
Come off it, Hen. It's been impossible!
I seen a fish.

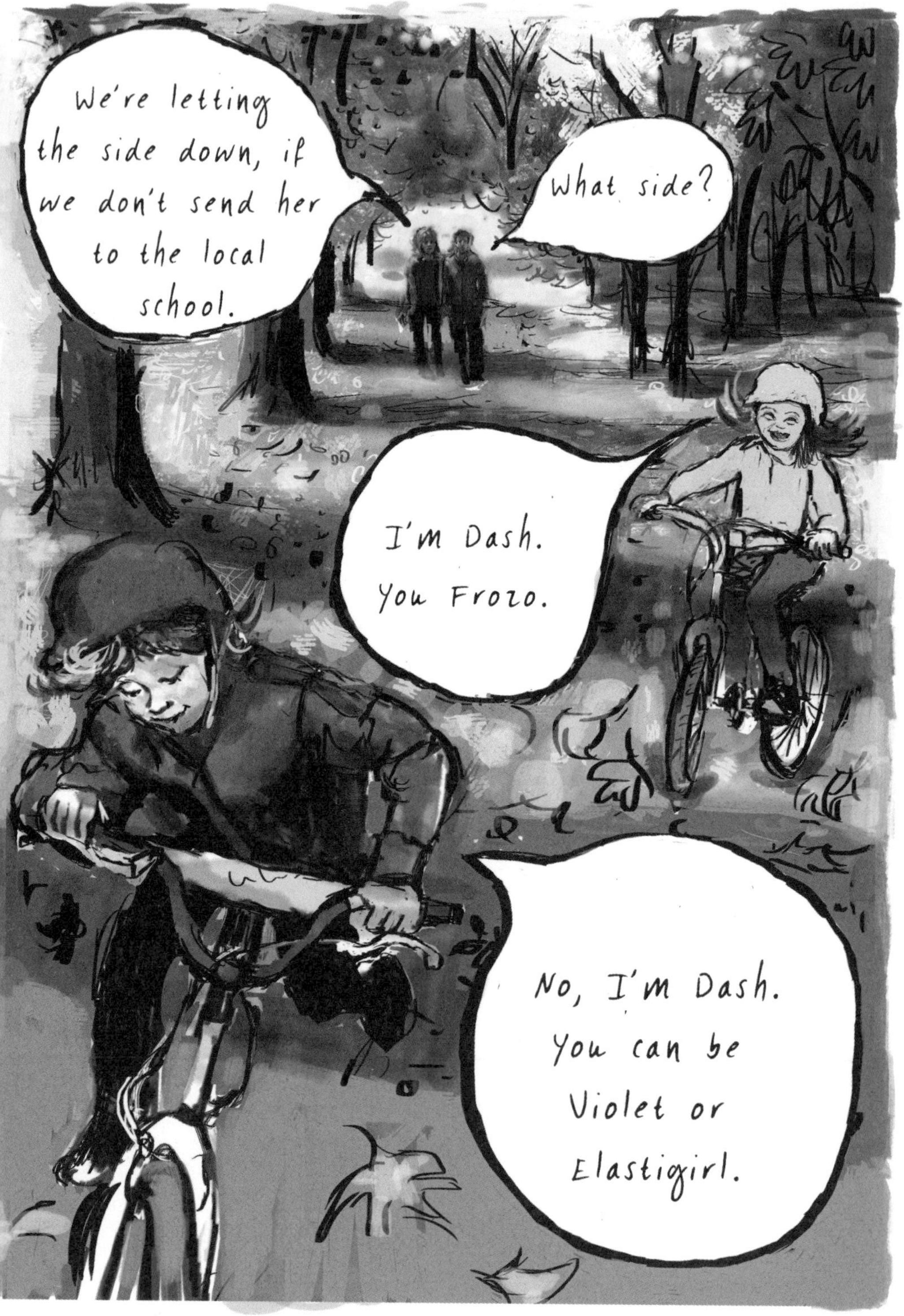
We're letting the side down, if we don't send her to the local school.
What side?
I'm Dash. You Frozo.
No, I'm Dash. You can be Violet or Elastigirl.

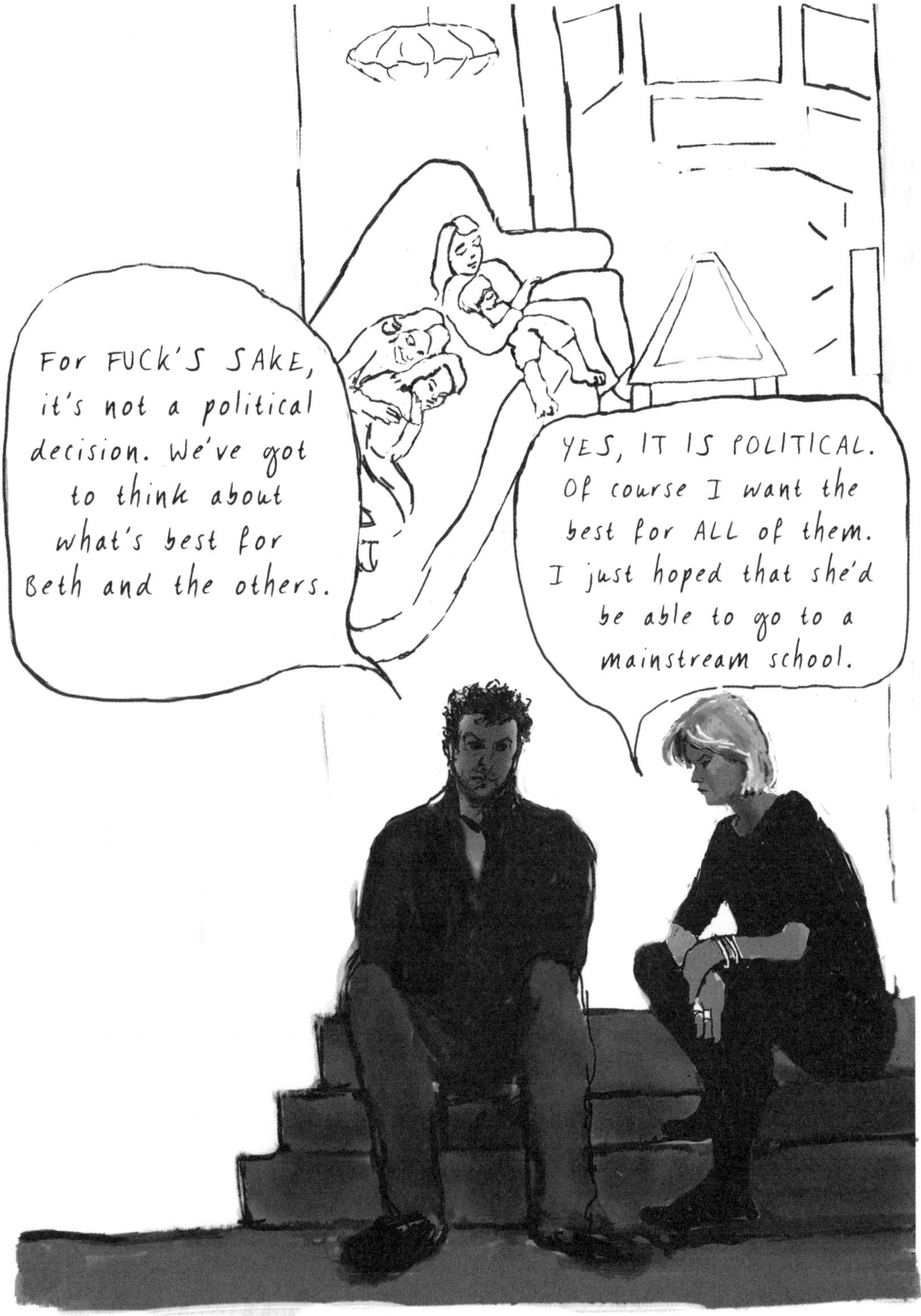
For FUCK'S SAKE, it's not a political decision. We've got to think about what's best for Beth and the others.
YES, IT IS POLITICAL. Of course I want the best for ALL of them. I just hoped that she'd be able to go to a mainstream school.

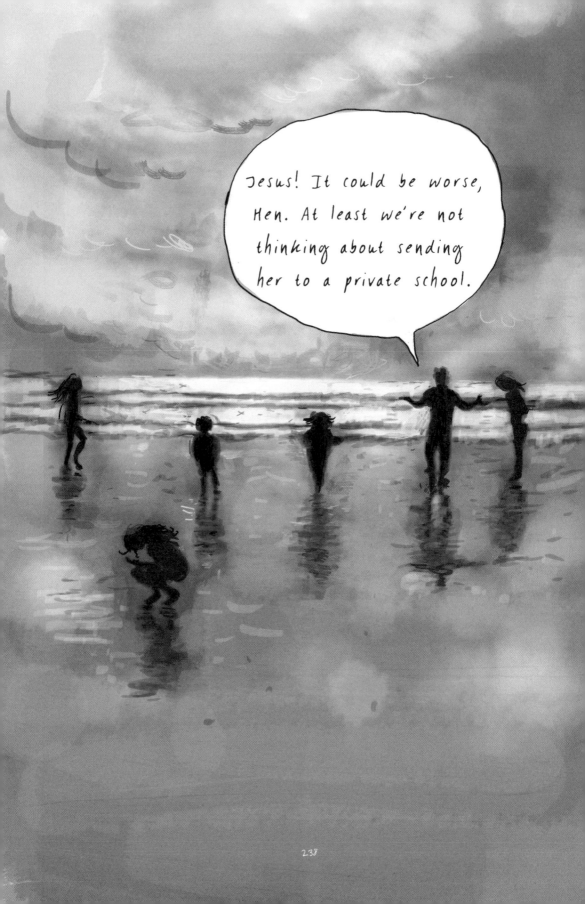

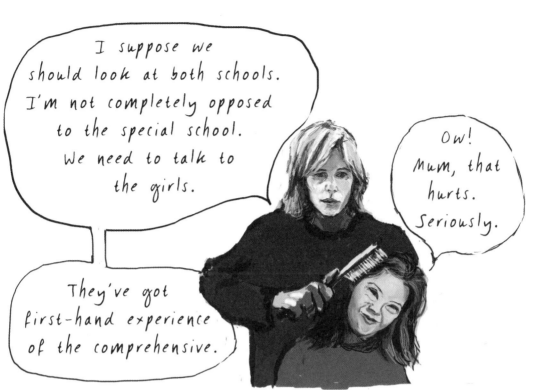

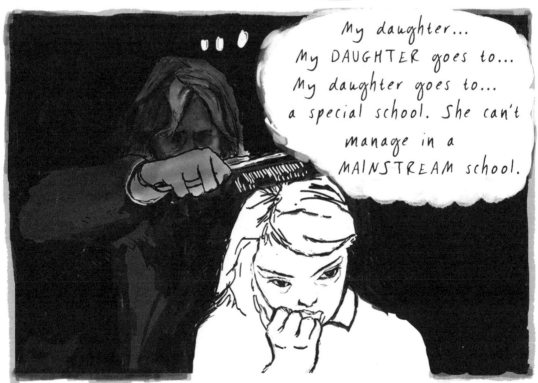

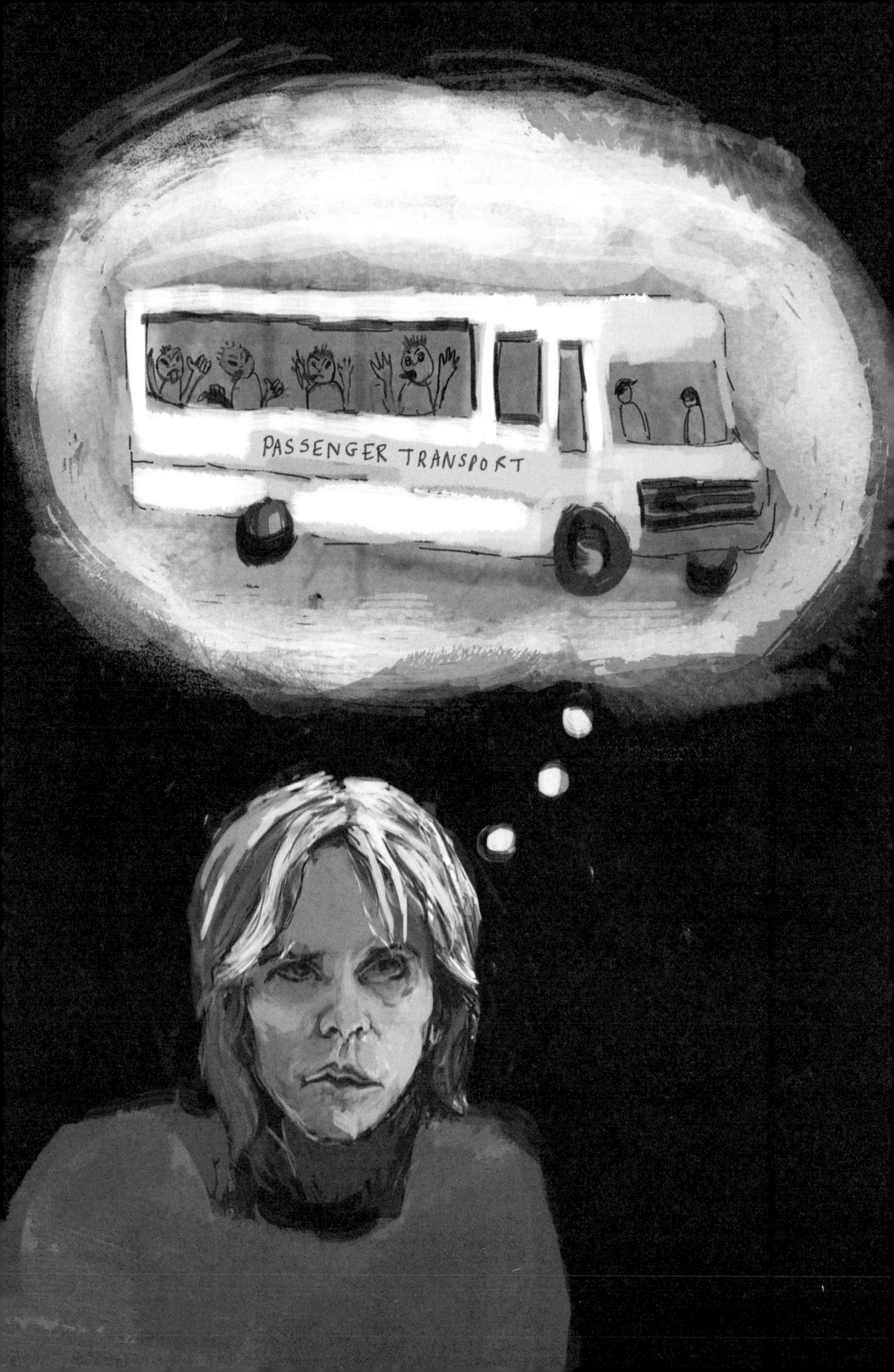
PASSENGER TRANSPORT

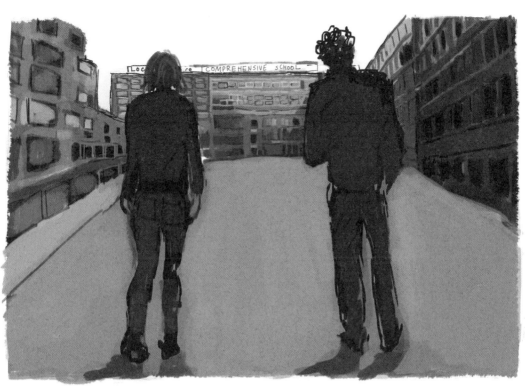

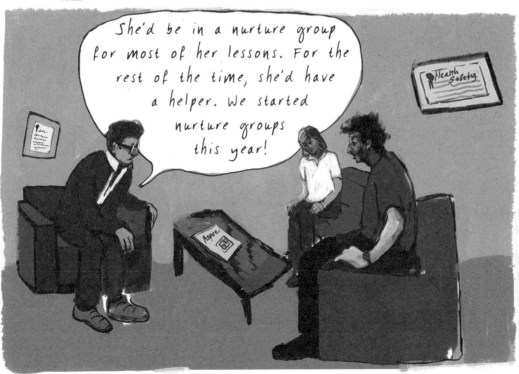

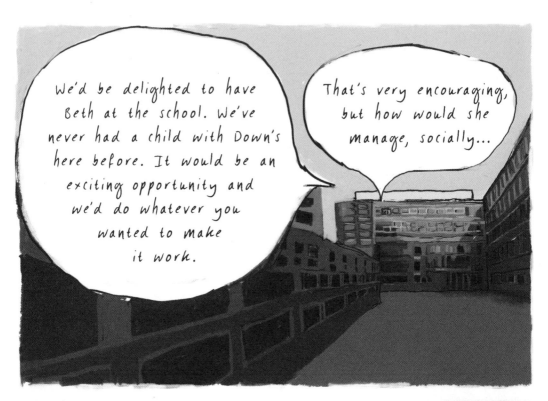

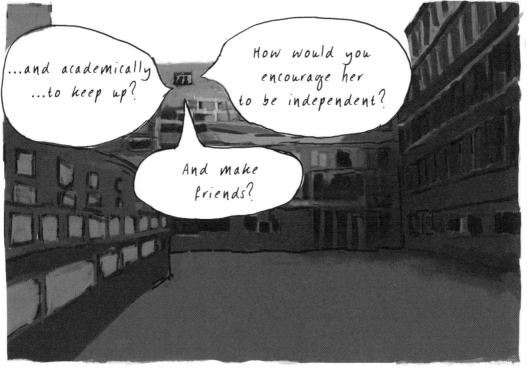

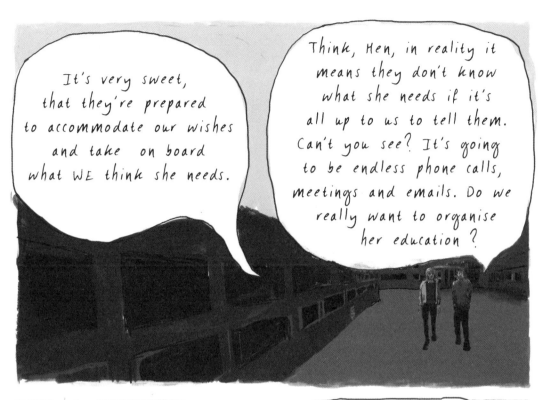

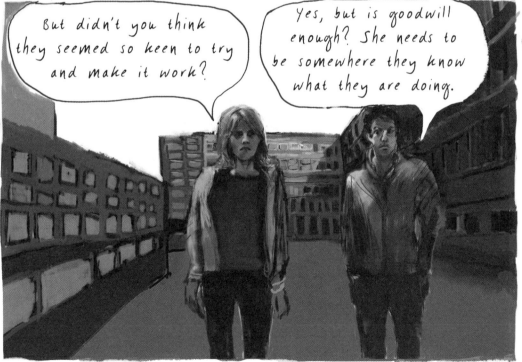

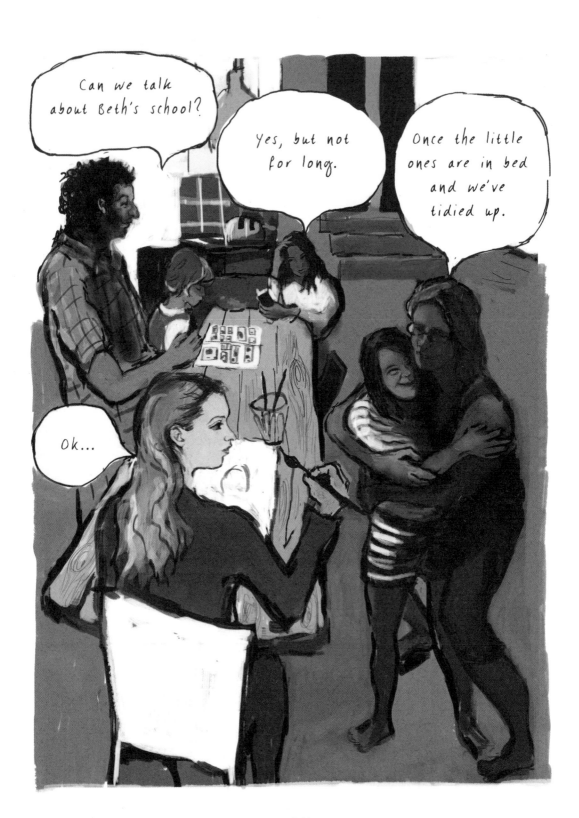

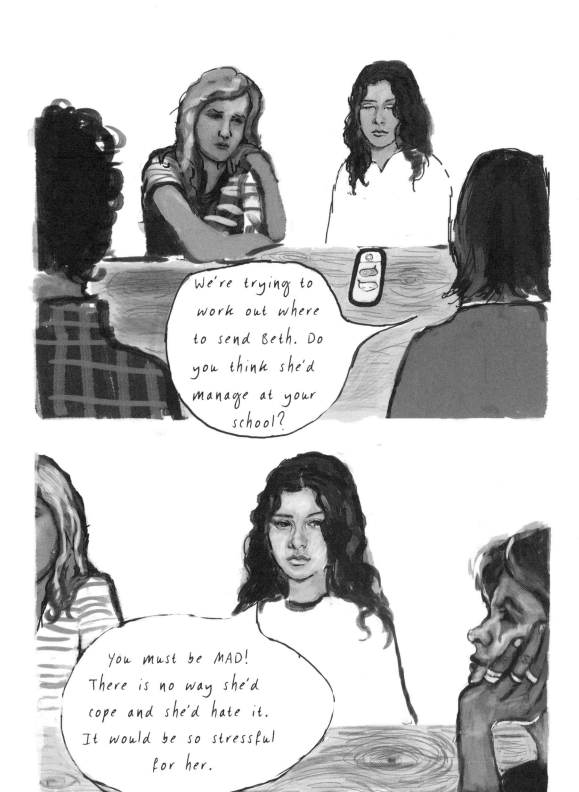

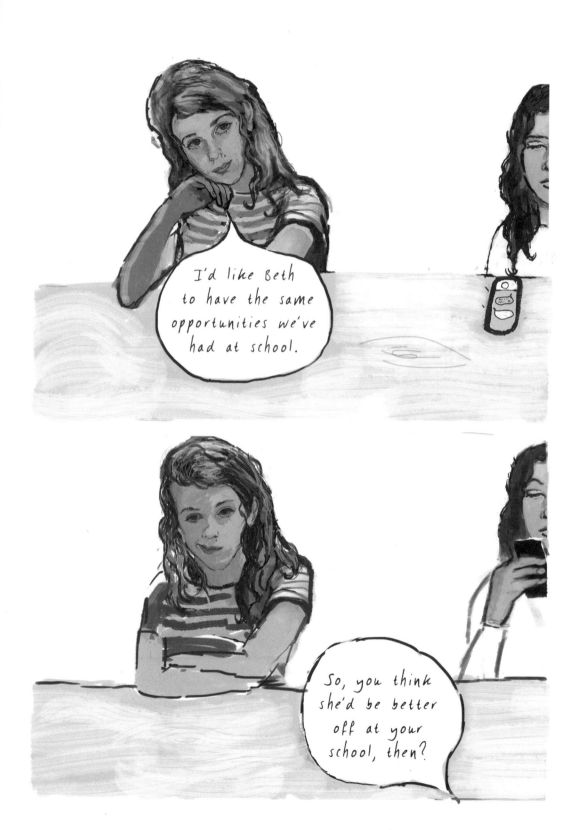

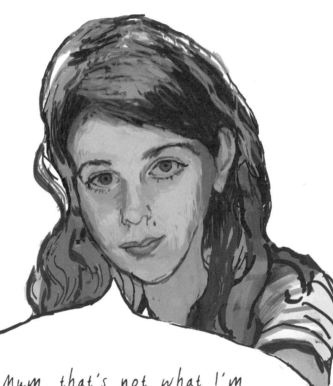

No, Mum, that's not what I'm saying. I want her to have the chance to be at the same level as the rest of her class, so she doesn't always feel she's at the bottom of the pile. She'll never get that at my school.

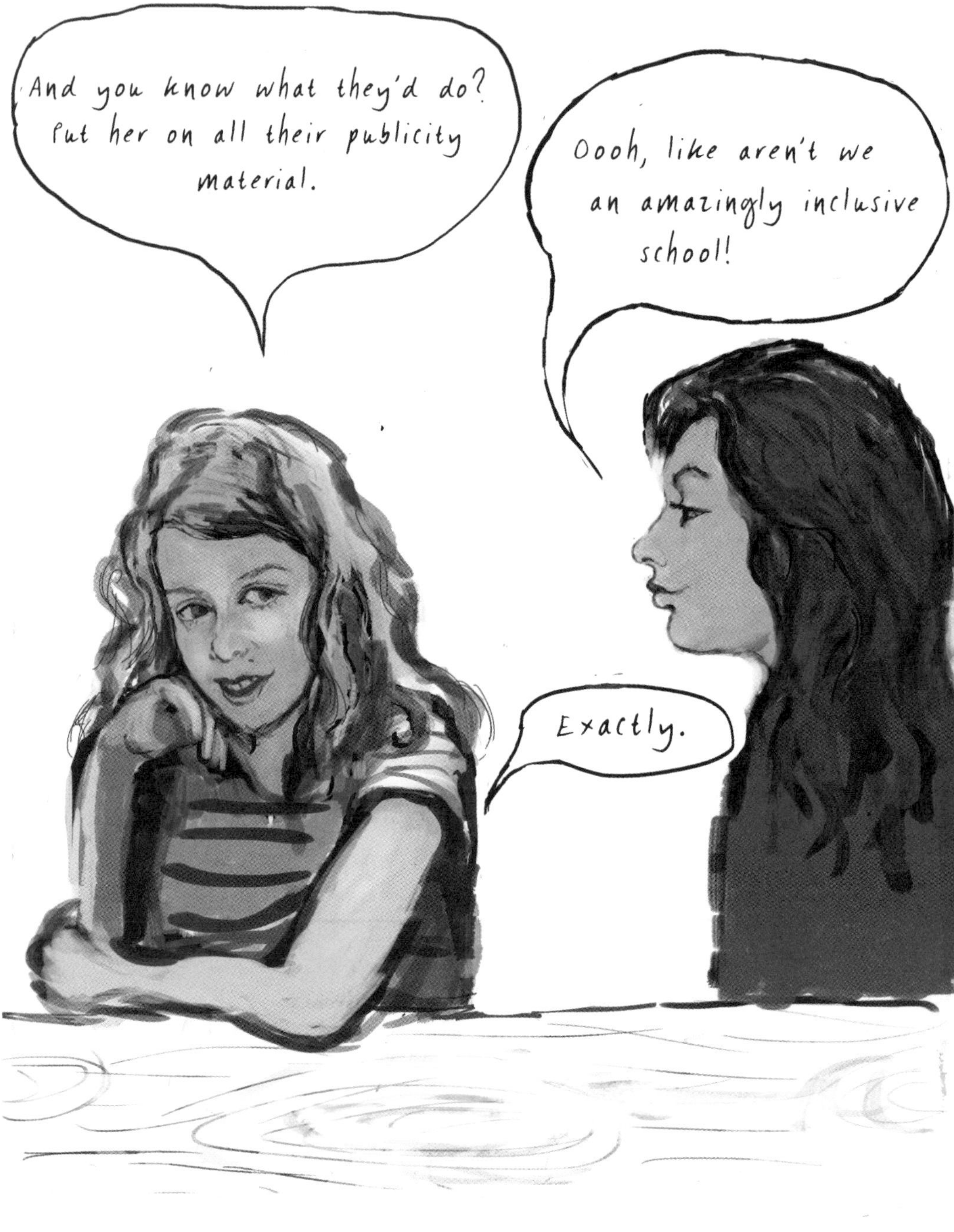
And you know what they'd do? Put her on all their publicity material.
Oooh, like aren't we an amazingly inclusive school!
Exactly.

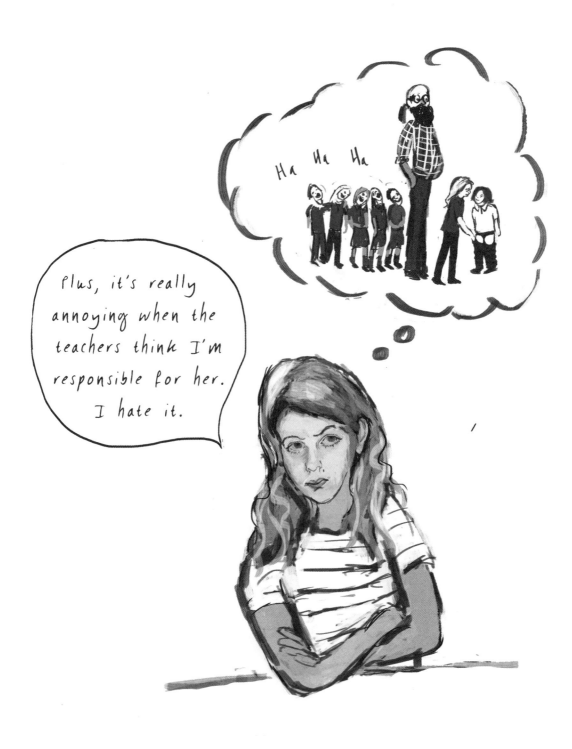

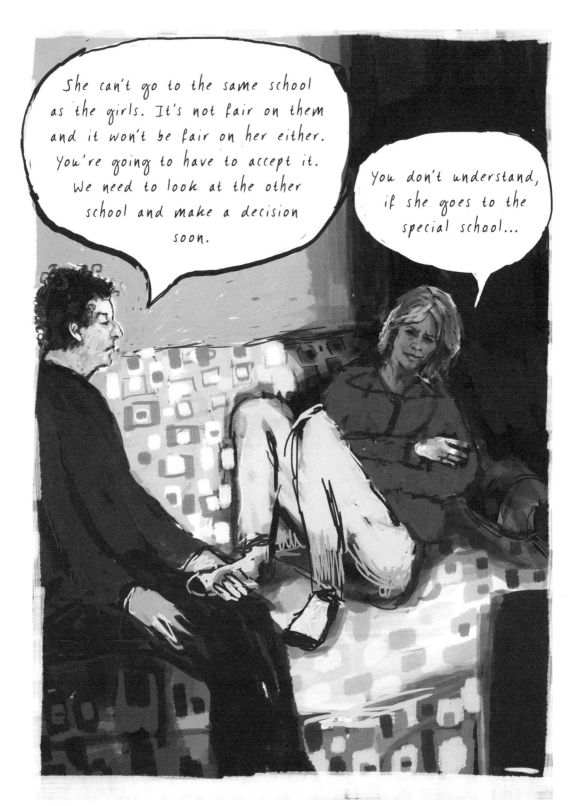

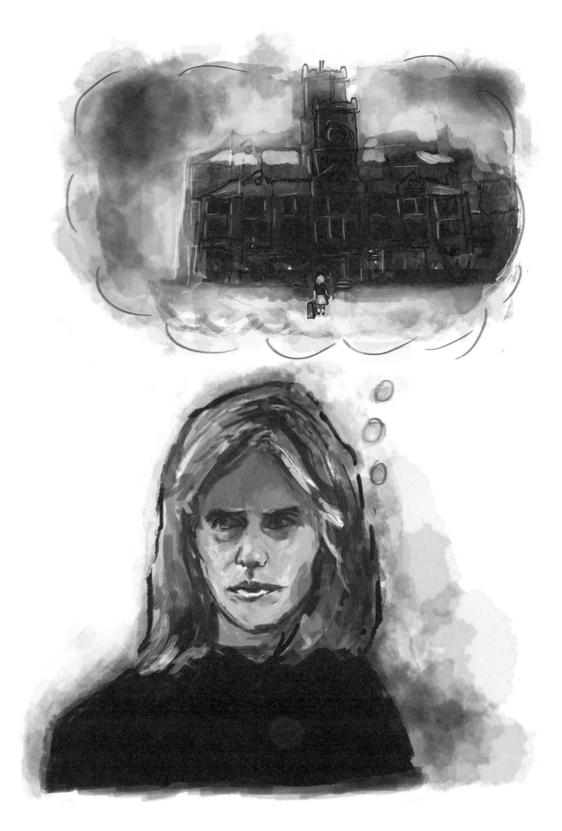

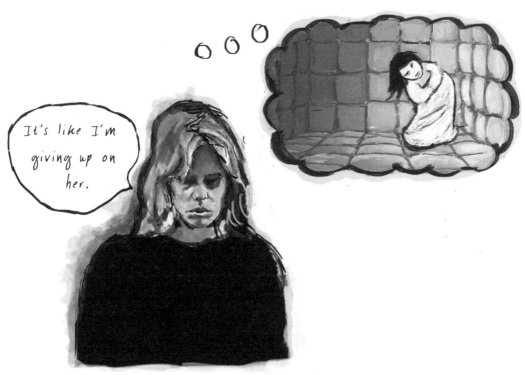

It's like I'm giving up on her.

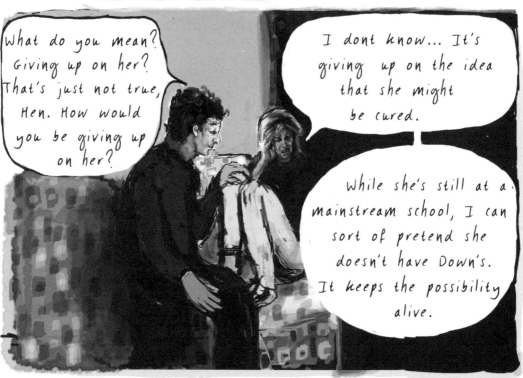

What do you mean? Giving up on her? That's just not true, Hen. How would you be giving up on her?

I don't know... It's giving up on the idea that she might be cured.

While she's still at a mainstream school, I can sort of pretend she doesn't have Down's. It keeps the possibility alive.

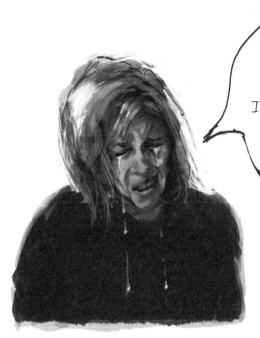

I can hope that she might miraculously get better. I know it doesn't make sense, Steve, but I can't bear the thought of sending her to a special school.

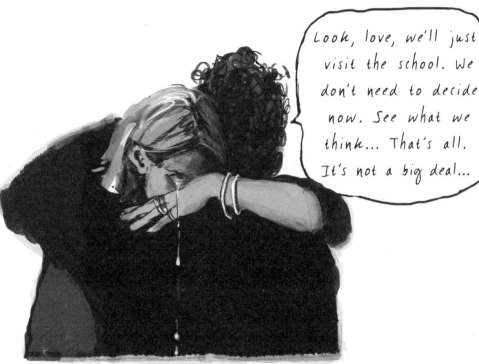

Look, love, we'll just visit the school. We don't need to decide now. See what we think... That's all. It's not a big deal...

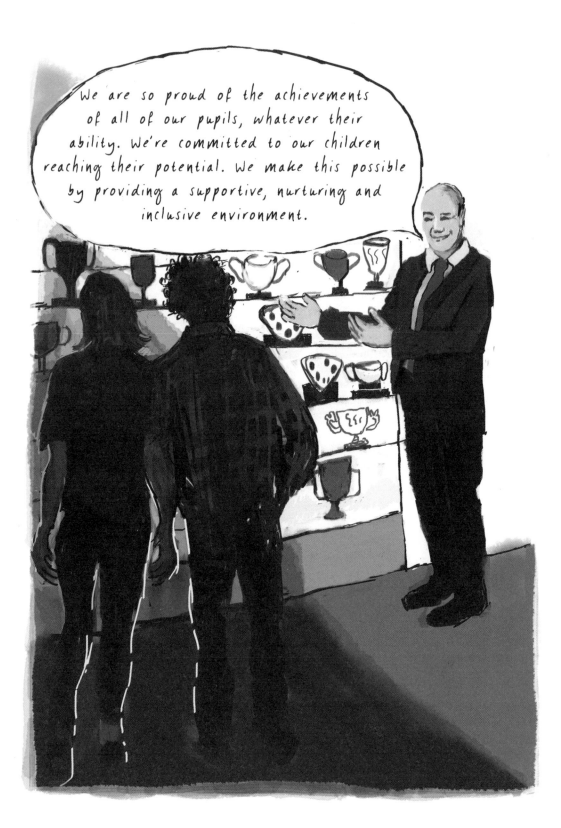

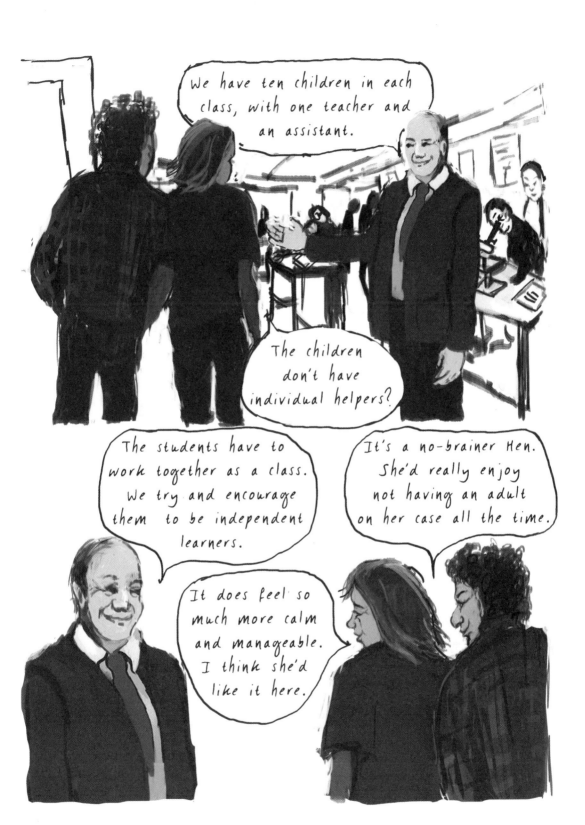

Part Five

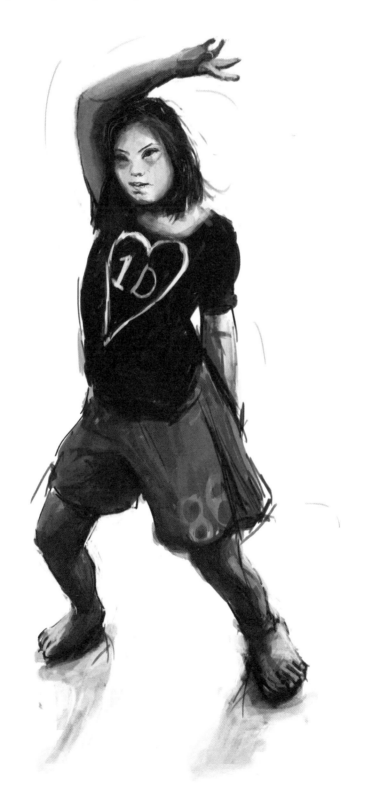

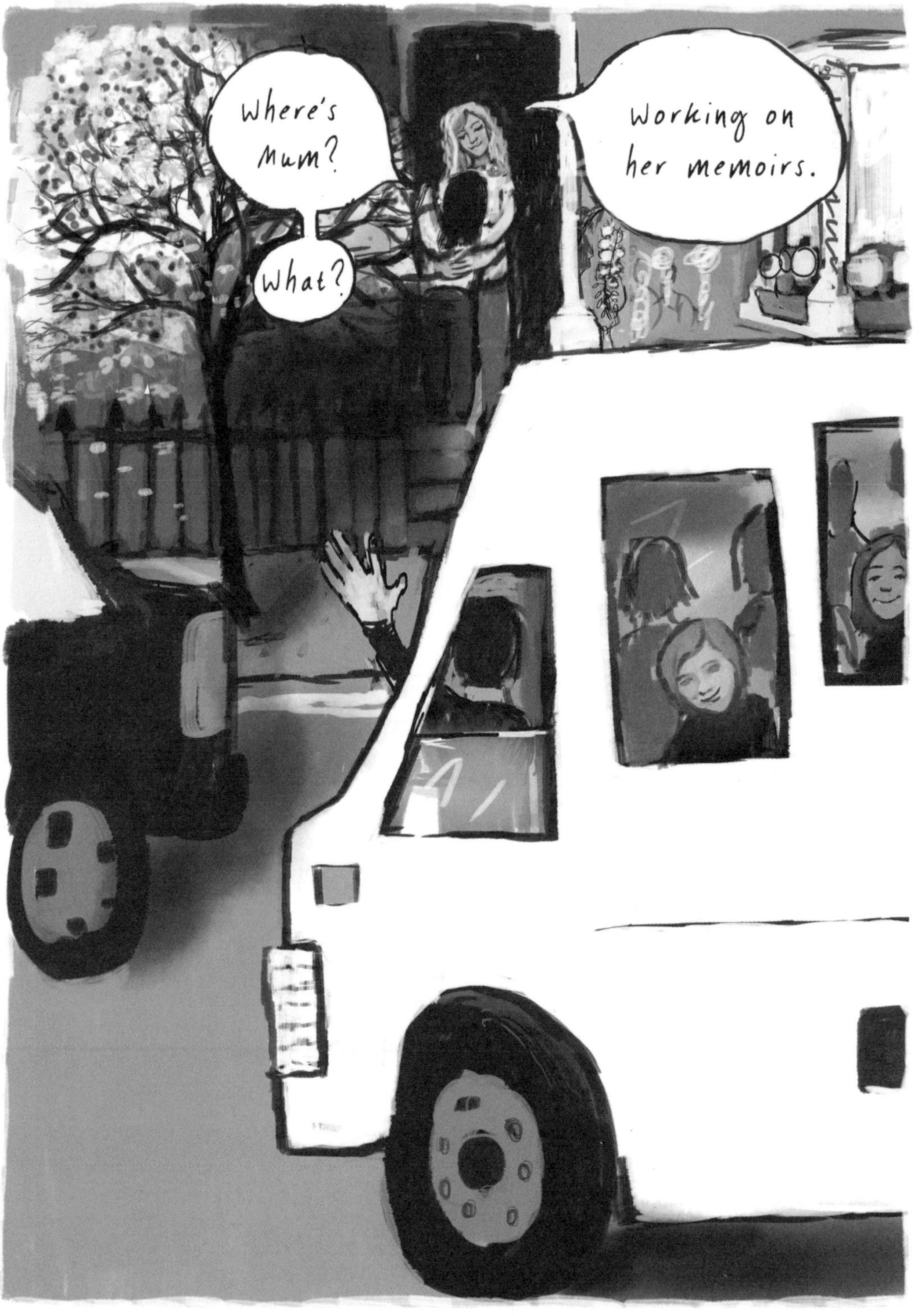
Where's Mum?
What?
Working on her memoirs.

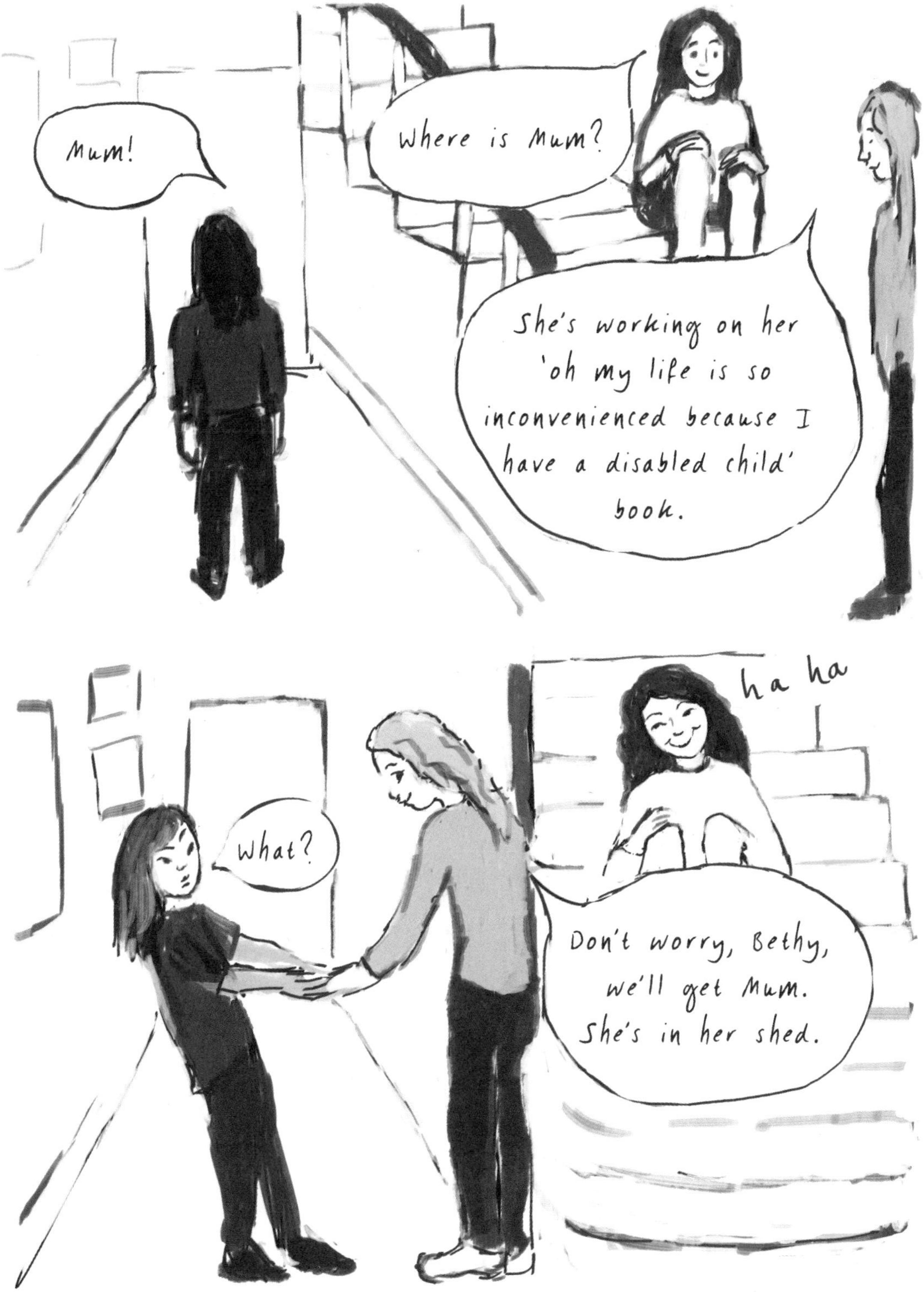
Mum!
Where is Mum?
She's working on her 'oh my life is so inconvenienced because I have a disabled child' book.
What?
ha ha
Don't worry, Bethy, we'll get Mum. She's in her shed.

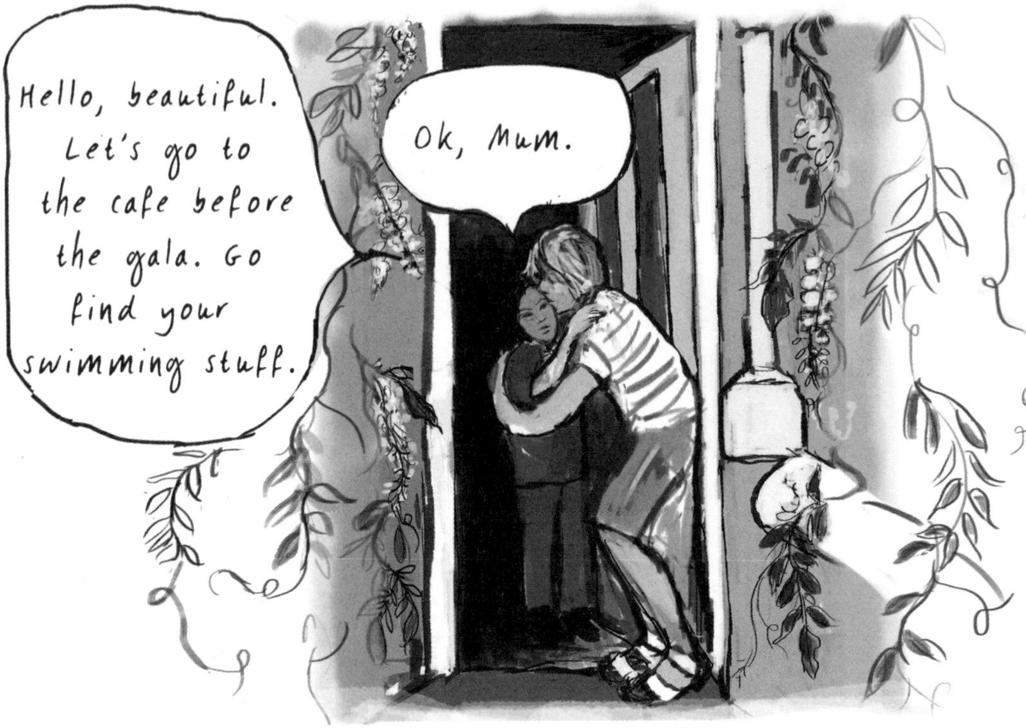
Hello, beautiful. Let's go to the cafe before the gala. Go find your swimming stuff.
Ok, Mum.

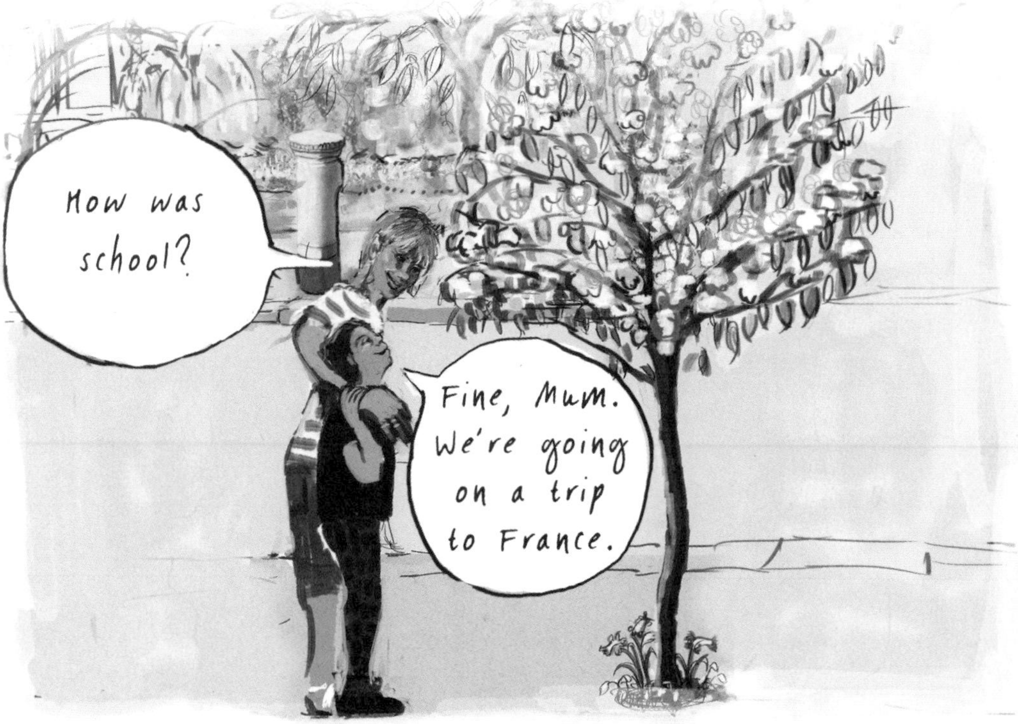
How was school?
Fine, Mum. We're going on a trip to France.

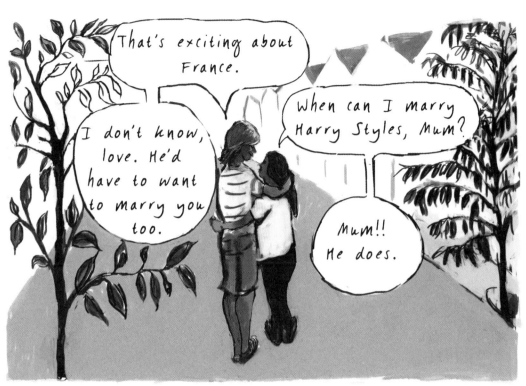

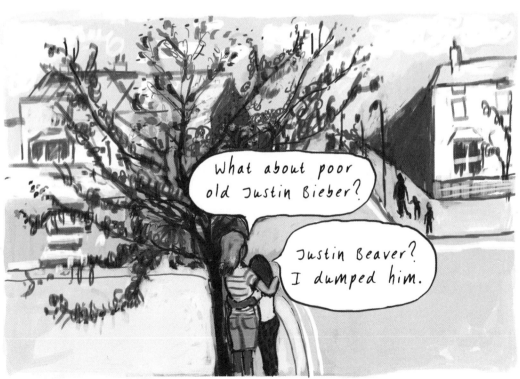

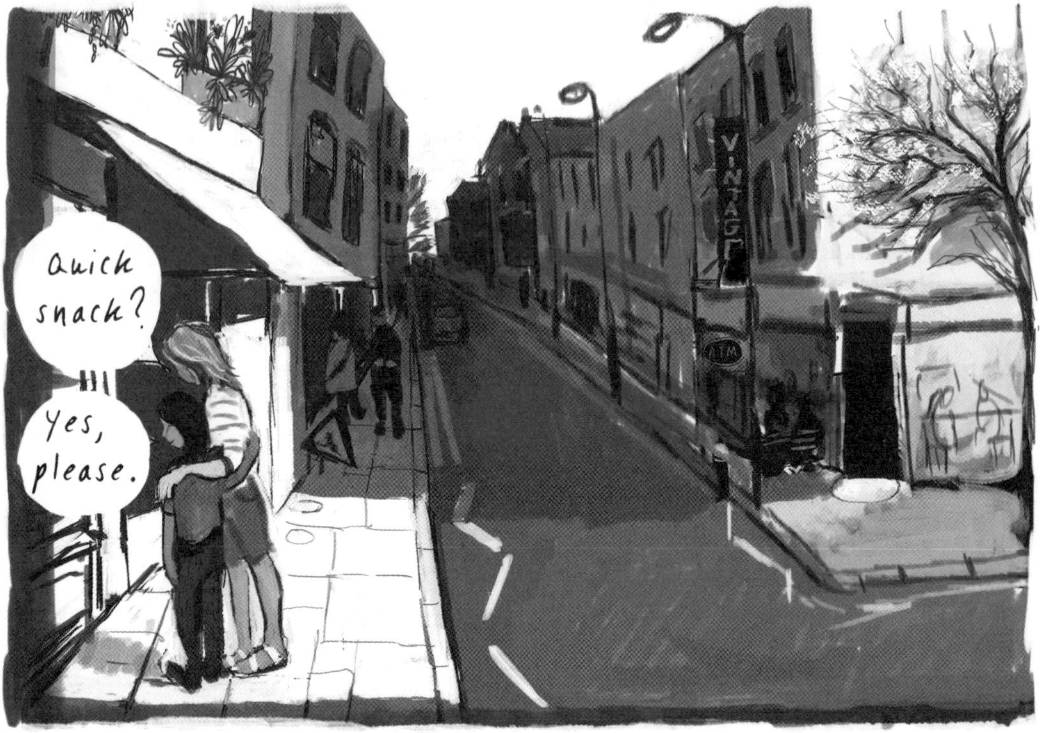
Quick snack?
Yes, please.
VINTAGE
ATM

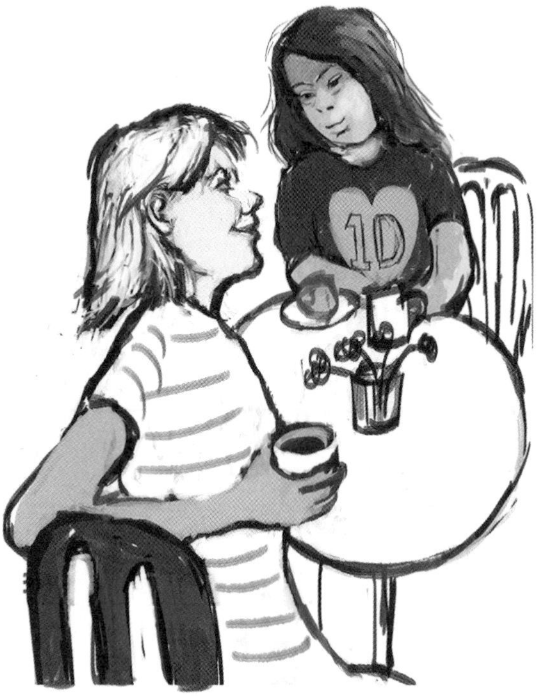
1D

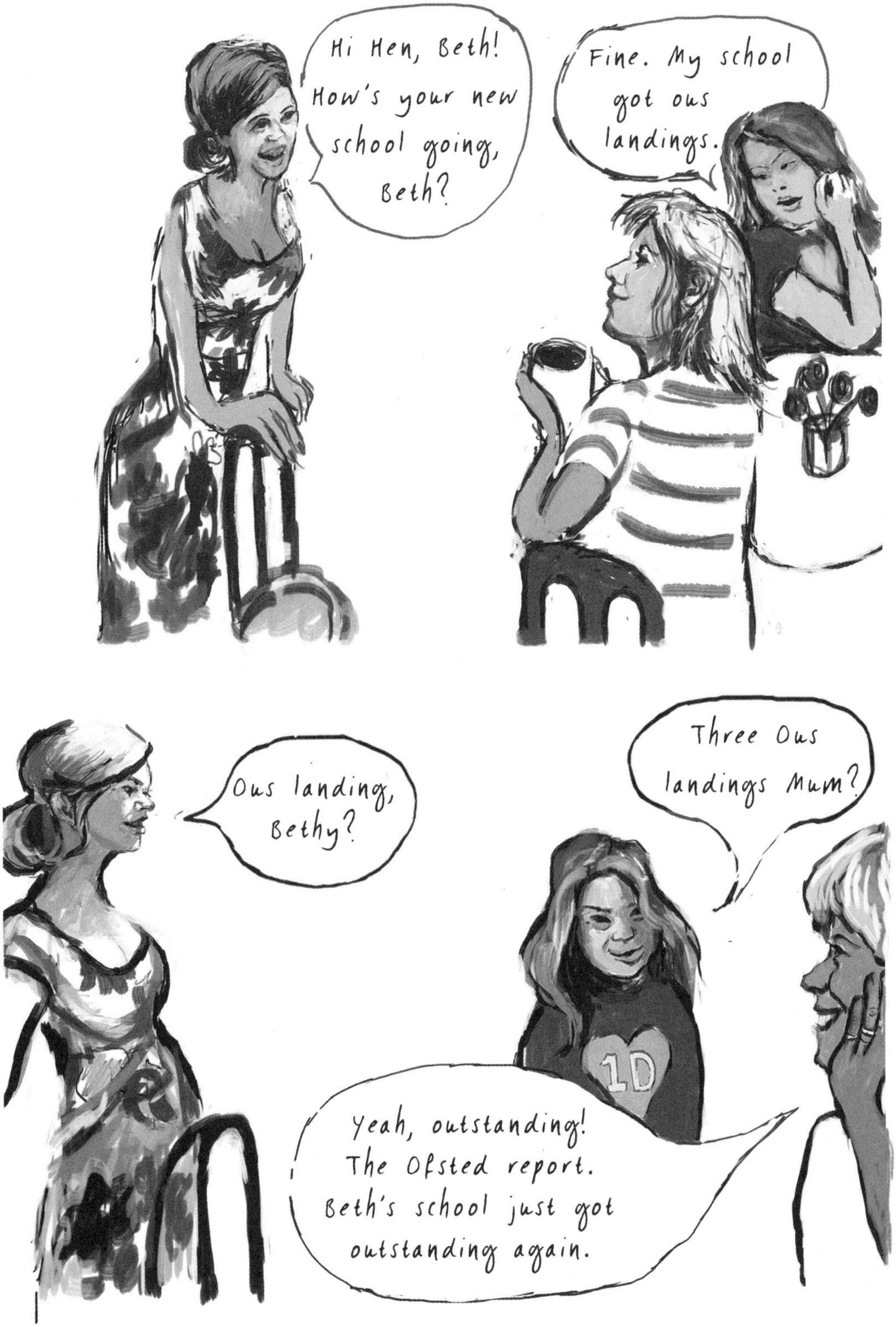
Hi Hen, Beth! How's your new school going, Beth?
Fine. My school got ous landings.
Ous landing, Bethy?
Three Ous landings Mum?
Yeah, outstanding! The Ofsted report. Beth's school just got outstanding again.

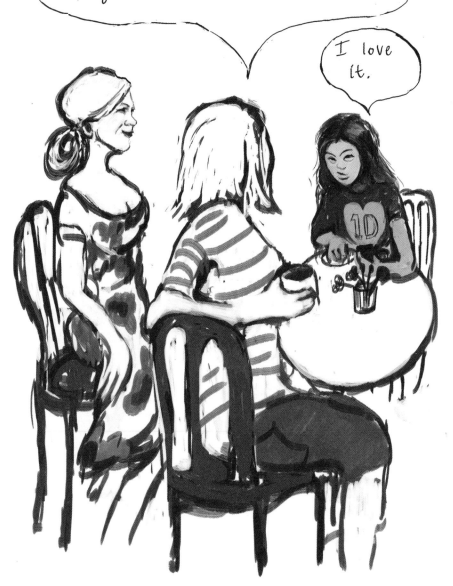

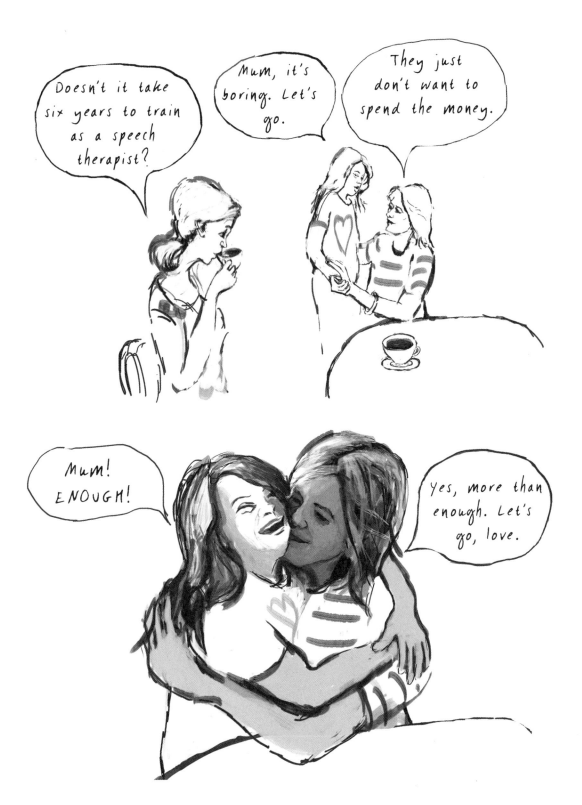

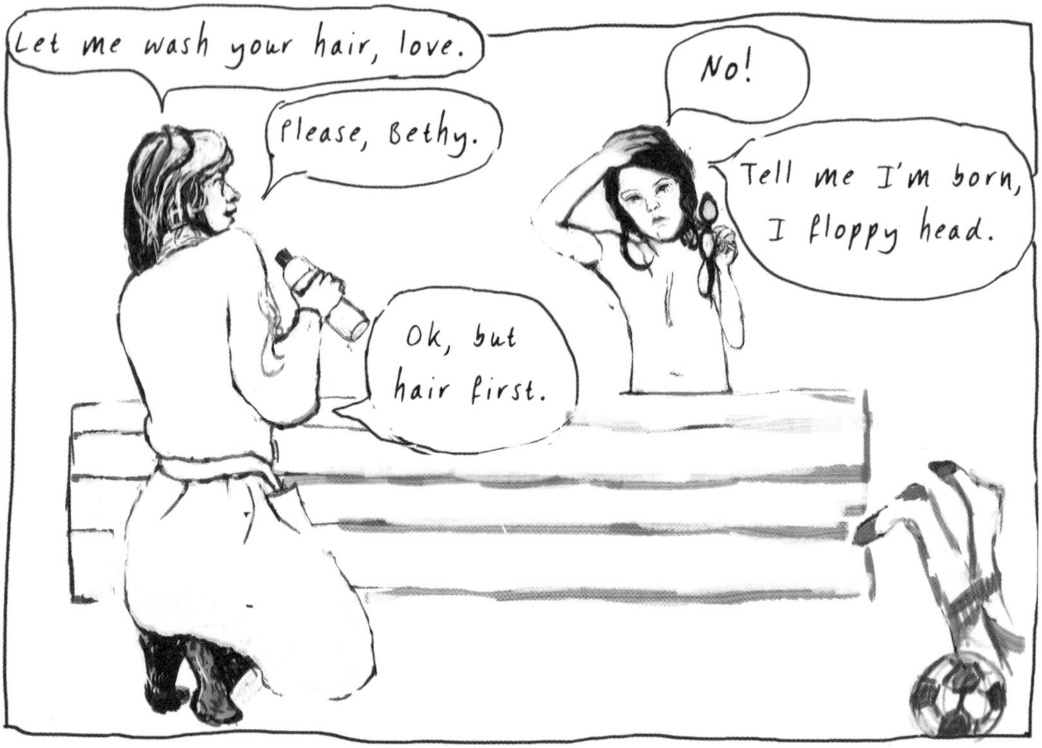
Let me wash your hair, love.
Please, Bethy.
No!
Tell me I'm born, I floppy head.
Ok, but hair first.

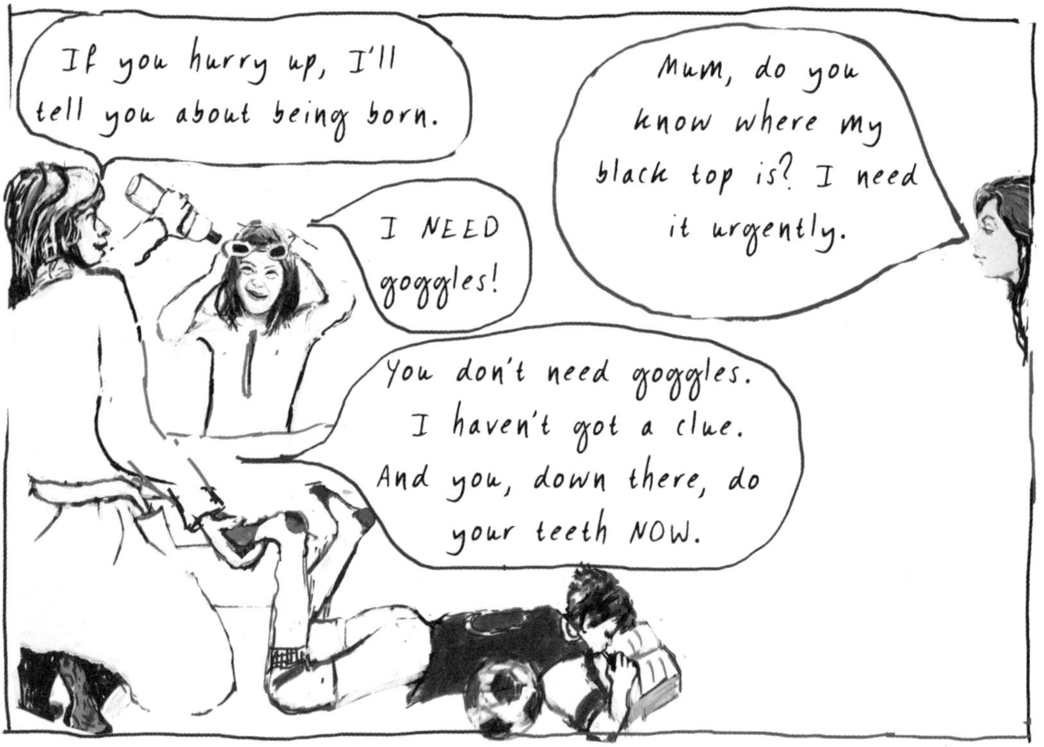
If you hurry up, I'll tell you about being born.
Mum, do you know where my black top is? I need it urgently.
I NEED goggles!
You don't need goggles. I haven't got a clue. And you, down there, do your teeth NOW.

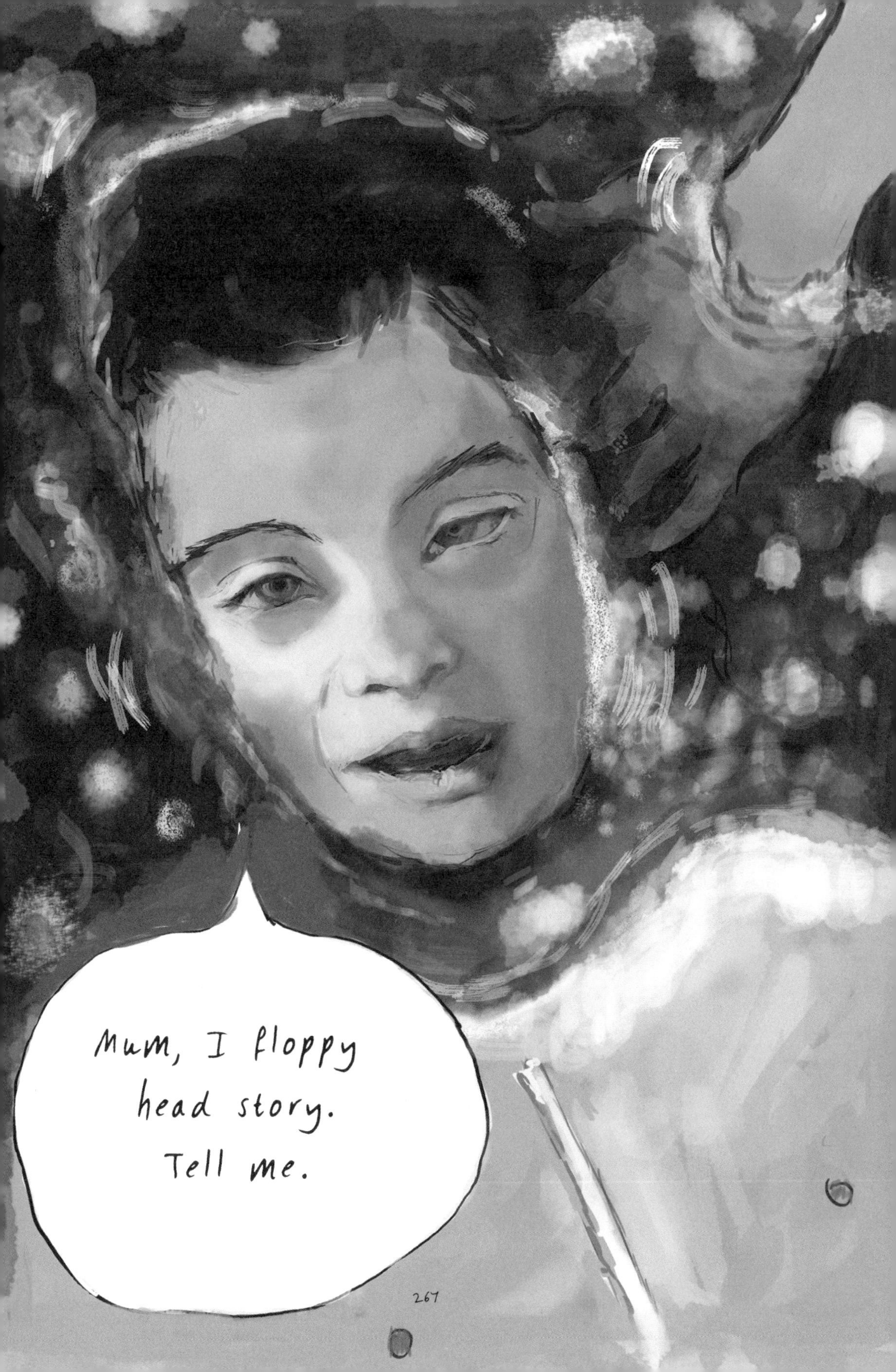
Mum, I floppy head story. Tell me.

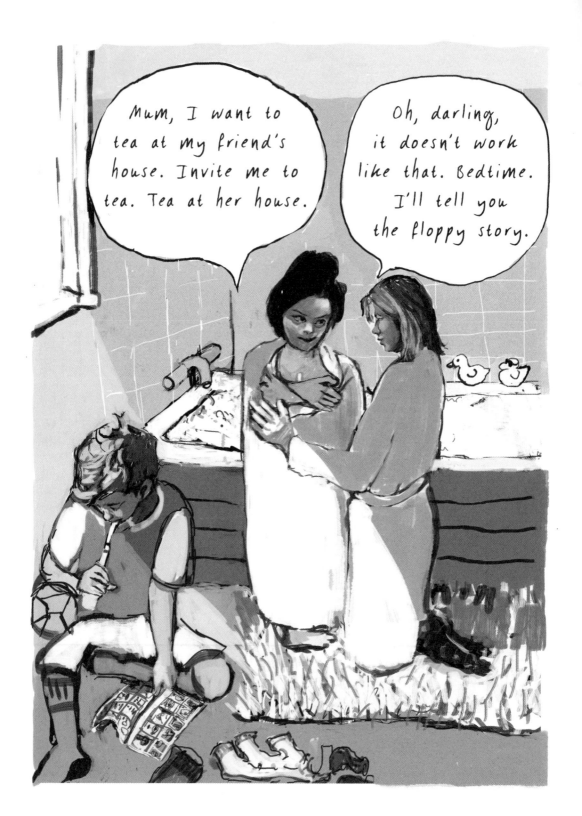

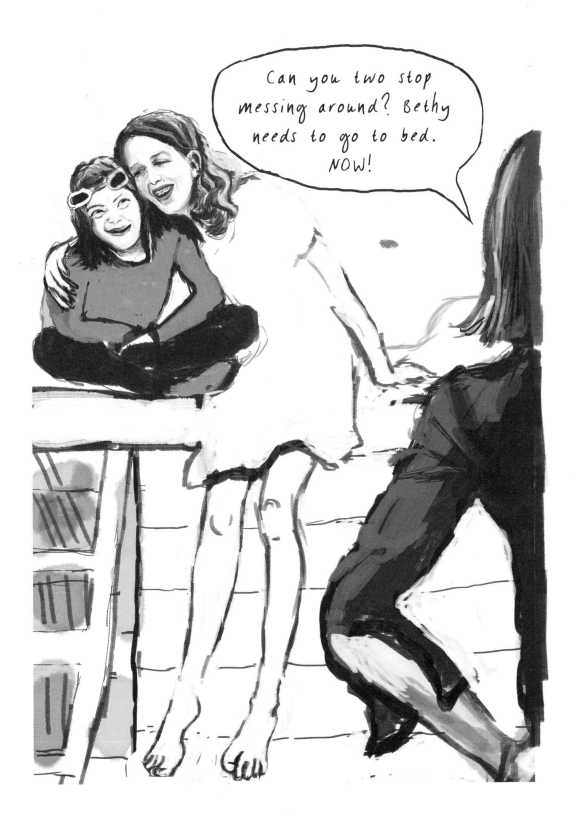

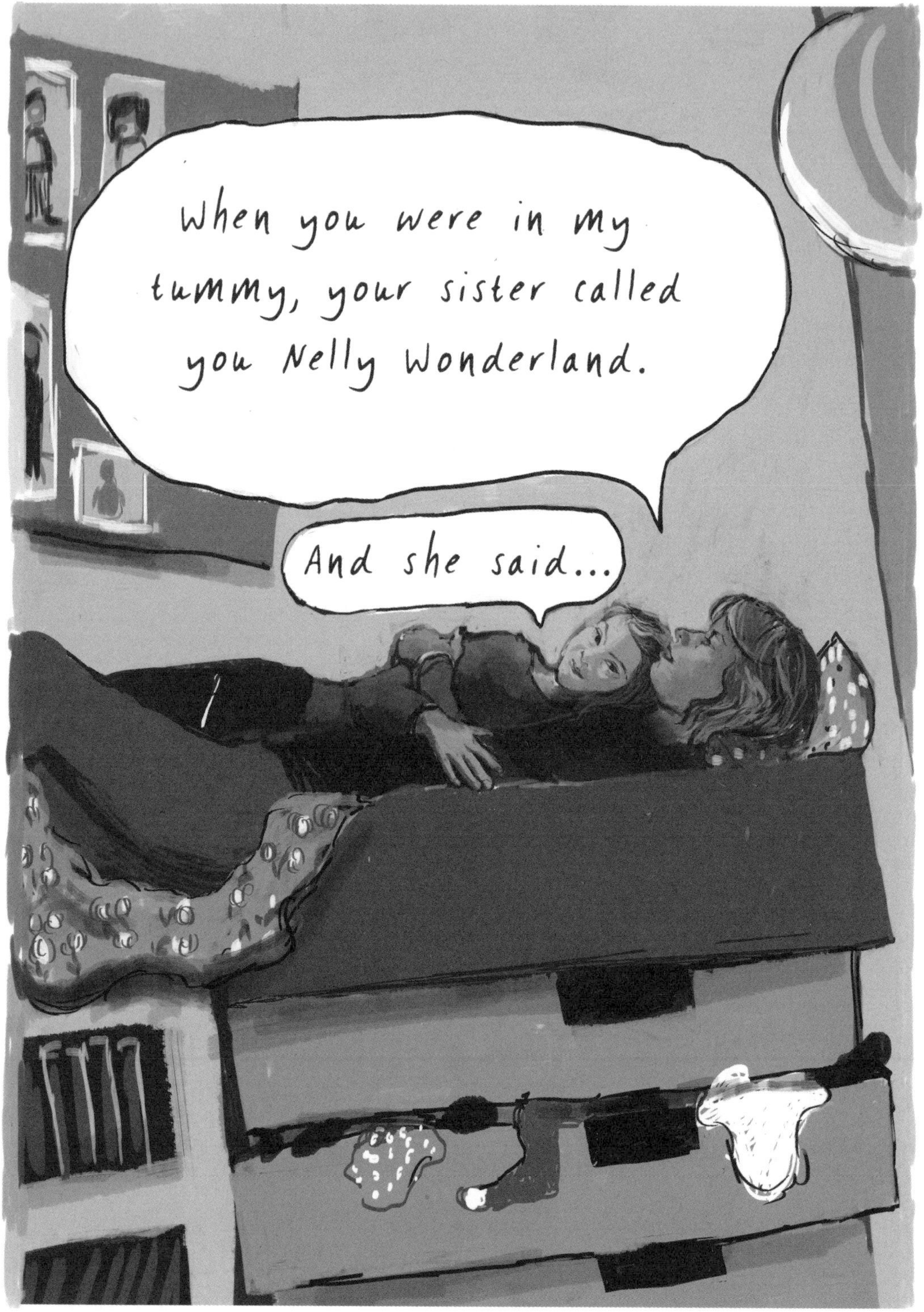
When you were in my tummy, your sister called you Nelly Wonderland.
And she said...

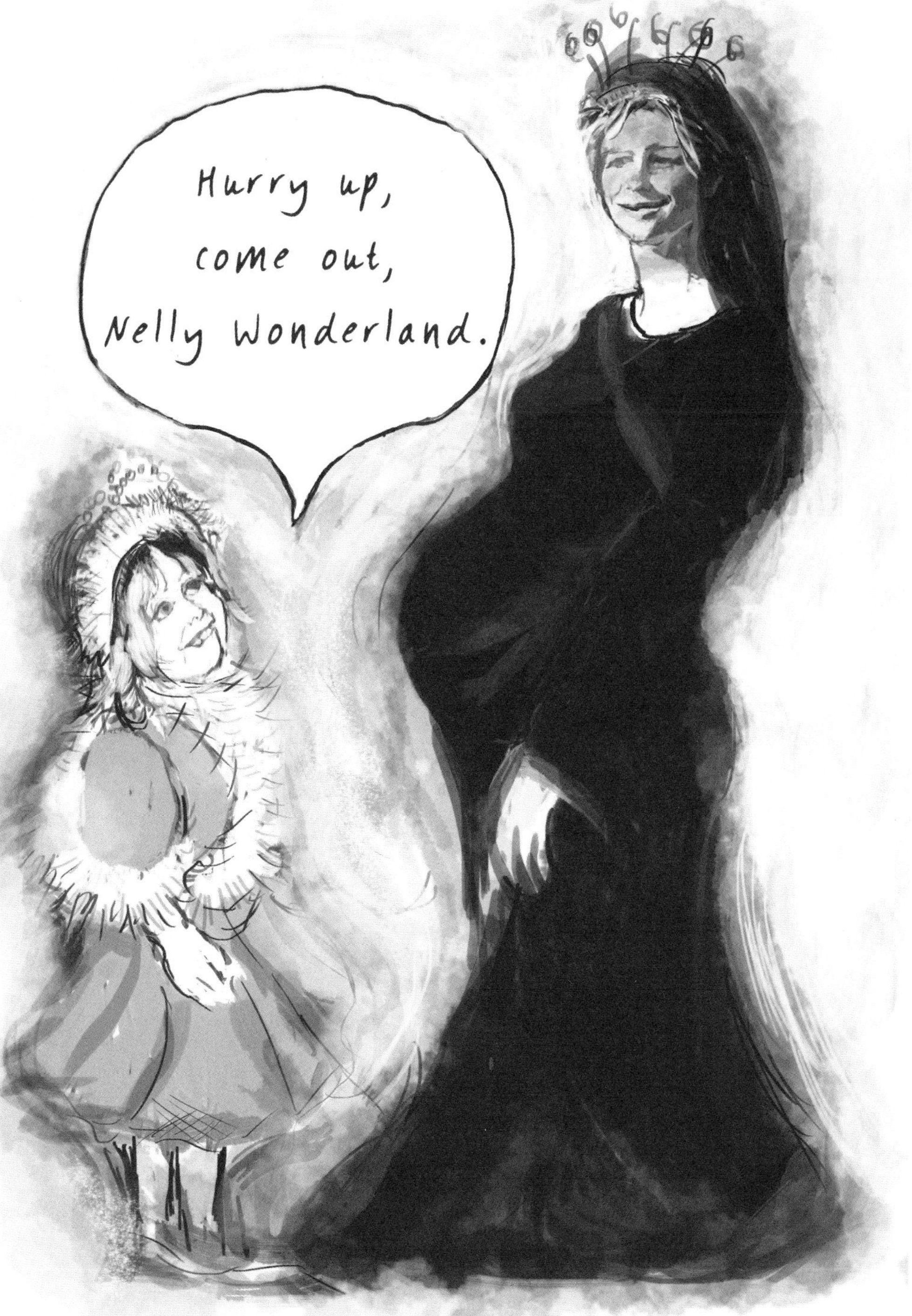
Hurry up, come out, Nelly Wonderland.

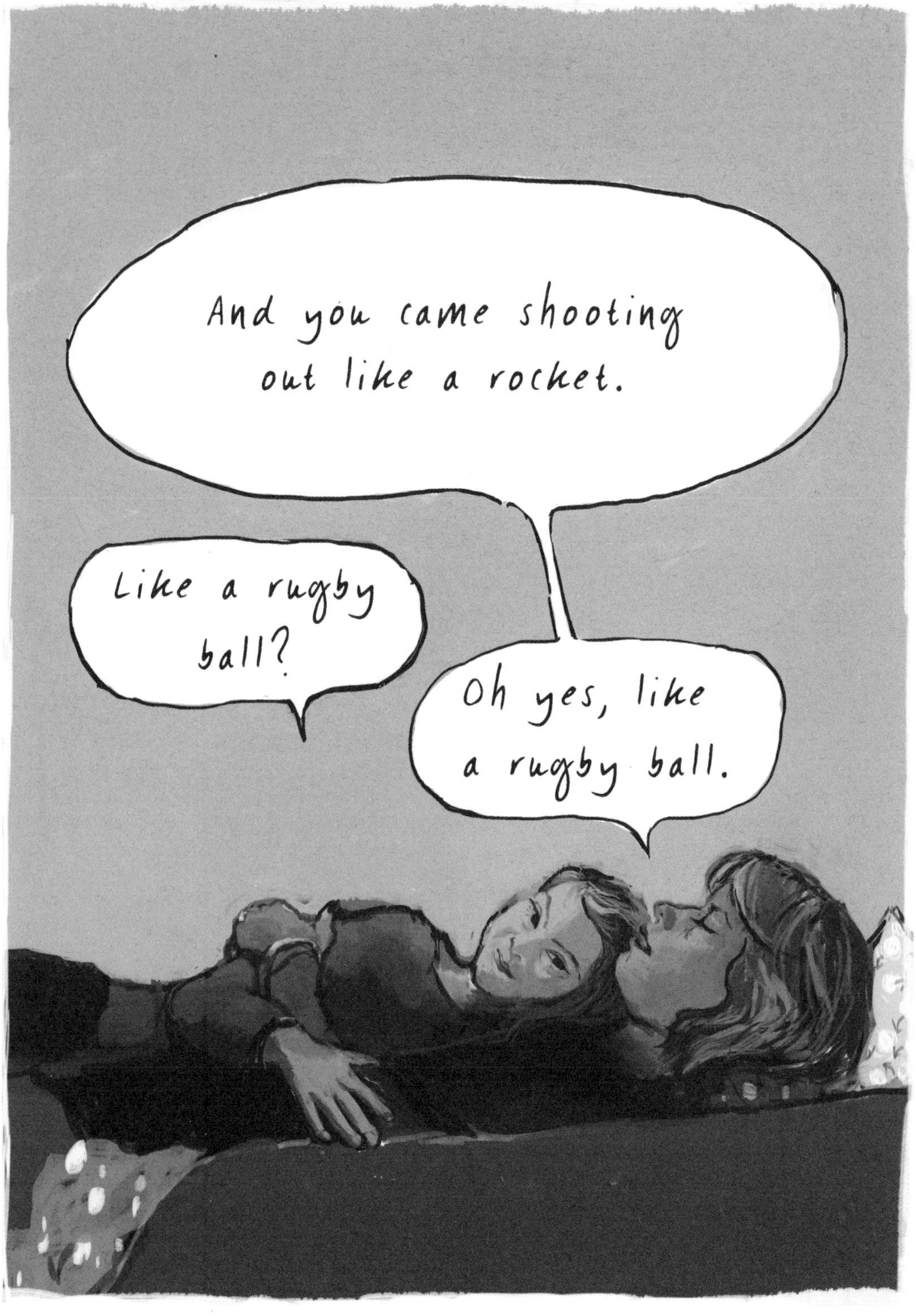
And you came shooting out like a rocket.
Like a rugby ball?
Oh yes, like a rugby ball.

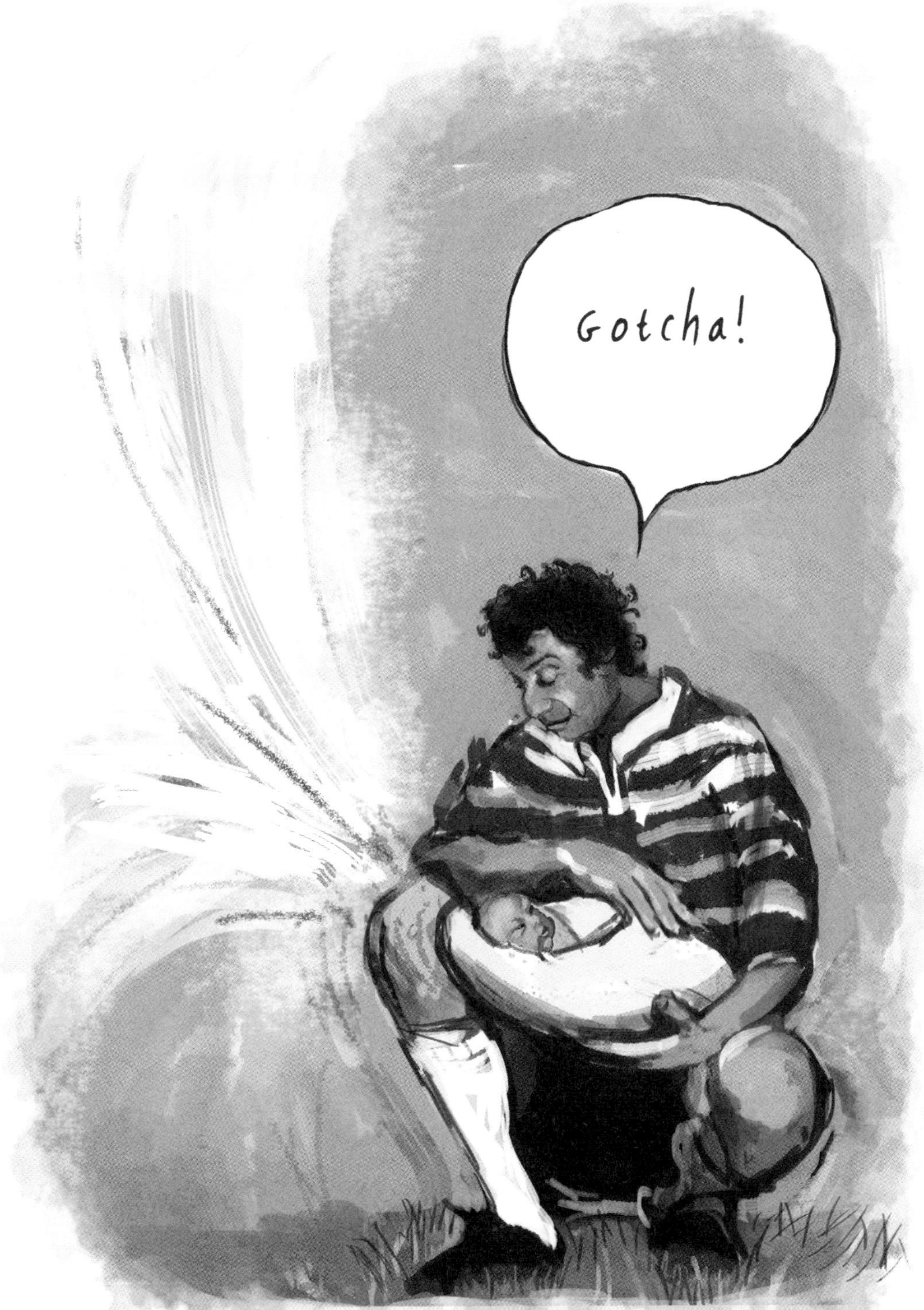
Gotcha!

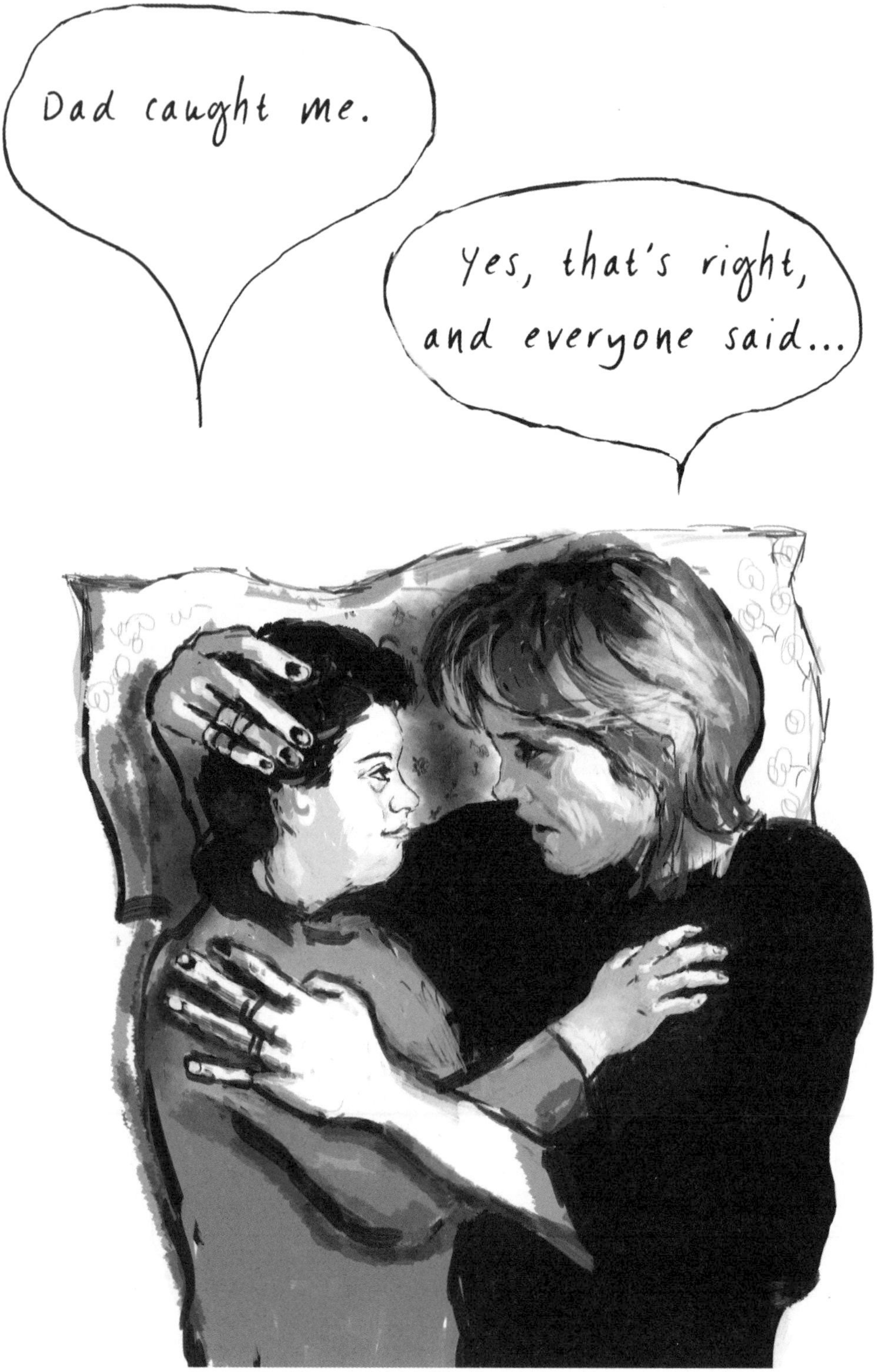
Dad caught me.
Yes, that's right, and everyone said...

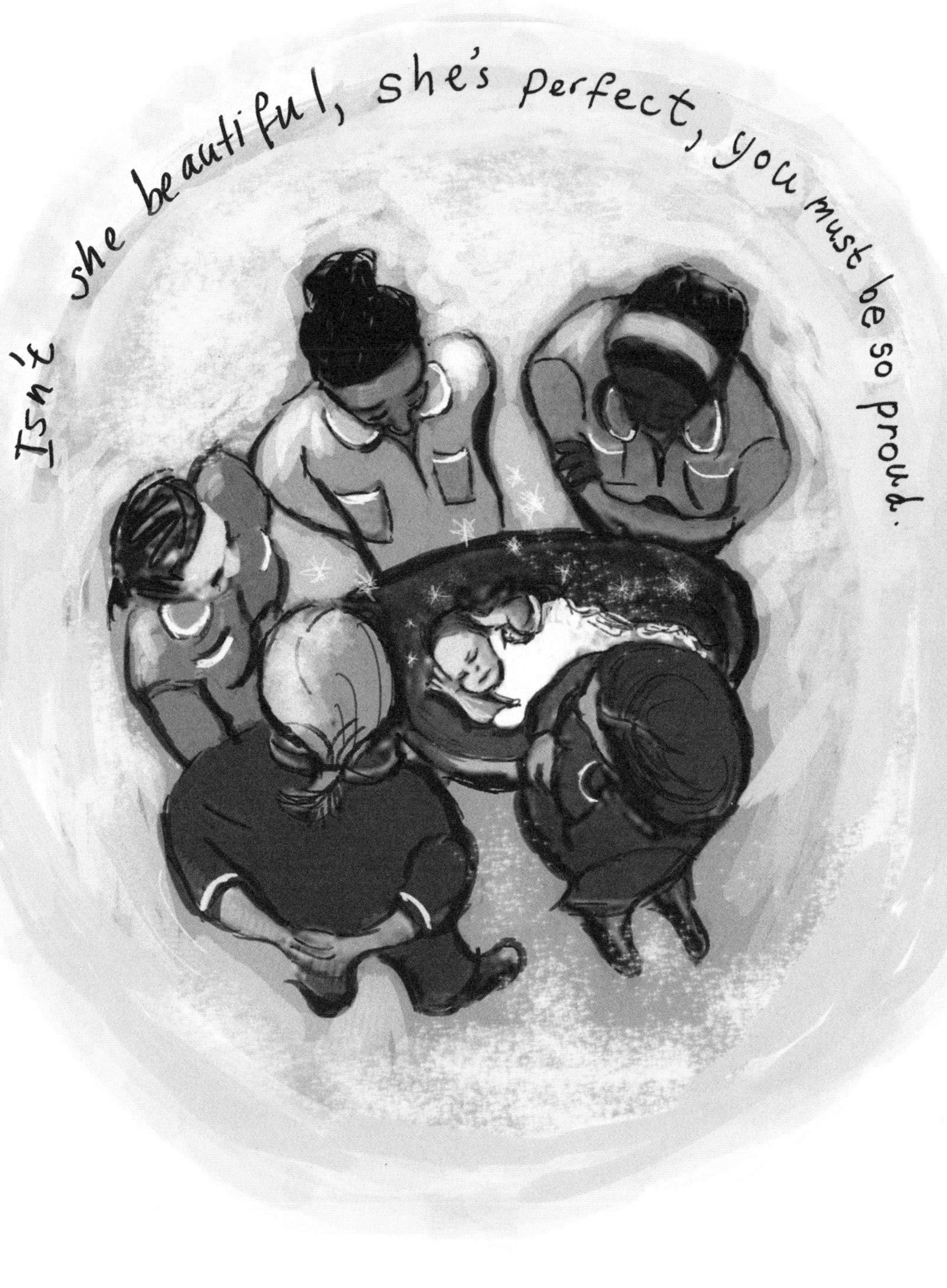
Isn't she beautiful, she's perfect, you must be so proud.

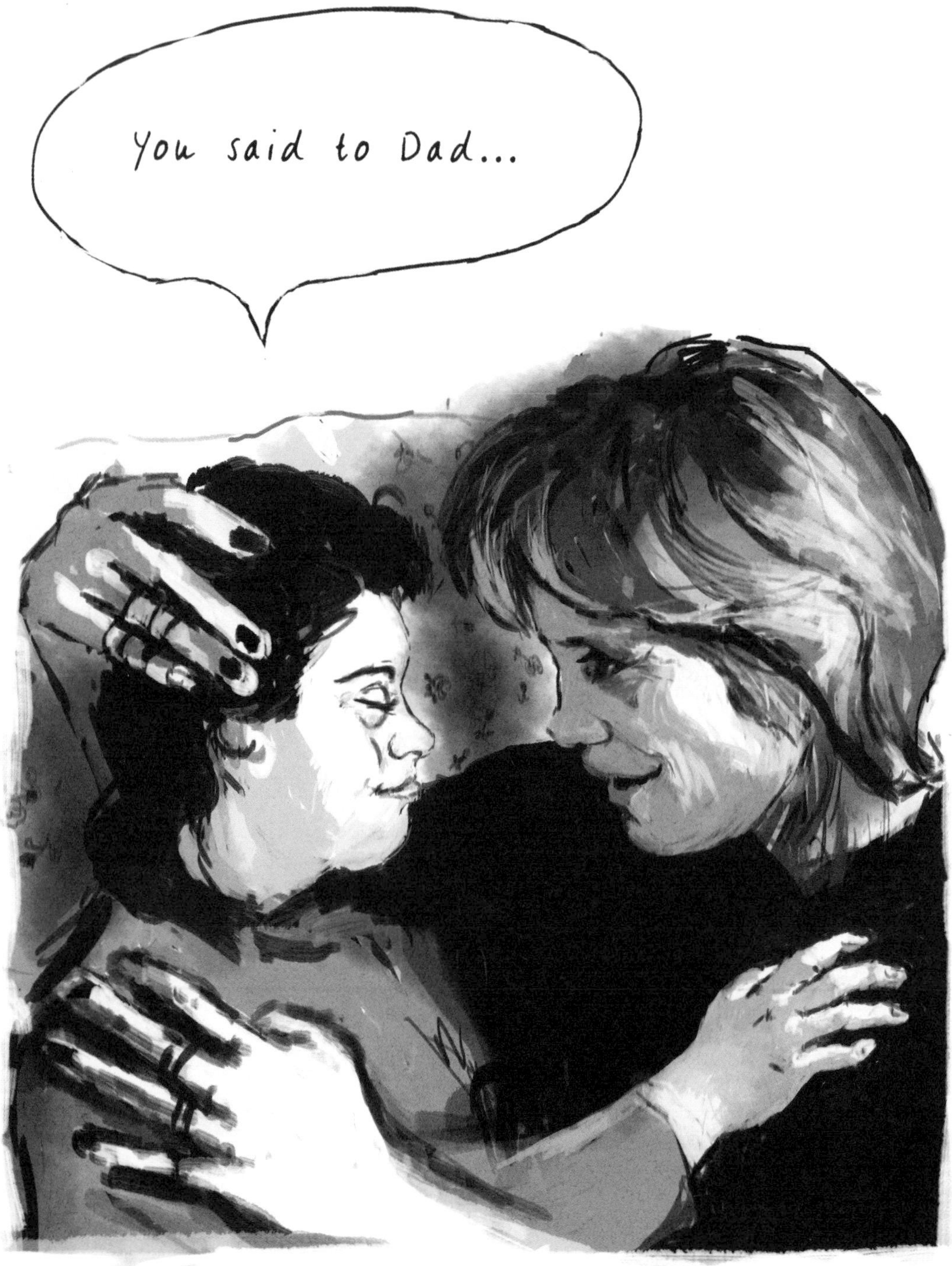
You said to Dad...

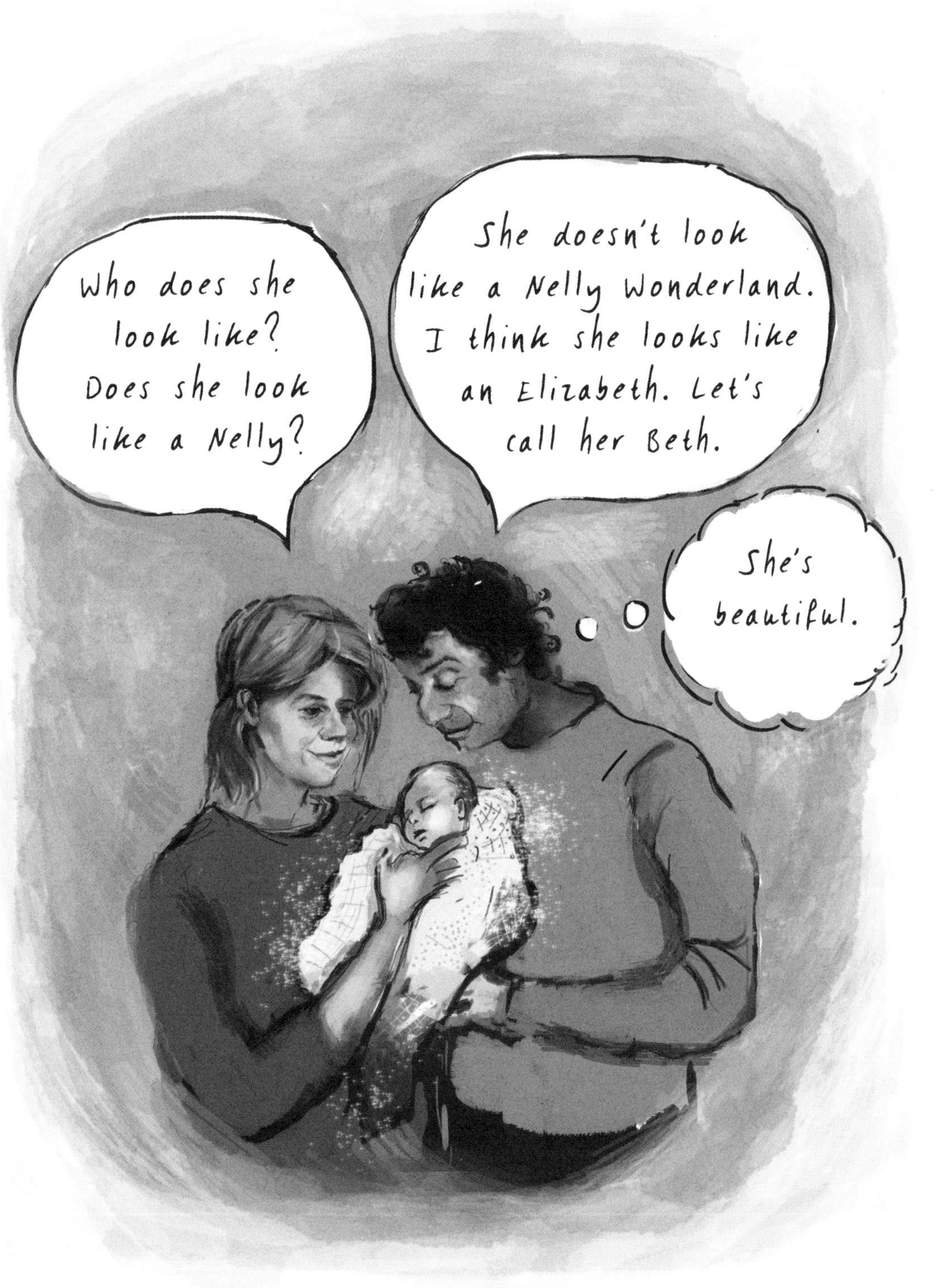
Who does she look like? Does she look like a Nelly?
She doesn't look like a Nelly Wonderland. I think she looks like an Elizabeth. Let's call her Beth.
She's beautiful.

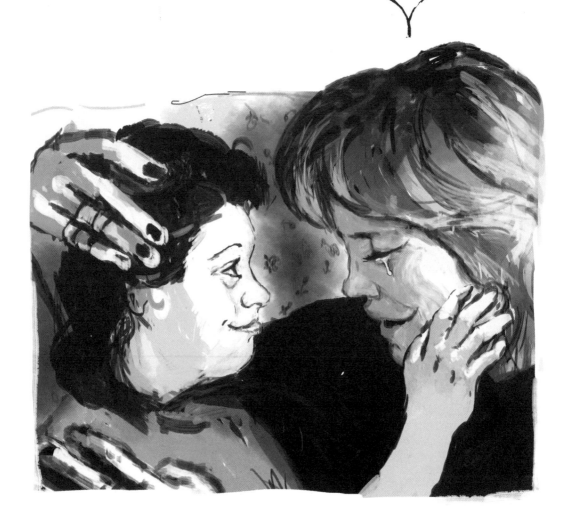

Mum, I need to hold her, I love her floppiness.

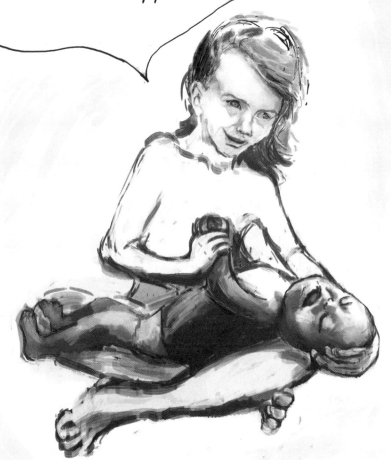

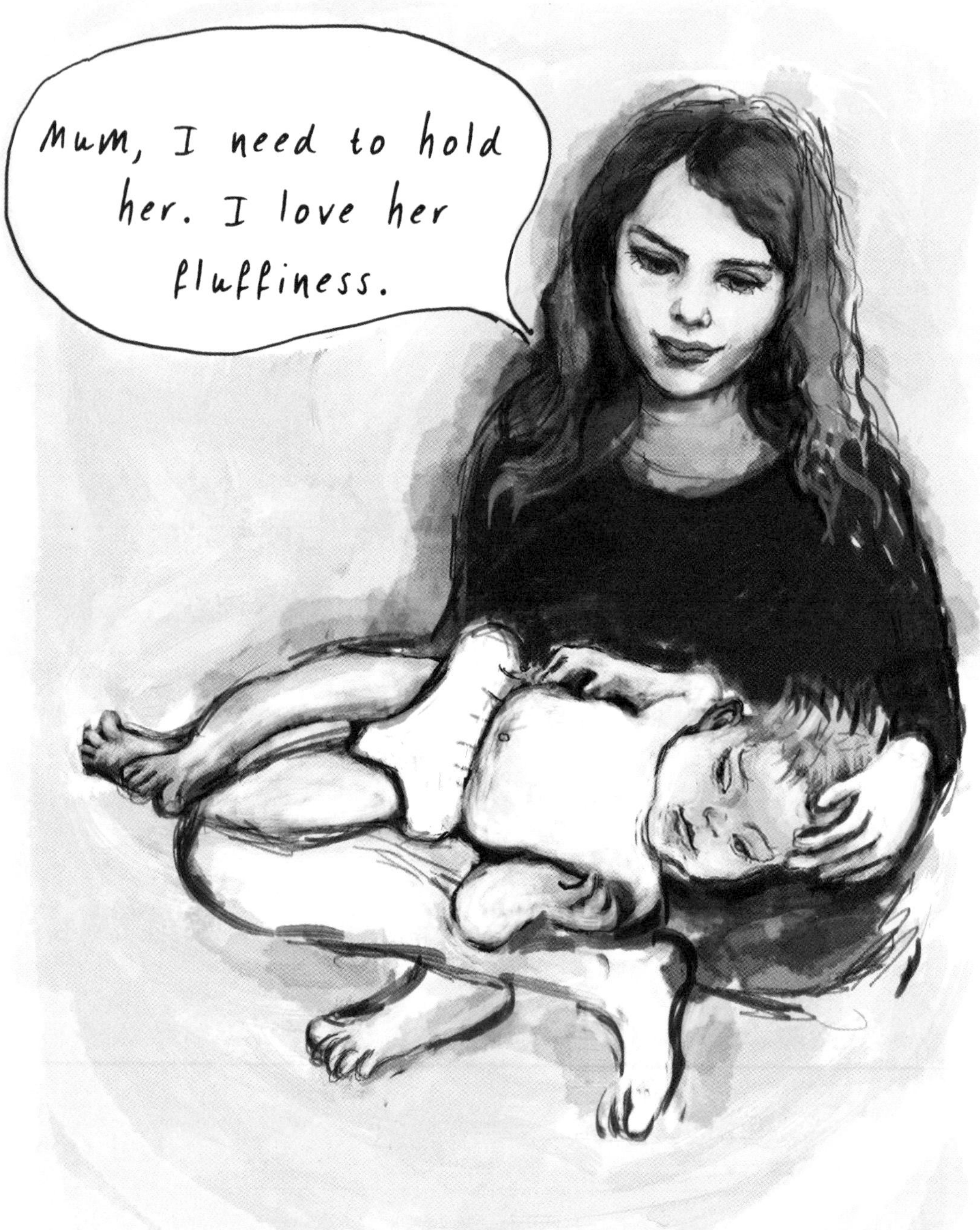
Mum, I need to hold her. I love her fluffiness.

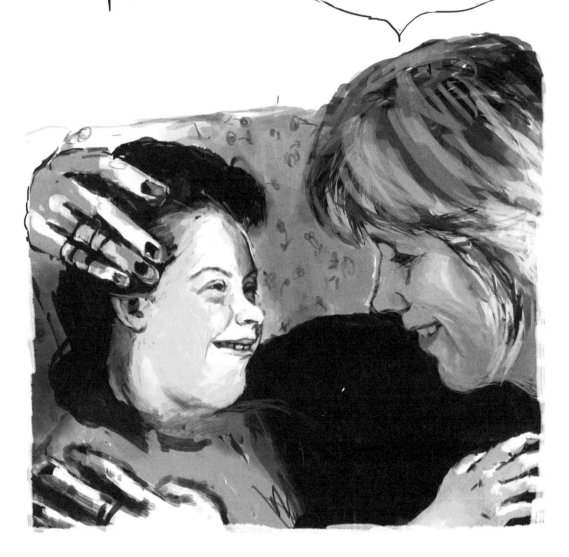

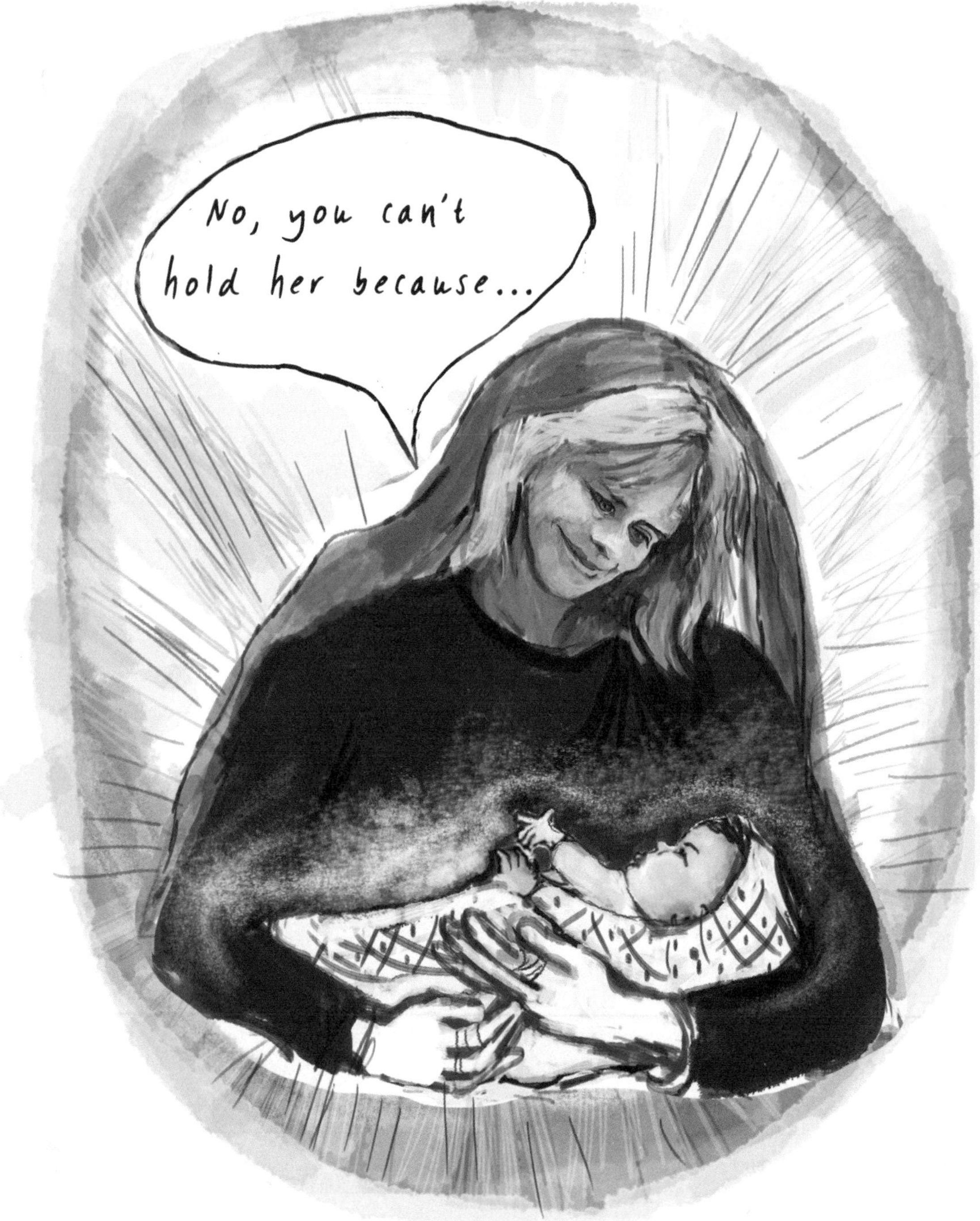
No, you can't hold her because...

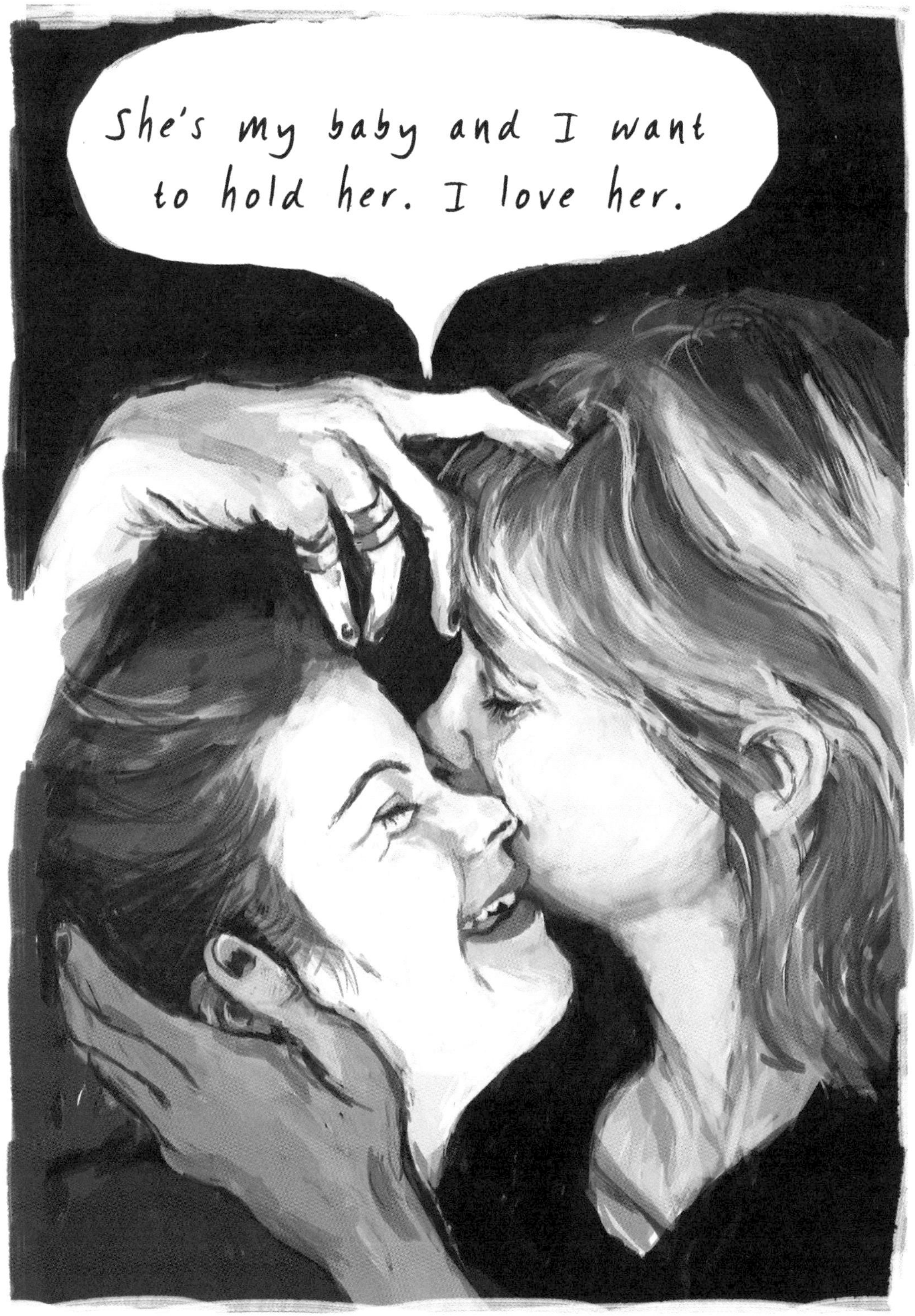
She's my baby and I want to hold her. I love her.

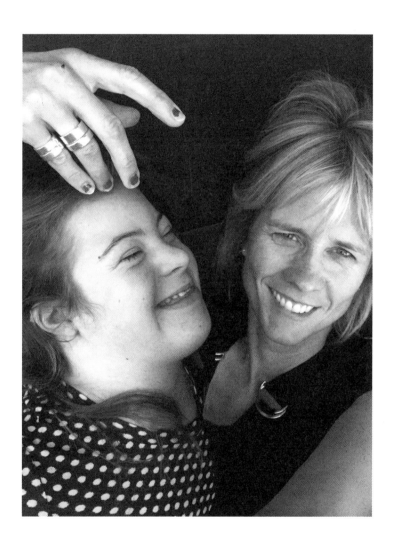

A C K N O W L E D G E M E N T S :

When I first started this book, I had no idea what a team effort it would become, and without the following people there would be no book.

Thank you to Myriad: Candida Lacey, Vicky Blunden, Emma Dowson, Dawn Sackett, Emma Grundy Haigh for all your invaluable help and advice.

My fantastic editor Corinne Pearlman for your unwavering patience, kindness and expertise.

Meg Rosoff for believing in and championing my work from the very beginning.

My agent Rebecca Carter from Janklow and Nesbit for being able to imagine that twenty drawings could become a book, and for your never-ending supply of support and wisdom, through every stage of the process.

To all my friends: Leslie Bookless for your unconditional love and humour, Brigit and Karen for the running and chats. Thank you: Philly Beaumont, Nick Coleman, Anna Hsiung, Juju Vail for looking at early drafts.

To Sophie Thomas and David Pearson for help with the cover.

Thank you to Lesley Caldwell.

To the Down's Syndrome Association and Great Ormond Street Hospital.

To Nicola Streeten and Laydeez Do Comics, Ian Williams and Graphic Medicine, for showing me the potential of graphic novels.

Thank you to my mum and dad.

To my siblings, Philly, Charlie and Chris and my extended family for your love and support.

To my other editors, Matty and Bridie, for helping me decide what to include and leave out, and for always coming up with the best lines. Thank you both for your honesty, humour and wisdom.

To Karl, for religiously keeping a count of how many drawings I did each week and dividing it by the amount of days I had left to make my deadline.

To Steve, the biggest thank you for all your support, understanding and love over the last thirty years and for posing for drawings when you really didn't want to.

And Bethy, last but not least, I couldn't have done it without you: thank you for being yourself.

GRAPHIC MEMOIR FROM MYRIAD

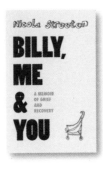
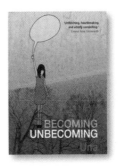
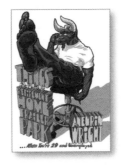

GRAPHIC FICTION FROM MYRIAD

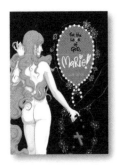
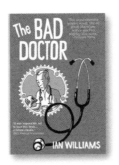
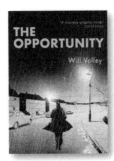
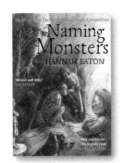
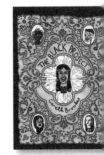

GRAPHIC NON-FICTION FROM MYRIAD

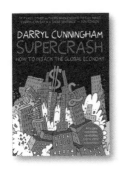
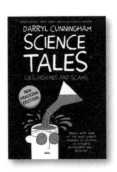
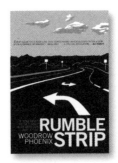
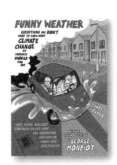

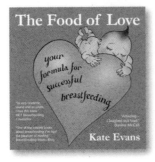
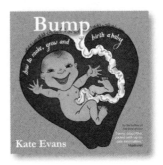

www.myriadeditions.com